D0934661

# Xenobiotic Metabolism: In Vitro Methods

**Gaylord D. Paulson,**
**D. Stuart Frear, and**
**Edwin P. Marks,** EDITORS

*U. S. Department of Agriculture*

A symposium sponsored

by the ACS Division

of Pesticide Chemistry

at the 176th Meeting of

the American Chemical Society,

Miami, Florida,

September 10–15, 1978.

ACS SYMPOSIUM SERIES 97

AMERICAN CHEMICAL SOCIETY

WASHINGTON, D. C.    1979

Library of Congress CIP Data

Xenobiotic metabolism, in vitro methods.
(ACS symposium series; 97 ISSN 0097-6156)

Includes bibliographies and index.

1. Xenobiotic metabolism—Congresses.
I. Paulson, Gaylord D. II. Frear, D. S., 1929-
III. Marks, Edwin P., 1925-  . IV. American Chemi-
cal Society. Division of Pesticide Chemistry. V. Series:
American Chemical Society. ACS symposium series; 97.

QH521.X46              615.9'02              79-789
ISBN 0-8412-0486-1    ASCMC 8      97 1-328 1979

# ACS Symposium Series

## Robert F. Gould, *Editor*

# FOREWORD

The ACS SYMPOSIUM SERIES was founded in 1974 to provide
a medium for publishing symposia quickly in book form. The
format of the Series parallels that of the continuing ADVANCES
IN CHEMISTRY SERIES except that in order to save time the
papers are not typeset but are reproduced as they are sub-
mitted by the authors in camera-ready form. Papers are reviewed under the supervision of the Editors with the assistance
of the Series Advisory Board and are selected to maintain the
integrity of the symposia; however, verbatim reproductions of
previously published papers are not accepted. Both reviews
and reports of research are acceptable since symposia may
embrace both types of presentation.

# CONTENTS

# PREFACE

The beneficial effects of a wide variety of pesticides and other xenobiotics in eliminating or controlling certain insects, plants, and disease processes have been demonstrated conclusively. The standard of living that we now enjoy is attributable, at least in part, to an increased use of xenobiotics. However, there is also a growing awareness and concern that some xenobiotics may have adverse effects on both man and his environment. This concern has resulted in more extensive testing and evaluation of xenobiotics to determine whether they can be used safely. One type of information that is important in making this evaluation is an understanding of the metabolic fate of the xenobiotic in both target and nontarget organisms.

In the past, most xenobiotic metabolism studies were conducted with the intact plant or animal. Such in vivo studies have generated a wealth of useful information and will continue to be the method of choice for many investigations. However, there is a growing realization that in vitro studies may be superior for generating certain types of information. For example, in vitro techniques are often the methods of choice when there is a need to isolate and identify intermediate products of a multistep metabolic sequence. Cofactor requirements and other factors (inhibitors, activators, etc.) affecting the enzymes involved in xenobiotic biotransformations usually are determined by in vitro studies. Comparative studies to determine the effect of factors such as species, sex, age, tissue, subcellular fraction, nutritional factors, disease states, etc. on xenobiotic metabolism often are conducted most quickly and easily in vitro. Usually the mode of action and selectivity of xenobiotics are investigated most effectively by in vitro studies.

Although in vitro techniques are extremely useful and have broad application in studying the metabolic fate of xenobiotics, they also have definite limitations. For example, many in vitro techniques are not applicable to long-term studies because of the buildup of end products, microbial contamination, and other problems. Some investigators have used in vitro conditions (temperature, substrate concentrations, etc.) that had little or no relationship to conditions in the intact organism; therefore, the results obtained were of limited value. Endogenous inhibitors that are retained in subcellular compartments (and therefore have no effect on the metabolism of a xenobiotic in vivo) may be released during the preparation of an in vitro system and result in misleading information. These and other potential problems cited in the proceedings of this symposium make it clear that in vitro methods must be used with caution. However, when properly used within the recognized limitations, in vitro techniques are extremely useful in studying the metabolism of xenobiotics.

This symposium was organized because of the growing interest in the use of in vitro techniques for xenobiotic metabolism studies. The primary objectives were to critically review, evaluate, and summarize: (1) how in vitro techniques are used in the laboratory with special emphasis on their application to xenobiotic metabolism studies; (2) advantages, disadvantages, and limitations of these techniques; and (3) examples of how in vitro techniques may be useful in future studies. It is our hope that the proceedings of this symposium will provide a point of departure for a more effective and efficient use of in vitro techniques in future research on the metabolism and fate of xenobiotics in the environment.

Metabolism and Radiation Research Laboratory    GAYLORD D. PAULSON

Agriculture Research,    D. STUART FREAR

Science and Education Administration    EDWIN P. MARKS

U.S. Department of Agriculture

Fargo, ND 58102

December 20, 1978

# Plants

# Xenobiotic Metabolism in Plants: In Vitro Tissue, Organ, and Isolated Cell Techniques[1]

R. H. SHIMABUKURO and W. C. WALSH

Metabolism and Radiation Research Laboratory, Agricultural Research, Science and Education Administration, U. S. Department of Agriculture, Fargo, ND 58105

Interest in xenobiotic metabolism in plants has centered primarily on the fate of pesticides in plants. Although herbicides have been of predominant interest in plant metabolism studies, the methods and techniques discussed in this report are equally applicable to other classes of pesticides including insecticides and fungicides. In this report, the term "xenobiotics" refers to synthetic pesticides and not to other unnatural compounds. However, the discussion on in vitro techniques for xenobiotic metabolism in plants is based primarily on research with herbicides.

The metabolism of pesticides in plants is discussed extensively in several publications (1, 2, 3). Much is known on the metabolism of organic pesticide chemicals in plants, but the fate of most pesticides in plants is still unknown. It is important to know the identity of transitory intermediate products and the ultimate fate of these chemicals in plants since the intermediate products may be toxic. Knowledge of chemical identity and quantity of intermediate products of a herbicide in plants at different times after treatment is essential for the elucidation of the mode of action and basis for selectivity.

Whole plants treated with pesticides through their roots or foliage have been used extensively for metabolism and "terminal" residue studies. Useful quantities of metabolites may be generated from large-scale treatments of whole plants; such metabolites can then be purified for chemical characterization. The development of various chromatographic techniques and improved UV, IR, NMR and mass spectroscopy instrumentation

[1] Mention of a trademark or proprietary product does not constitute a guarantee or warranty of the product by the U. S. Department of Agriculture and does not imply its approval to the exclusion of other products that may also be suitable.

has made it possible to characterize chemically small amounts
of metabolites. Excised plant tissues and organs and isolated
cells may be used for pesticide metabolism studies for short
periods where limited quantities of metabolites are generated.
Results from selected reports are presented to illustrate the
techniques and methods that may be used.

## Metabolism of Xenobiotics

The successful isolation and chemical characterization of
any xenobiotic biotransformation product require the generation
of sufficient quantities of the metabolite. The degradation
mechanisms in plants may be slower than those in animals (1).
Plants also lack an excretory system comparable to the renal
excretion system in mammals. Therefore, intermediate degradation products of pesticides cannot be concentrated from normal
excretion products as with mammals. Plants metabolize significant amounts of pesticides ultimately to insoluble residues (3).
The chemical nature and quantities of the metabolites in a
plant are influenced by the site of absorption of the pesticide,
translocation, and the residence time in the plant. The use of
excised plant tissues, organs, and isolated cells for studies
of xenobiotic metabolism is an attempt to modify the influence
of the above physiological functions in order to optimize the
conditions for maximum metabolite generation. Fundamental
functions of the whole plant, including absorption, translocation, cell functions and senescence should be considered when
in vitro techniques with isolated plant parts are used. The
physiological significance of metabolism in isolated plant
parts must be evaluated ultimately in terms of results in
intact plants.

Absorption. Regardless of how a pesticide is applied
to the plant, the chemical must penetrate the plant and be
absorbed specifically into the cells where biotransformation
reactions occur. The leaf surfaces and root tips are the
primary sites of penetration into the plant (4, 5). The
cuticle, a thin, lipoidal membrane that covers the entire
surface area of the above ground parts of a plant, is the
primary barrier to penetration by organic pesticides.
The penetration of nonpolar organic pesticides into leaves
and roots is believed to be a two-stage process (4, 6). The
first stage in leaf absorption involves passive penetration or
partitioning of the nonpolar compound into the cuticle and
desorption into the cell walls (apoplast) of the underlying
cells. In roots, the first stage involves the inactive diffusion of the compound into the root "free space" (apoplast).
The second stage in leaves is the active transport of the
pesticides across the plasmalemma (cell membrane) into leaf
cells (symplast), and in some cases into the phloem for

symplastic transport.  Symplastic transport is an active, energy-requiring process occurring in the living cytoplasmic continuum of the plant.  In roots, the second stage involves an active transport of the pesticides across the endodermis and into the stele where the differentiated vascular structure is located.  Therefore, symplastic intercellular transport of pesticides occurs at one stage during the transport of pesticides from the external root solution into the xylem vessels in the stele for apoplastic transport to the shoot.  Apoplastic transport from the root to shoot is an inactive, physical process occurring in the non-living extra-protoplasmic component of the plant under the influence of the transpiration stream.  The symplast-apoplast concept is applied as defined by Crafts and Crisp (7).  Unfortunately, little is known about the mechanisms of absorption and transport of organic pesticide molecules in roots.  The above hypothesis is based mainly on information regarding the absorption of inorganic ions by roots.

Translocation.  Once penetration into leaf cells or root tips is accomplished, the pesticide must be translocated symplastically from leaves and apoplastically from roots to different plant organs and distributed to specific tissues and cells where the target sites for biological activity may be located.  The target sites of the pesticide may or may not be located in the same tissues or cells as the biotransformation sites.  Detailed discussions on structure of the vascular system and mechanisms of transport are discussed in several publications (5, 7, 8).

It is generally recognized that phloem or symplastic transport occurs from "sources to sinks" or in broad terms from green leaves to active centers of growth and storage. This results in differential or selective translocation and accumulation of photosynthates in young leaves, buds, and meristematic regions of the plant.  Most herbicides, and probably other pesticides, do not appear to translocate very readily in the symplast (2) although exceptions are known (5). Nonspecific translocation and uniform distribution to all parts of plants occur by apoplastic transport.  This is generally observed when herbicides are translocated in the xylem from roots to shoots under the influence of the transpiration stream (9).  The rates of pesticides translocated in the xylem appear to depend on the amount of material released by parenchyma cells to the xylem (9).  Factors affecting transpiration also influence apoplastic transport of pesticides from roots to shoots.

The absorption and translocation functions in a whole plant reflect the functions of specific organs, tissues, and cells organized and integrated in their activities to meet the requirements of growth and maintenance.  The implications of separating the organs, tissues, and cells for use in in vitro xenobiotic metabolism studies are clearly evident.

      Senescence. Senescence of plant tissues is a major
factor that must be considered in xenobiotic metabolism studies
with isolated plant organs and cells. In contrast to mammals,
senescence in plants is not due to irreversible changes in the
genome (DNA breakdown), but due to internal plant factors that
inhibit cell metabolism or alter its direction toward autolytic
pathways (10). Plant senescence is a hormonally controlled
phenomenon (10, 11) that may be induced, retarded or reversed
under different circumstances.

      The process of leaf senescence begins as soon as leaves
are excised or detached from the whole plant. Protein synthesis and chlorophyll content decline, and protease activity,
respiration, and RNase levels increase in detached leaves
(12, 13, 14, 15). In wheat leaves the levels of lipase,
esterase, and acid phosphatase declined after detachment.
However, the decline in the enzyme levels was retarded by
treatment of leaves with kinetin (15). Light retards senescence in excised leaves (12). Light-induced retardation of
senescence was not linked to phytochrome action, but was
related directly to photosynthesis (12). However, evidence
indicates that light retardation of senescence is not linked
to $CO_2$ fixation or photochemical activity of PS II. Diuron
[3-(3,4-dichlorophenyl)-1,1-dimethylurea] did not eliminate or
reduce the effectiveness of light in retarding chlorophyll loss
(16). Addition of sucrose also had no effect on chlorophyll
loss when $CO_2$ fixation was inhibited by diuron (16). Glucose
inhibited significantly the loss of chlorophyll in the dark
(14). However, the effectiveness of glucose at the optimum
concentration of 100 μM was still only half the effectiveness
of kinetin at 10 μM (14). If a high-energy intermediate is
required to delay senescence, the results indicate that light
may be acting through its action on cyclic photophosphoryla-
tion, a system that is not inhibited by diuron.

      Total protein synthesis declines in senescence but a
specific proteinase with L-serine in its active center increases in activity as senescence progresses (17). Most of
the total soluble protein lost in early senescence was accounted for by a decrease in ribulose-1,5-biphosphate carboxylase
(13). Therefore, the chloroplast appears to be the organelle
in which the initial senescence sequence begins.

      Excised leaves or leaf discs have been utilized exten-
sively to study senescence in plants. These systems have two
advantages: 1) detached tissues senesce at a faster rate than
when they are attached to the plant, and 2) regulatory compounds
can be fed conveniently to the tissues through the cut surfaces.
However, it is uncertain whether the biochemical and physiological changes in an excised leaf resemble those in attached
leaves. These considerations in the study of senescence are

relevant also to studies on metabolism of xenobiotics in
isolated plant tissues.

## Isolated Plant Part and Cell Methods

Whole plants with pesticides applied through their roots
or leaves or injected into stems and fruits are the most commonly used experimental material for xenobiotic metabolism
studies.  However, studies with intact plants are complicated
by variables related to root and leaf absorption, translocation
and transpiration.  To overcome some of these variables,
researchers have used excised plant parts and enzymatically
separated mesophyll cells.  Isolated plant protoplasts also
may be useful for xenobiotic metabolism studies.

Results of xenobiotic metabolism studies and observed
biochemical and physiological responses in separated plant
parts or cells are usually extrapolated to reflect reactions
occurring in complex whole plants.  This may or may not be
appropriate and caution must be exercised in evaluating results
from separated systems.  The different methods used for xenobiotic metabolism studies with plant parts and isolated cells
together with results from selected reports are presented here.

Excised Leaves and Roots.  Whole organs separated
from the intact plant are used in this method.  The leaves of
both di- and monocotyledonous plants may be used.

Method.  Dicotyledonous plants such as cotton (Gossypium
hirsutum L.) (18, 19, 20), peanut (Arachis hypogaea L.) (21,
22), carrot (Daucus carota L.) (20) and soybean [Glycine max
(L.) Merr.] are grown until their first true leaves are fully
expanded.  The petioles of the true leaves are excised under
water to prevent disruption of the water column in the xylem by
the introduction of air.  This precautionary step minimizes
permanent wilting of leaves due to the interruption of the
transpiration stream.

Leaves of monocotyledonous plants lack petioles.  Therefore, selected leaves may be excised near the base of the
lamina or blade as described for the petioles of dicots.
Leaves from corn (Zea mays L.), sorghum (Sorghum vulgare Pers.),
and sugarcane (Saccharum officianarum L.) have been excised
and used successfully (23, 24).  Excised leaf blades of barley
(Hordeum vulgare L.) and rice (Oryza sativa L.) have been used
to study the metabolism of detergents (25).  The entire shoot
of young (2- to 3-leaf stage) barley, wheat (Triticum aestivum
L.) and wild oat (Avena fatua L.) seedlings may be excised at
the soil level by the same method and used for metabolism
studies.  Morphologically, the shoots of young cereals and
other grasses consist of overlapping leaf sheaths of emerged
and younger leaves.  The vascular anatomy of the leaf sheath

would be comparable to that of the petiole. Excising the shoot
of young cereal plants is nearly equivalent to excising several
leaf blades.

The cut edges of either petioles or leaf blades are
immersed in a solution of the xenobiotic compound (18, 25).
Excised leaves are normally treated in a controlled-environment
chamber with a definite photoperiod. Light not only retards
senescence but it stimulates transpiration and increases the
uptake of treatment solution.

Excised whole roots, separated from the shoots, have not
been used extensively for metabolism studies. The root, a
heterotrophic plant organ, is more conducive for use in tissue
culture where a carbon source may be provided. Corn roots
supplied with glucose in aseptic culture metabolized atrazine
(2-chloro-4-ethylamino-6-isopropylamino-s-triazine) over a 72-
hr period (26). Excised roots of several species, including
corn, wheat, soybean, oats (Avena sativa L.) and barley were
incubated with simazine [2-chloro-4,6-bis(ethylamino)-s-
triazine] in Hoagland's nutrient solution for 6 hours (27).
Excised roots and hypocotyls of soybean were incubated for 24
hours in the dark in a 0.1% $Na_2CO_3$ or distilled water solution
of amiben (3-amino-2,5-dichlorobenzoic acid). The amiben
metabolite, N-glucosyl amiben [N-(3-carboxy-2,5-dichlorophenyl)-
glucosylamine], was isolated and characterized from these
tissues (28).

Roots of dicotyledonous seedlings with large endogenous
sources of carbon in their cotyledons may be cultured successfully after removal of their epicotyls (immature shoots). The
growth of roots from pea (Pisum sativum L.) seedlings with
their epicotyls removed was similar to growth of roots from
intact seedlings for 11 days in nutrient solution (29). These
roots were treated with atrazine for 9 days. The endogenous
reserve in the cotyledons was the only carbon source for the
roots.

Discussion. The use of excised leaves for xenobiotic
metabolism has several advantages: 1) ease of treating plant
material with the xenobiotic chemical, 2) rapid uptake of the
chemical into plant tissues, and 3) elimination of root and
leaf surface absorption as barriers. Some limitations of this
technique include: 1) the treatment period for metabolism must
be short, 2) senescence of the plant organ begins upon excision
from the intact plant, and 3) reactions in excised plant organ
may not be the same as those occurring in intact plants.

A relatively large number of excised leaves can be treated
with a minimum volume of treatment solution to obtain maximum
uptake and distribution of a xenobiotic in leaf tissues.
Metabolites of fluorodifen (2,4'-dinitro-4-trifluoromethyl
diphenylether) (22) and perfluidone [1,1,1-trifluoro-N-{2-
methyl-4-(phenysulfonyl)phenyl}methanesulfonamide] (21) were

isolated and characterized from 300 and 3000 excised peanut leaves, respectively. Treatment solutions were prepared at physiological concentrations of 1 to 100 μM and sparingly soluble compounds may be prepared as aqueous solutions containing up to 1% acetone (22). Acetone at 1% did not cause severe injury to excised leaves. The use of surfactants and emulsifiers common to leaf surface applications is not necessary.

Absorption and transport of xenobiotics to cellular biotransformation sites are fairly rapid in excised leaves. Absorption by dicot leaves is rapid, usually within the first 3 to 5 hours of treatment. Peanut leaves absorbed approximately 3 to 4 ml of fluorodifen solution per leaf within 5 hours (22), and cotton leaves absorbed up to 5 ml of cisanilide (cis-2,5-dimethyl-1-pyrrolidinecarboxanilide) solution per leaf within 3 hours (20). Additional distilled water is required to maintain excised leaves for treatment periods exceeding 5 to 6 hours. The distilled water may be added as a pulse-chase and to replace treatment solution lost through transpiration by excised leaves. Generally, the rate of xenobiotic absorption declines significantly after the initial 3 to 5 hours.

Absorption of treatment solution by excised leaf blades of monocots is not as rapid as with excised leaves of dicots. The rate of treatment solution lost per unit leaf area was not determined, but excised leaf blades generally required little additional distilled water. Sufficient quantities of s-triazines (23), propachlor (2-chloro-N-isopropylacetamide) (24), and diclofop-methyl [methyl-2-{4-(2',4'-dichlorophenoxy)phenoxy}propanoate] (30) were absorbed within 24- to 48-hour periods by excised corn and sorghum leaves and wheat shoots, respectively, for metabolite isolation and characterization.

Excised leaves may be useful for investigating pesticide interactions. Rapid pulse-chase treatment of excised leaves is possible with a xenobiotic preceded or followed by a second compound. The pulse-chase technique with excised leaves also is useful in studies on product-precursor relationships. Isolated metabolites may be used in treatments. Simultaneous treatment with xenobiotics may be appropriate if the compounds are compatible as a mixture. However, before any treatments with two or more compounds are made, the absorption and translocation characteristics of each compound in excised leaves should be determined to insure proper evaluation of results.

Absorption and translocation in excised leaves. Absorption of a xenobiotic in solution occurs predominantly through the cut edges of petioles or leaf blades or sheaths. Therefore, any influence exerted by roots on the absorption and translocation of a xenobiotic is circumvented by the excised leaf method. This method allows direct uptake of the xenobiotic into the xylem (apoplast) and transport throughout the leaf under the influence of the transpiration stream. Maximum

number of degradation sites in the mesophyll cells of leaves
should be exposed to the xenobiotic.  This is often a distinct
advantage of the excised leaf method.  However, the apoplastic
transport of xenobiotics, even when introduced directly into
the xylem, may not be solely a function of transpiration.
Several herbicides were selected (Figure 1) to illustrate
translocation differences in excised leaves.

Figures 2 to 5 show the translocation of [$^{14}$C-ring]
amitrole (3-amino-1,2,4-triazole) (A), [$^{14}$C-ring]atrazine (B),
[$^{14}$C-phenyl]diclofop-methyl (C), and [$^{14}$CF$_3$]fluorodifen (D) in
root-treated intact plants and excised leaves of soybean and
oat.  All herbicides were applied at 10 μM (spec. act. 0.54
mCi/mmol) concentration.  Two excised soybean leaves and oat
shoots were treated with 10 ml and 5 ml, respectively, of each
herbicide for 24 hours (Figures 2 and 4).  The roots of a
soybean and oat plant were treated with 50 ml and 30 ml,
respectively, of each herbicide for 48 hours (Figures 3 and 5).
All plant materials were exposed to a 14-10-hour light-dark
cycle at 13 klux light intensity, 26 C day and 20 C night
temperatures.  The relative absorption date of soybean and oat
plants (Tables I and II) cannot be compared directly since the
surface areas and the $^{14}$C applied differed between the two
species.  However, apparent differences between a dicot (soybean) and monocot (oat), as discussed previously, are evident.

Table I.  Absorption and translocation of [$^{14}$C]herbicides by
          excised soybean leaves and excised shoots of oat.[a]

| Herbicide | % of applied $^{14}$C absorbed[b] | | Distribution of absorbed $^{14}$C(%) | | | |
| | | | soybean | | oat | |
| | soybean | oat | immersed[c] | leaf | immersed[c] | shoot |
|---|---|---|---|---|---|---|
| Amitrole(A) | 99 | 32 | 6 | 94 | 53 | 47 |
| Atrazine(B) | 99 | 28 | 1 | 99 | 22 | 78 |
| Diclofop-methyl(C) | 92 | 77 | 36 | 64 | 75 | 25 |
| Fluorodifen(D) | 94 | 56 | 49 | 51 | 81 | 19 |

[a] Quantitative data for plants in Figures 2 and 4.

[b] $^{14}$C remaining in post-treatment solution: A, B, D - 100%
    parent herbicide; C - soybean - 100% parent herbicide; oat -
    30% parent herbicide, 70% acid metabolite (diclofop).

[c] Lower 3 cm of soybean petiole and excised oat shoot immersed
    in [$^{14}$C]herbicide solution.  Length of soybean petioles was
    8 cm.

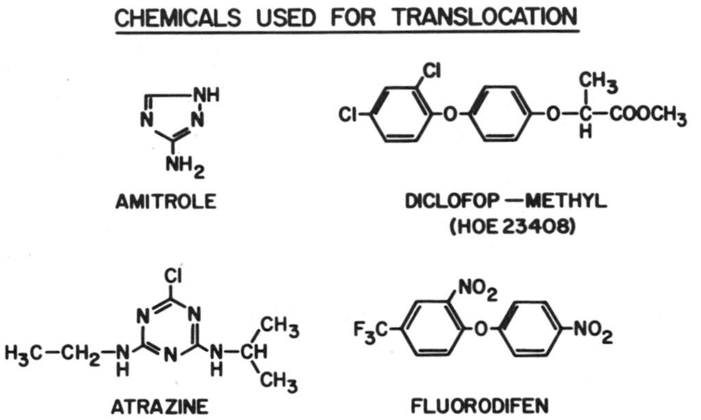

Figure 1.   *C-14 herbicides applied to excised soybean leaves, excised oat shoots, and roots of both species for absorption and translocation*

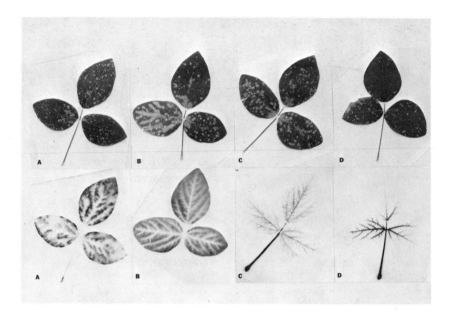

Figure 2. Radioautographs of excised soybean leaves treated with (A), $^{14}$C-labeled amitrole; (B), atrazine; (C), diclofop-methyl; and (D), fluorodifen. The bottom are radioautographs of the leaves above. The lower 3-cm section of each petiole was immersed in $^{14}$C herbicide solution for 24 hr.

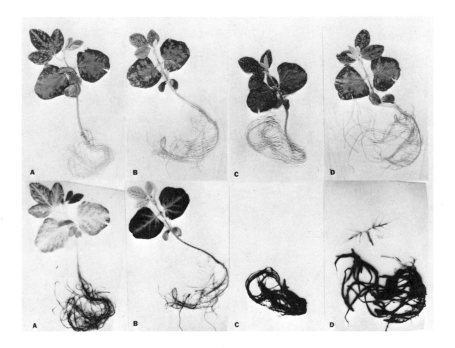

*Figure 3.   Radioautographs of soybean plants root-treated with (A), $^{14}$C-labeled amitrole; (B), atrazine; (C), diclofop-methyl; and (D), fluorodifen.  The bottom are radioautographs of the plants above.  Plants were root-treated for 48 hr.*

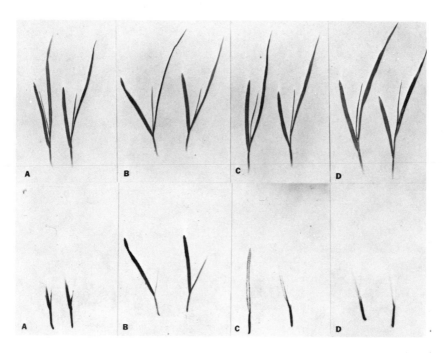

Figure 4.   Radioautographs of excised oat shoots treated with (A), [14]C-labeled amitrole; (B), atrazine; (C), diclofop-methyl; and (D), fluorodifen. The bottom are radioautographs of the excised shoots above. The lower 3-cm section of each shoot was immersed in [14]C herbicide solution for 24 hr.

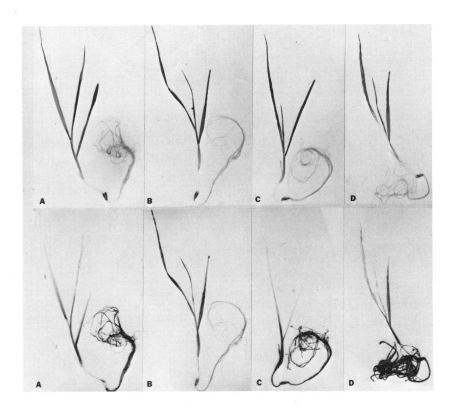

*Figure 5.  Radioautographs of oat plants root-treated with (A), ¹⁴C-labeled ami-trole; (B), atrazine; (C), diclofop-methyl; and (D), fluorodifen. The bottom are radioautographs of the plants above. Plants were root-treated for 48 hr.*

Table II.  Absorption and translocation of [$^{14}$C]herbicides by
root-treated intact soybean and oat plants.[a]

| | % of applied $^{14}$C absorbed[b] | | Distribution of absorbed $^{14}$C(%) | | | |
| | | | soybean | | oat | |
| Herbicide | soybean | oat | root | shoot | root | shoot |
|---|---|---|---|---|---|---|
| Amitrole(A) | 27 | 14 | 52 | 48 | 60 | 40 |
| Atrazine(B) | 29 | 8 | 20 | 80 | 31 | 69 |
| Diclofop-methyl(C) | 34 | 16 | 98 | 2 | 63 | 37 |
| Fluorodifen(D) | 77 | 48 | 83 | 17 | 78 | 22 |

[a] Quantitative data for plants in Figures 3 and 5.

[b] $^{14}$C remaining in post-treatment solution:  A, B, D - 100%
parent herbicide; C - 100% acid metabolite (diclofop).


Rapid transpiration rates increased the uptake of [$^{14}$C]
herbicides in excised leaves, especially in soybean (Table I).
Distilled water was added to excised soybean leaves after 5
hours.  Excised oat shoots required no additional water over
the 24-hour period.  Root uptake varied according to the
herbicide (Table II).  No additional distilled water was added
to root-treated plants over the 48-hour period.

The $^{14}$C from atrazine was uniformly distributed in excised
leaves and root-treated plants.  This is typical of apoplastic
transport under the influence of the transpiration stream.  The
distribution of $^{14}$C from amitrole was less uniform than that
from atrazine in both species.  The differential localization
of $^{14}$C from amitrole in younger leaves and apex of soybean
plants (Figure 3) indicates retranslocation or symplastic transport of $^{14}$C out of older leaves.  This contrasts to $^{14}$C from
atrazine which localized in the two unifoliate primary leaves
with little $^{14}$C in the younger developing leaves.  Symplastic
transport of [$^{14}$C]atrazine and/or its metabolites from older
leaves does not occur as with amitrole (Figure 3).  Retranslocation from leaves following initial apoplastic transport from
roots is not as evident in a monocot (Figure 5) as in a dicot
(Figure 3).  The vascular transport of material into and out of
leaves, a normal physiological process, is altered when leaves
are excised (Figures 2 and 4).  Therefore, the significance of
results from excised leaves must be evaluated in terms of what
may be occurring in an intact plant.

Diclofop-methyl and fluorodifen were readily absorbed by
excised leaves and root-treated plants (Tables I and II).

Uptake was enhanced by transpiration, especially in excised leaves of soybean (Table I). However, transpiration appeared to have very little influence on transport. Unlike amitrole and atrazine, much of the [14]C from diclofop-methyl and fluorodifen was immobilized in the petiole of soybean leaf and the immersed section of excised oat shoot and the roots of both species (Tables I and II, Figures 2 to 5). Atrazine is not metabolized in significant amounts in soybean (26, 31) and probably in oat, an atrazine-susceptible species. Amitrole metabolism in soybean may be as rapid as in bean (Phaseolus vulgaris L.) (32) and oat (33). Fluorodifen metabolism is rapid in soybean (20) whereas diclofop-methyl metabolism is rapid in both oat and soybean (30).

Immobilization of xenobiotics in the xylem may be due to adsorption by xylem vessels or uptake and retention by parenchyma cells. The extent of immobilization may be a function of the physical and chemical properties of the molecular entities being translocated with only limited influence by the transpiration stream. Therefore, metabolism of a xenobiotic and the formation of products with differing physical and chemical properties may be a greater factor influencing translocation than species differences in the translocation mechanisms per se. The greater translocation of [14]C from [[14]C]dipropetryn [2-ethylthio-4,6-bis(isopropylamino)-s-triazine] to the leaf tips in oat than in corn excised leaves was reported to be a factor in the higher susceptibility of oat to dipropetryn (34). This difference in translocation between excised leaves of oat and corn was attributed to an inherent mechanism regulating translocation of dipropetryne within the leaves of these species (34). However, such a conclusion is questionable since the molecular forms of the [14]C being translocated were not determined. The translocation differences between a resistant and susceptible species may simply reflect differences in metabolism of the xenobiotic and immobilization of its metabolites as a function of their physical and chemical properties.

Translocation of [14]C-labeled xenobiotics in excised leaves must be determined and not assumed to be typical of apoplastic transport. If immobilization occurs in specific parts of excised leaves, extraction of metabolites from these parts will maximize the concentration of metabolites and minimize the impurities and natural products that must be removed in the purification procedure.

Xenobiotic metabolism in excised leaves. The metabolism of xenobiotics in excised leaves appears to be similar qualitatively to metabolism in shoots of intact plants, but may differ quantitatively. The same water-soluble metabolites of perfluidone were detected in excised peanut leaves and leaves or shoots of intact peanut plants treated through their roots (21). However, excised leaves tolerated treatment with twice the highest

concentration used for root-treatment with 62% uptake of applied
[$^{14}$C]perfluidone versus 25% uptake by roots.  Only 31% of the
root uptake was translocated to the shoots.  Two water-soluble
conjugates of perfluidone accounted for 31% of the $^{14}$C in
excised peanut leaves after 48 hours but the same metabolites
accounted for only 8% of the $^{14}$C in the shoots of root-treated
intact plants after 8 days (21).  Ethylenethiourea (ETU), a
decomposition product of ethylenebis(dithiocarbamate) fungicides, was metabolized similarly by excised leaves and shoots
of root-treated tomato (Lycopersicon esculentum Mill.) (35).
However, metabolism in tomato shoots was slower than in excised
leaves when ETU was stem-injected into intact plants.  The
metabolism of diclofop-methyl, a post-emergence herbicide, in
wheat and wild oat was qualitatively similar in excised shoots
and root-treated intact plants (29).  Excised shoots of wheat
and wild oat absorbed 81% and 87% of the applied [$^{14}$C]diclofop-
methyl, respectively, and metabolized 77% and 72% of the
absorbed $^{14}$C to water-soluble conjugates within 24 hours.
Intact root-treated wheat and wild oat absorbed 68% and 37%
of applied [$^{14}$C]diclofop-methyl, respectively, but only 8% and
11% of the root uptake was translocated to the shoots.  Therefore, the use of excised leaves (dicots) or shoots (monocots)
to study metabolism of foliarly-applied xenobiotics such as
diclofop-methyl may have distinct advantages over root application or stem-injection.

Metabolites of monuron [3-(4-chlorophenyl)-1,1-dimethy-
lurea] were isolated and characterized from excised cotton
leaves (18, 19).  Within 24 hours, two β-D-glucosides consti-
tuted 20 to 25% of the methanol-soluble metabolites (18).
These were identified as conjugates of the hydroxymethyl intermediates.  Longer treatments of up to 4 days indicated that the
rapid oxidative N-demethylation of monuron, occurring within
the first 24 hours, was followed by slow oxidative aryl hydroxylation and subsequent conjugation (19).  Both rapid and slow
biotransformation reactions of monuron were elucidated by the
use of excised leaves.

Qualitative differences in the metabolism of a xenobiotic
between roots and shoots are not common.  However, such differences have been observed for some herbicides (36, 37).  Little
or no glutathione conjugates of atrazine (GS-atrazine) and its
derivatives were detected in the roots of intact root-treated
corn plants (36).  The major metabolite in corn roots was
hydroxyatrazine (2-hydroxy-4-ethylamino-6-isopropylamino-s-
triazine).  Significant concentrations (10 to 20% of $^{14}$C in
intact plant) of GS-atrazine were found only in the shoots.
GS-atrazine and its derivatives accounted for 60 to 70% of the
atrazine absorbed directly into excised corn leaf blades within
24 hours.  Very little hydroxyatrazine was detected (36).  The
qualitative differences in atrazine metabolism between roots and
shoots of corn were due to the localization of glutathione S-

transferase in the shoots and not roots of corn (37). The
metabolites of chlorpropham (isopropyl-m-chlorocarbanilate)
differed between roots and shoots in root-treated intact soybean plants (38). Conjugates of 2-hydroxy-chlorpropham and
4-hydroxy-chlorpropham were present in the shoots, but only the
conjugate of 2-hydroxy-chlorpropham was found in root tissue
(38). This suggests that leaf tissue probably formed both
hydroxylated derivatives, but root tissues formed only 2-
hydroxy-chlorpropham. Studies on chlorpropham metabolism in
excised soybean leaves should confirm the above conclusion.

Leaf Discs and Leaf Sections. Leaf discs of uniform
size, leaf sections of lamina (leaf blade) from grasses or thin
leaf strips may be used for xenobiotic metabolism studies. The
structural and metabolic integrity of the leaf tissues is maintained, but the normal vascular transport of materials to and
from the leaf tissues is eliminated. Penetration of xenobiotics
into the mesophyll and palisade cells is predominantly through
the cells along the cut edges of leaf discs or sections (39).
The cuticle, a major barrier to leaf penetration by surface-
applied chemicals, is circumvented by the use of leaf discs or
sections as in the use of excised leaves or shoots described
previously. The uptake and efflux of organic compounds in plant
cells are not well understood (40). The mechanism of uptake
involving physico-chemical interactions at the plasmalemma and
tonoplast (vacuole membrane) (41) is applicable to leaf discs
and leaf sections.

Method. The size of leaf discs and leaf sections used,
the incubation medium for the leaf tissue, and the method of
applying the test chemicals vary according to the objectives of
the specific experiments. Leaf discs are usually cut with a
cork borer (8 to 15 mm diameter) from interveinal areas of the
leaf blade (41, 42, 43, 44). Leaf sections or slices from
monocots varied from barley leaves cut transversely at 0.75 mm
wide strips (45) to sorghum lamina cut into 1 cm x 1 cm sections
(46). Dicotyledonous cotton leaves were cut into 0.4 mm wide
strips (47).
The incubation medium for leaf discs or sections may or may
not contain an osmoticum. Sucrose (0.25 M, pH 6.2) (41) and
mannitol at 0.26 M (pH 4 to 6) (45) and 0.35 M (42, 48) are
commonly used osmoticums. Leaf tissues were also incubated in
water (43, 44, 46, 49, 50). Other than an osmoticum and buffer,
inorganic salts are not commonly added to the incubation medium.
The simplicity of the incubation medium for leaf discs or sections is in marked contrast to the medium required for separated
cells or aseptic tissue culture.
The leaf discs or sections are treated with xenobiotics
or other test compounds by vacuum infiltration (41, 42, 43, 48)
or by either floatation or submersion of the leaves in solutions

of the compounds (44, 45, 46, 50). Infiltration of the test
chemical into leaf tissue may be accomplished by evacuating the
leaf tissue in a solution of the compound to a given pressure
(20 cm Hg) (49) before releasing the vacuum or maintaining a
given pressure (40 cm Hg) for a specific period (15 min) (41).
The most common practice is to evacuate to the maximum pressure
with a water aspirator (42) and either maintain the vacuum or
release it immediately. Successful infiltration of the solution into the intercellular air spaces of the mesophyll cells
can be checked visually by the darker, water-soaked appearance
of the leaf tissue.

    Discussion. Leaf discs or sections have been used exten-
sively for basic research on the uptake of inorganic salts and
organic compounds by plant cells, and on photosynthesis and
photorespiration. Use of this method to study metabolism of
xenobiotics has been limited. Little is known about the penetration of plant cell membranes by xenobiotics (51). Unlike
inorganic ions, amino acids, and sugars that appear to have
specific membrane transport systems, the predominantly lipophilic and neutral xenobiotics, such as herbicides, probably
cross cell membranes by diffusion (51). Therefore, vacuum
infiltration of the xenobiotic should enhance penetration of
the compound into mesophyll cells. The xenobiotic will penetrate more cells than without vacuum infiltration, thereby
increasing the concentration of metabolites formed in leaf
discs.
    Vacuum infiltration of leaf discs has some detrimental
effects. Although respiration in wheat, barley, and bean leaf
discs was unaffected by vacuum infiltration of water, $CO_2$
fixation and $O_2$ evolution were totally inhibited (49). Carrier-
mediated uptake of amino acids into leaf sections was dependent
on respiration and photosynthesis for ATP as its energy source
(45, 52). Amino acid uptake was inhibited by 2,4-dinitrophenol
or anaerobic conditions in the dark. Light stimulated amino
acid uptake under anaerobic conditions, but this stimulation
was totally inhibited by 10 μM diuron (45). If uptake of
compounds such as 2,4-D (2,4-dichlorophenoxyacetic acid) is an
active process in leaf discs as it appears to be in root tissue
(53), then vacuum infiltration of leaf discs may not be advisable for studies with such compounds. However, for compounds
such as monuron which is taken up passively by diffusion in
roots (53), vacuum infiltration for uptake by leaf discs may be
advantageous. This may be true for metabolism studies but not
for experiments on inhibition of photosynthesis by monuron.
Studies comparable to those on amino acid uptake by plant cells
have not been reported for herbicides and other pesticides.
Therefore, the effect of vacuum infiltration on the uptake of
specific herbicides in leaf discs is only speculative.
    Little is known of the effects of senescence on uptake and

metabolism of xenobiotics by leaf discs or sections.  The
senescence processes described earlier may have significant
effects on the processes described above.

<u>Metabolism in leaf discs or sections</u>.  Selected examples
are presented to illustrate the versatility of the leaf disc or
section technique.  The use of this method permits:  1) rapid
assessment of pesticide degradation in plant tissues, 2) determination of physiological factors that influence metabolism of
pesticides, and 3) evaluation of interaction effects between
pesticides.  A thorough study on the metabolism of phenylurea
herbicides in leaf discs of resistant and susceptible plants
(54, 55) demonstrates the above points.  A time-course study on
the metabolism of monuron showed rapid N-demethylation and
metabolism to water-soluble conjugates within 3 hours after pre-
incubation of resistant cotton and plantain (<u>Plantago</u> <u>major</u> L.)
leaf discs in a buffered solution of monuron (54).  Leaf discs
of monuron-sensitive soybean and corn metabolized monuron to a
much lesser extent over the same period than cotton or plantain.
Active photosynthesis was not required for monuron metabolism
since the rate of degradation was similar in the dark and light
under $CO_2$-free conditions.
  A flux of a chemical into and out of leaf discs may be
expected (41, 51).  The kinetics of uptake and efflux of non-
electrolytes have been described (41).  However, in most of
these studies it was assumed that the chemical was not altered
between its uptake and efflux by leaf discs.  Some evidence
indicates that this may not be necessarily true.  The efflux
from monuron-resistant plantain leaf discs was nearly one-half
of the initially absorbed herbicide within 2 to 3 hours (54).
Subsequent reabsorption and metabolism occurred but 37% of the
total [14]C was present in the efflux after 7.6 hours.  More than
50% of the [14]C in the efflux was three metabolites with parent
monuron accounting for the remainder (54).  However, polar
water-soluble conjugates, which constitute the major metabolites
of monuron in leaf discs, were not detected in the efflux.
Similarly, major water-soluble conjugates of atrazine (56) in
corn leaf discs and diclofop-methyl (30) in wheat leaf sections
were not detected in the efflux from these tissues.  Therefore,
a selective efflux of non-polar parent compounds or their
metabolites appears to occur in leaf discs or sections with some
xenobiotics.  Any relationship between the efflux characteristics
of leaf discs and release of material from parenchyma cells into
the vascular system of intact plants is still obscure.  However,
efflux characteristics of specific compounds from leaf discs may
be related to their immobilization or translocation in intact
plants.
  The evaluation of xenobiotic metabolism as a factor in
selectivity, antagonism, or synergism is possible because of the
rapid determination of metabolism in leaf discs.  Metabolism and

detoxication of herbicides in plants is probably the most important single factor in herbicide selectivity. Physiological responses coupled to time-course metabolism may be readily demonstrated in leaf discs for photosynthetic inhibitors such as monuron (55) and atrazine (44, 48, 56). Inhibition of photosynthesis and recovery within 8 hours was correlated with glutathione conjugation of atrazine in sorghum (44), corn (56), and several species of the subfamilies, Festucoideae and Panicoideae (48). Recovery of photosynthesis to nearly the control level occurred in monuron-treated cotton leaf discs within 4 to 5 hours with rapid N-demethylation of monuron (55).

The nature of interaction between xenobiotics at the molecular level may be demonstrated readily in leaf discs. The application of a mixture of the herbicide, propanil (3,4-dichloropropionanilide), with a carbamate or phosphate insecticide caused injury to resistant rice (57). The injury was due to the inhibition of an aryl acylamidase in rice by carbamate insecticides that prevented detoxication of propanil in the resistant species (58, 59). In resistant cotton leaf discs, certain carbamate insecticides such as carbaryl (1-napthyl-methylcarbamate) strongly inhibited the degradation of the photosynthetic inhibitor, monuron. The inhibition of photosynthesis was enhanced and normal recovery to control levels of photosynthetic activity was delayed (55).

The interactions between several organophosphate and carbamate insecticides and herbicides were tested in leaf discs of several species (60, 61). Organophosphate insecticides, dyfonate (O-ethyl-S-phenyl ethylphosphonodithioate) and malathion [O,O-dimethyl-S-(1,2-bis-carbethoxy)-ethyl phosphorodithioate], strongly inhibited the metabolism of substituted phenylurea herbicides. Several carbamates [carbaryl, carbofuran (2,3-dihydro-2,2-dimethyl-7-benzofuranyl methylcarbamate), PCMC (p-chlorophenyl-N-methylcarbamate)] strongly inhibited propanil metabolism (60). The effects of several herbicides on the degradation of carbaryl, dyfonate, and malathion were not as severe as the effects of the insecticides on herbicide metabolism (61). Carbaryl metabolism was stimulated by chlorpropham while metabolism of dyfonate and malathion was inhibited by propanil (61). The nature of the interaction between carbofuran and the herbicides, alachor (2-chloro-2',6'-diethyl-N-methoxymethyl acetanilide) (62), chlorbromuron [3-(4-bromo-3-chlorophenyl)-1-methoxy-1-methylurea] (63), and butylate (S-ethyldiisobutylthiocarbamate) (64) was explained on the basis of whole-plant experiments. Carbofuran increased the absorption and inhibited slightly the metabolism of the herbicides. If the inhibition of herbicide metabolism by carbofuran is significant, it should be readily demonstrated in leaf discs over much shorter periods than is possible with whole plants.

Isolation and characterization of metabolites. The
identification of metabolites extracted from leaf discs is
generally based on thin-layer cochromatography with known
standards. Limited numbers of leaf discs or sections are
treated with radiolabeled xenobiotics, extracted, and the radioactive metabolites are separated and quantitated. Leaf discs
or sections also may be used to generate sufficient quantities
of metabolites for purification and chemical characterization.
However, use of leaf discs or sections for such a purpose has
been limited.

The identification of glutathione conjugation as one of
the major pathways for herbicide detoxication in plants was
made through the use of sorghum leaf discs and sections. A
water-soluble metabolite of atrazine was detected as a major
metabolite in sorghum leaf discs during recovery of atrazine-
inhibited photosynthesis (44). This metabolite was generated
from a large-scale treatment of sorghum leaf sections bathed in
a solution of atrazine for 20 hours (46). The metabolites,
S-(4-ethylamino-6-isopropylamino-s-triazinyl-2)glutathione (III)
and γ-glutamyl-S-(4-ethylamino-6-isopropylamino-s-triazinyl-
2)cysteine (IV), were successfully isolated and characterized
from sorghum leaf sections (46). Subsequent studies with whole
plants elucidated the mercapturic acid-like pathway for atrazine
metabolism in plants (65).

The limited periods that leaf discs or sections may be
allowed to metabolize xenobiotics could be a disadvantage.
Metabolites that are formed over longer periods cannot be
generated in leaf discs or sections. The metabolite of atrazine,
N-(4-ethylamino-6-isopropylamino-s-triazinyl-2)lanthionine
(VII), was present in significant quantities in leaves of root-
treated sorghum plants only after 5 days (65). Metabolites
III and IV were major metabolites in sorghum shoots of whole
plants after 14.4 hours of treatment but declined thereafter
(65). Therefore, due to temporal requirements it is doubtful
if metabolites such as VII can be successfully generated and
isolated from leaf discs or sections.

Separated Leaf Cells. In this method the mesophyll
and palisade cells from leaves are separated to give a homogenous liquid suspension of cells that can be manipulated much
like unicellular algae. The separated cell system is useful
for studying biochemical, physiological and cytochemical processes in plants. Use of individual cells in suspension permits
equal exposure of all cells to test chemicals. This is unlike
the techniques involving leaf discs or sections in which cells
along the cut edges are exposed preferentially to the test
chemicals. The presence of rigid cell walls permits repeated
washing and centrifugation of cells with minimal damage. The
metabolic function of the leaf tissue is maintained in the cell
suspension but the structural integrity of the leaf and the

normal function of vascular transport are no longer retained.

   Method.  Morphologically intact mesophyll cells may be
separated by: 1) gently grinding leaf tissue and separating
individual cells from leaf debris by selective filtration and
centrifugation (66, 67); and 2) digestion of leaf tissue with
enzyme preparations containing polygalacturonase and cellulase
(68, 69, 70, 71, 72).  The enzyme separation methods presently
used are basically modifications of those developed by Takebe
et al. (68) and Jensen et al. (69).
   Separated leaf cells are prepared by cutting leaves into
strips (69) or squares (72) and vacuum infiltrating these
tissues with a maceration medium containing the enzyme (0.5 to
3.0%), inorganic salts, buffer (pH 5.8), potassium dextran
sulfate, a hypertonic solution of sorbitol (0.7 to 0.8 M),
anti-senescent agents (2,4-D, benzyladenine), and antibiotics.
The infiltrated tissue is digested with additional maceration
medium for 10 to 30 min.  The cells separated during this first
and a second similar maceration periods are discarded.  The
cells obtained during the third maceration period (30 to 45
min) are most active metabolically and are used for experimentation.  The wash and assay media contain similar salts as the
maceration medium, 0.6 to 0.7 M sorbitol and are buffered at a
higher pH (6.7 to 7.2).

   Discussion.  The discussion is limited to enzymatically
separated cells since this is the system that has been used to
study the effects of xenobiotics (herbicides) on separated
plant cells.
   Maceration of leaf tissue in a hypertonic environment
that results in cell plasmolysis was necessary to yield photo-
synthetically active cells (69).  Plasmolyzed cells with intact
plasmalemmas were detected by phase contrast microscopy (69).
Separated cotton mesophyll cells fixed $CO_2$ at linear rates of
50 to 100 μmoles/mg chlorophyll /hour for 4 to 8 hours (71).
Uptake of $^{14}C$-leucine and $^{14}C$-uracil and incorporation into
protein and RNA, respectively, occurred in separated tobacco
(Nicotiana tabacum L.) cells (73).  Uptake and incorporation of
the percursors into macromolecules required light and active
photosynthesis.  Addition of ATP only partially substituted for
the light requirement.  A smaller percentage of the absorbed
percursors was incorporated into macromolecules when cells were
incubated in the dark than in light (73).  Efflux of photosynthetic products amounted to 1 to 2% of total carbon fixed per
hour (71).  Efflux was inhibited by the addition of $Ca^{2+}$ in
the incubation medium.
   The metabolic activity is similar between separated cells
and cells of intact leaves and leaf discs described earlier.
The separated cells were metabolically active for 20 to 30
hours (69, 73).  However, critical experimental periods should

not exceed 5 to 12 hours since the metabolic activity in the cells may not be sustained beyond this period.

Metabolism in separated cells. Separated cells have been used to study primarily the effects of herbicides and surfactants on plant cell membranes (74, 75, 76) and selected metabolic reactions (70, 72, 77, 78, 79). The biochemical and physiological changes observed in the above studies were not correlated with metabolism of the xenobiotics in separated cells. Therefore, the studies are not complete. However, the potential usefulness of this technique has been demonstrated in the limited number of reports.

Cationic surfactants increased significantly the efflux of $^{14}CO_2$ fixation products in separated soybean, wild onion (Allium canadense L.) and cotton mesophyll cells (74, 75). In wild onion, $CO_2$ fixation was also inhibited by the same surfactants. Nonionic surfactants had relatively less effect on membrane permeability and photosynthesis than the cationic surfactants (74, 75). Wild onion cells were less sensitive to the action of a cationic surfactant than were soybean cells (75). Mixtures of oryzalin (3,5-dinitro-$N^4$,$N^4$-dipropylsulfanilamide) with selected surfactants enhanced efflux in soybean cells above that of cells treated with oryzalin or surfactant alone (74). Oryzalin and surfactants caused greater efflux of intracellular material from cotton cells than from soybean cells (74). The synergistic effects between oryzalin and surfactants were not observed in cotton as with soybean cells. The differences observed between cells from different species in response to treatment with a chemical may not be due to inherent differences in their membranes. Such differences may be only a reflection of the differences in metabolism and detoxication of the biologically active compound between cells from different species. Nonionic surfactants like Triton X-100 are rapidly metabolized in plants when taken up by excised leaves or absorbed from leaf surfaces (25, 80).

The concept that herbicides have multiple sites of action rather than a single site has been supported by results from separated cells (72, 77, 78). A time-course effect of 13 major herbicides on photosynthesis, respiration, protein synthesis, RNA synthesis, and lipid synthesis was measured in separated kidney bean cells at various concentrations (72). Photosynthetic inhibitors such as atrazine, monuron, bromacil (5-bromo-3-sec-butyl-6-methyluracil), and dinoseb (2-sec-butyl-4,6-dinitrophenol) inhibited photosynthesis significantly but stimulated lipid synthesis at physiological concentrations of 0.1 to 1.0 µM. RNA synthesis also was inhibited at the same concentrations. At 100 µM, the same herbicides strongly inhibited lipid synthesis. The inhibition of macromolecule synthesis by photosynthetic inhibitors is probably a secondary effect since the uptake and incorporation of percursors require

active photosynthesis (73). The physiological significance
of the reported effects on metabolic processes may be evaluated
better if information on the metabolism and intracellular
localization of the herbicides were known.

The metabolism of differentially labeled [$^{14}$C]fluorodifen
in separated mesophyll cells from resistant peanut is shown in
Table III. The cells were prepared using the method of Jensen
et al. (69) except that Pectinol 41-P (crude pectinase and
cellulase) was used in place of macerozyme, no 2,4-D was added
to any media, K$_2$SO$_4$ was substituted for potassium dextran
sulfate and the assay medium contained 0.6 M sorbitol buffered
with 0.05 M HEPES (pH 7.0). Assays were conducted in 2 ml
photosynthetic medium (69) that contained 10 μM [$^{14}$C]fluoro-
difen, 1% acetone, 7.5 mM NaHCO3, and separated cells (238 μg
chlorophyll per reaction flask). Reaction flasks were incubated in a differential respirometer at 25 C and illuminated
from below with incandescent lamps (5000 lux). The cells were
separated from the assay medium and extracted with 80% methanol.
The cell extract and the assay medium were analyzed for
fluorodifen and its metabolites as reported previously (22, 81,
82).

The uptake of fluorodifen by peanut mesophyll cells
occurred readily in light or dark (Table III). The ratio of
$^{14}$C in the cell pellet to that in assay medium decreased with
decreasing cell concentrations in repeated experiments. Maximum uptake and metabolism of fluorodifen occurred within 2
hours. Light appeared to have no influence on the uptake of
fluorodifen. However, fluorodifen metabolism was enhanced by
light in the 2-hour treatment period. Efflux of water-soluble
metabolites (glucosides and peptide conjugates) occurred from
separated cells. However, efflux of fluorodifen could not be
determined. The role of light in the enhanced metabolism of
fluorodifen is not clear. Oxygen evolution was not inhibited
by fluorodifen and ATP was not a required co-factor for glutathione S-transferase, the enzyme that catalyzes the ether
cleavage of fluorodifen (83).

Separated zinia (Zinia elegans Jacq.) cells absorbed
[$^{14}$C]fluorodifen and [$^{14}$C]trifluralin (α,α,α-trifluoro-2,6-
dinitro-N,N-dipropyl-p-toluidine) within 2 hours (70). After
washing cells with solutions of the unlabeled herbicides,
[$^{14}$C]trifluralin appeared to be bound more strongly than
[$^{14}$C]fluorodifen. However, the significance of the results is
not clear since metabolism of the two compounds was not determined.

The single example of xenobiotic metabolism in a separated
cell system illustrates the importance of metabolism when
studying the mechanism of action and selectivity of a compound.
Separated cells can be used to measure rapid biochemical and
physiological changes in response to treatment with a xenobiotic. However, the dynamic changes in uptake, metabolism,

Table III. Metabolism of [14CF3]- and [14C-p-NO2-phenyl]-labeled fluorodifen in separated peanut mesophyll cells.

| | Distribution of total 14C (%) | | | | | |
| | 2-hour treatment | | | | 4-hour treatment | |
| | [14CF3]a/ | | [14C-p-NO2-phenyl]a/ | | | (light) |
| | light | dark | light | dark | [14CF3] | [14C-p-NO2-phenyl] |
|---|---|---|---|---|---|---|
| Assay medium: | | | | | | |
| fluorodifen | 18 | 31 | 15 | 29 | 16 | 13 |
| conjugates b/ | 9 | 1 | 11 | 5 | 10 | 16 |
| Cell Pellet: | | | | | | |
| fluorodifen | 29 | 58 | 30 | 58 | 27 | 26 |
| conjugates b/ | 40 | 9 | 39 | 7 | 40 | 40 |
| MeOH-insoluble residue: | 4 | 1 | 5 | 1 | 7 | 5 |
| Total | 100 | 100 | 100 | 100 | 100 | 100 |

a/ Specific activities: [14CF3 fluorodifen] - 2.95 mCi/mmol; [14C-p-NO2-phenyl] fluorodifen - 2.7 mCi/mmol.

b/ [14CF3]fluorodifen: predominantly S-(2-nitro-4-trifluoromethylphenyl)-gluthathione with small amounts of S-(2-nitro-4-trifluoromethylphenyl)-N-malonylcysteine (82); [14C-p-NO2-phenyl]fluorodifen: mixture of p-nitrophenyl-β-D-glucoside and p-nitrophenyl-6-O-malonyl-β-D-glucoside (81).

and efflux of the xenobiotic and its metabolites in plant cells
also should be known before conclusions on mechanisms of action
and selectivity are made.

Plant Protoplasts.  Protoplasts are naked cells
obtained by removal of their cell walls.  This may be accomplished by: 1) microdissection, or 2) enzymatic digestion.
The latter is the more effective and commonly used procedure.
The exposed plasmalemma differentiates protoplasts from
isolated mesophyll cells whose rigid primary cell walls are
still intact.  The same advantages described for isolated
mesophyll cells apply to protoplasts.  Because of the exposed
plasmalemma, it is possible to study membrane absorption and
permeability effects without interference by the cell wall (84).
Protoplasts have been useful for studies on cell ultrastructure and functions.  They have not been used for studies
on metabolism of xenobiotics or their mechanisms of action.
This may be due to the difficulties of preparing and maintaining
protoplasts; they are extremely fragile and must be stabilized
by osmotic stabilizers (sorbitol or mannitol) and $Ca^{2+}$ salts
(85, 86).

Method.  Numerous methods for the isolation of plant
protoplasts have been published, but no standard method exists
since each species, type of tissue, cell-strain, environmental
growth conditions, etc., require new adjustments in the isolation procedures (85, 86).  Generally, the methods are modifications of that originally published by Cocking (87).  Each
special problem appears to require empirical adjustments to a
general scheme outlined as follows (85):  Leaves are selected
from plants exposed to specific growth regimes and surface
sterilized.  All operations are performed aseptically.  The
lower epidermis of leaves is removed to expose mesophyll cells;
the leaves are cut into sections and transferred to an enzyme
solution.  The enzyme solution for cell wall digestion may
contain pectinase and/or cellulase and/or hemicellulase with
an osmotic stabilizer and $Ca^{2+}$.  Protoplasts, usually released
within 6 to 24 hours, are washed with a solution of the osmoticum and used for experimentation or cultured under aseptic
conditions for subsequent studies.  Modifications to this basic
procedure are illustrated in recent publications (88, 89, 90).

Discussion.  Isolated plant protoplasts are generally
spherical in appearance with cellular components arranged along
the cell periphery (91).  Protoplasts may undergo wall rejuve-
nation, cell division, and differentiation to produce new
plants under suitable conditions (86, 92).  One of the greatest
potentials of protoplasts is the production of intra- and
inter-generic hybrids through cell fusion.  Fusion of naked
protoplasts from two tobacco species has been reported (93).

Protoplasts may not be suitable for large scale generation, purification, and characterization of metabolites from xenobiotics at present. However, if the techniques for preparation of protoplasts are further improved and standardized, protoplasts may become another important tool for the pesticide chemist.

Protoplasts may be useful for studying physiological and biochemical effects of xenobiotics in plant cells. Oat mesophyll protoplasts incorporated uridine and leucine up to 6 hours and thymidine up to 21 hours. Kinetin inhibited leucine incorporation with increasing concentration of the growth hormone, but 2,4-D, abscisic acid and gibberellic acid had no effect on the same process (94). Uridine incorporation was inhibited by 2,4-D at concentrations above 0.1 μM. None of the growth hormones had any effect on thymidine incorporation (94). The differential susceptibility of resistant and susceptible oat varieties to the phytotoxin, victorin, was demonstrated with isolated protoplasts (95). The cytokinin-like action of methyl-2-benzimidazole carbamate (MBZ), the fungitoxic metabolite of benomyl [methyl-1-(butylcarbamoyl)-2-benzimidazole carbamate], was confirmed in oat protoplasts (96). The decrease in nuclease activity, increase in leucine incorporation and decrease in uridine and thymidine incorporation were similar in protoplasts treated with kinetin or MBZ (96). The effect of MBZ on the plasmalemma of protoplasts was not resolved.

Tomato fruit protoplasts absorbed and retained significant amounts of fluorodifen and trifluralin (70). The short-term structural integrity of the plasmalemma from tomato protoplasts was unaffected by fluorodifen, trifluralin, fluometuron [1,1-dimethyl-3-(α,α,α-trifluoro-m-tolyl)urea], and chlorbromuron. However, complete membrane breakage and collapse of the protoplasts occurred after 30 minutes of treatment with paraquat (1,1'-dimethyl-4,4'-bypyridinium dichloride) (97).

The protoplasts have not been used to investigate metabolism of xenobiotics. However, it appears to be a convenient system to determine the metabolism of xenobiotics concurrently with a study on the phytotoxic and selective action of these compounds in plant cells.

Conclusion.

The survey of the literature on in vitro organ, tissue, and isolated cell techniques for xenobiotic metabolism in plants is not complete. Selected reports indicate that isolated plant systems may be used successfully by pesticide chemists to elucidate degradation pathways and interactions of xenobiotic compounds in plants.

Isolated plant systems are most useful for short-term investigations on metabolism, mechanism of action and selectivity.

One of the major advantages of the techniques discussed in
this report is the ability to measure rapid biochemical and
physiological changes in response to a chemical coupled to its
metabolism under carefully controlled conditions.  This may
not be possible in whole-plant experiments.  Reduced growth
and other visible manifestations of injury in whole plants are
usually much delayed secondary responses to a chemical.  However, results from isolated plant systems must be carefully
evaluated before they are extrapolated to intact whole plants.
Also, conclusions based only on whole-plant experiments should
be confirmed by in vitro techniques.

Abstract.

     Whole plants have been used for xenobiotic metabolism
and "terminal" residue studies.  However, in vitro techniques
using isolated leaves or roots, leaf discs or sections, and
separated mesophyll cells have proven to be more useful for
short-term investigations on xenobiotic metabolism, mechanism
of action and selectivity.  The in vitro techniques allow the
treatment of large amounts of plant material with a minimum of
chemical and facilitate rapid uptake of the chemical into plant
tissues.  The influence of root and leaf surface absorption
is also circumvented by the use of in vitro techniques.  Quantitative differences in xenobiotic metabolism between whole
plants and isolated plant systems have been observed, but
qualitative differences are not common.  Results from isolated
plant systems must be carefully evaluated before extrapolation
to intact plants because of the unknown influence of senescence,
absorption, and translocation on in vitro systems.

Literature Cited

1.  Casida, J. E. and Lykken, L., Annu. Rev. Plant Physiol.
    (1969) 20, 607.
2.  Kearney, P. C. and Kaufman, D. D., eds., "Herbicides -
    Chemistry, Degradation and Mode of Action," Vol. 1 and 2,
    Marcel Dekker, Inc., New York, NY (1975).
3.  Frear, D. S., Hodgson, R. H., Shimabukuro, R. H. and
    Still, G. G., Advan. Agron. (1972) 24, 328.
4.  Bukovac, M. J., "Herbicides - Physiology, Biochemistry,
    Ecology," Audus, L. J., ed., Vol. 1, p. 335, Academic
    Press, New York, NY (1976).
5.  Hay, J. R., "Herbicides - Physiology, Biochemistry,
    Ecology," Audus, L. J., ed., Vol. 1, p. 365, Academic
    Press, New York, NY (1976).
6.  Haynes, R. J. and Goh, K. M., Scien. Hort. (1977) 7, 291.
7.  Crafts, A. S. and Crisp, C. E., "Phloem Transport in
    Plants," W. H. Freeman and Co., San Francisco, CA (1971).

8. Zimmerman, M. H. and Milburn, J. A., eds., "Transport in Plants I: Phloem Transport," Encyclopedia Plant Physiol. (N.S.), Vol. 1, Springer-Verlag, Heidelberg, West Germany (1975).

9. Crafts, A. S., in "The Physiology and Biochemistry of Herbicides," Audus, L. J., ed., p. 75, Academic Press, New York, NY (1964).

10. Woolhouse, H. W., Sci. Prog. (1974) 61, 123.

11. Thimann, K. V., "Hormone Action in the Whole Life of Plants," p. 357, University of Massachusetts Press, Amherst, MA (1977).

12. Goldthwaite, J. J. and Laetsch, W. M., Plant Physiol. (1967) 42, 1757.

13. Peterson, L. W. and Huffaker, R. C., Plant Physiol. (1975) 55, 1009.

14. Tetley, R. M. and Thimann, K. V., Plant Physiol. (1974) 54, 294.

15. Sodek, L. and Wright, S. T. C., Phytochem. (1969) 8, 1629.

16. Haber, A. H., Thompson, P. J., Walne, P. L. and Triplett, L. L., Plant Physiol. (1969) 44, 1619.

17. Martin, C. and Thimann, K. V., Plant Physiol. (1972) 49, 64.

18. Frear, D. S. and Swanson, H. R., Phytochem. (1972) 11, 1919.

19. Frear, D. S. and Swanson, H. R., Phytochem. (1974) 13, 357.

20. Frear, D. S. and Swanson, H. R., Pest. Biochem. Physiol. (1975) 5, 73.

21. Lamoureux, G. L. and Stafford, L. E., J. Agric. Food Chem. (1977) 25, 512.

22. Shimabukuro, R. H., Lamoureux, G. L., Swanson, H. R., Walsh, W. C., Stafford, L. E. and Frear, D. S., Pestic. Biochem. Physiol. (1973) 3, 483.

23. Lamoureux, G. L., Stafford, L. E. and Shimabukuro, R. H., J. Agric. Food Chem. (1972) 20, 1004.

24. Lamoureux, G. L., Stafford, L. E. and Tanaka, F. S., J. Agric. Food Chem. (1971) 19, 346.

25. Stolzenberg, G. E. and Olson, P. A., 173rd Amer. Chem. Soc. Meeting (1977) Abst. Pest. 42.

26. Shimabukuro, R. H., Masteller, V. J. and Walsh, W. C., Weed Sci. (1976) 24, 336.

27. Hamilton, R. H., J. Agric. Food Chem. (1964) 12, 14.

28. Swanson, C. R., Kadunce, R. E., Hodgson, R. H. and Frear, D. S., Weeds (1966) 14, 319.

29. Shimabukuro, R. H., J. Agric. Food Chem. (1967) 15, 557.

30. Shimabukuro, R. H., Walsh, W. C. and Hoerauf, R. A., (unpublished data).

31. Shimabukuro, R. H., Plant Physiol. (1967) 42, 1269.

32. Carter, M. C., "Herbicides - Chemistry, Degradation and Mode of Action," Kearney, P. C. and Kaufmann, D. D., eds., Vol. 1, p. 377, Marcel Dekker, Inc., New York, NY (1975)

33. Lund-Höie, K., Weed Res. (1970) 10, 367.

34.  Basler, E., Murray, D. S. and Santelmann, P. W., Weed Sci.
     (1978) 26, 358.
35.  Hoagland, R. E. and Frear, D. S., J. Agric. Food Chem.
     (1976) 24, 129.
36.  Shimabukuro, R. H., Frear, D. S., Swanson, H. R. and Walsh,
     W. C., Plant Physiol. (1971) 47, 10.
37.  Frear, D. S. and Swanson, H. R., Phytochem. (1970) 9, 2123.
38.  Still, G. G. and Mansager, E. R., Pestic. Biochem. Physiol.
     (1973) 3, 87.
39.  Shtarkshall, R. A., Reinhold, L. and Harel, H., J. Exp. Bot.
     (1970) 21, 915.
40.  Nissen, P., Annu. Rev. Plant Physiol. (1974) 25, 53.
41.  Morrod, R. S., J. Exp. Bot. (1974) 25, 521.
42.  Jensen, K. I. N., Banden, J. D., and SouzaMachado, V.,
     Can. J. Plant Sci. (1977) 57, 1169.
43.  Miflin, B. J., Planta (1972) 105, 225.
44.  Shimabukuro, R. H. and Swanson, H. R., J. Agric. Food Chem.
     (1969) 17, 199.
45.  Lien, R. and Rognes, S. E., Physiol. Plant. (1977) 41, 175.
46.  Lamoureux, G. L., Shimabukuro, R. H., Swanson, H. R. and
     Frear, D. S., J. Agric. Food Chem. (1970) 18, 81.
47.  Jones, H. G., Aust. J. Biol. Sci. (1973) 26, 25.
48.  Jensen, K. I. N., Stephenson, G. R. and Hunt, L. A., Weed
     Sci. (1977) 25, 212.
49.  MacDonald, I. R., Plant Physiol. (1975) 56, 109.
50.  Chollet, R., Plant Physiol. (1978) 61, 929.
51.  Morrod, R. S., "Herbicides - Physiology, Biochemistry,
     Ecology," Audus, L. J., ed., Vol. 1, p. 281, Academic
     Press, New York, NY (1976).
52.  Cheung, Y. K. S. and Nobel, P. S., Plant Physiol. (1973)
     52, 633.
53.  Donaldson, T. W., Bayer, D. E. and Leonard, O. A., Plant
     Physiol. (1973) 52, 638.
54.  Swanson, C. R. and Swanson, H. R., Weed Sci. (1968) 16,
     137.
55.  Swanson, C. R. and Swanson, H. R., Weed Sci. (1968) 16,
     481.
56.  Shimabukuro, R. H., Swanson, H. R. and Walsh, W. C., Plant
     Physiol. (1970) 46, 103.
57.  Bowling, C. C. and Hudgins, H. R., Weeds (1966) 14, 94.
58.  Matsunaka, S., Science (1968) 160, 1360.
59.  Frear, D. S. and Still, G. G., Phytochem. (1968) 7, 913.
60.  Chang, F-Y., Smith, L. W. and Stephenson, G. R., J. Agric.
     Food Chem. (1971) 19, 1183.
61.  Chang, F-Y., Stephenson, G. R. and Smith, L. W., J. Agric.
     Food Chem. (1971) 19, 1187.
62.  Hamill, A. S. and Penner, D., Weed Sci. (1973) 21, 330.
63.  Hamill, A. S. and Penner, D., Weed Sci. (1973) 21, 335.
64.  Hamill, A. S. and Penner, D., Weed Sci. (1973) 21, 339.

65. Lamoureux, G. L., Stafford, L. E., Shimabukuro, R. H. and Zaylskie, R. G., J. Agric. Food Chem. (1973) 21, 1020.
66. Gnanam, A. and Kulandaivelu, G., Plant Physiol. (1969) 44, 1451.
67. Edwards, G. E. and Black, C. C. Jr., Plant Physiol. (1971) 47, 149.
68. Takebe, I., Otsuki, Y. and Aoki, S., Plant Cell Physiol. (1968) 9, 115.
69. Jensen, R. G., Francki, R. I. B. and Zaitlin, M., Plant Physiol. (1971) 48, 9.
70. Boulware, M. A. and Camper, N. D., Weed Sci. (1973) 21, 145.
71. Rehfeld, D. W. and Jensen, R. G., Plant Physiol. (1973) 52, 17.
72. Ashton, F. M., DeVilliers, O. T., Glenn, R. K. and Duke, W. B., Pestic. Biochem. Physiol. (1977) 7, 122.
73. Francki, R. I. B., Zaitlin, M. and Jenson, R. G., Plant Physiol. (1971) 48, 14.
74. Towne, C. A., Bartels, P. G. and Hilton, J. L., Weed Sci. (1978) 26, 182.
75. St. John, J. B., Bartels, P. G. and Hilton, J. L., Weed Sci. (1974) 22, 233.
76. Davis, D. G. and Shimabukuro, R. H., Weed Sci. Soc. Abst. No. 157 (1973).
77. Porter, E. M. and Bartels, P. G., Weed Sci. (1977) 25, 60.
78. Radosevich, S. R. and DeVilliers, O. T., Weed Sci. (1976) 24, 229.
79. DeVilliers, O. T. and Ashton, F. M., Agroplantae (1976) 8, 87.
80. Stolzenberg, G. E. and Olson, P. A., 175th Amer. Chem. Soc. Meeting (1978) Abst. Pest. 67.
81. Shimabukuro, R. H., Walsh, W. C., Stolzenberg, G. E. and Olson, P. A., Weed Sci. Soc. Am. (1975) Abst. No. 171.
82. Shimabukuro, R. H., Walsh, W. C., Stolzenberg, G. E. and Olson, P. A., Weed Sci. Soc. Am. (1976) Abst. No. 196.
83. Frear, D. S. and Swanson, H. R., Pestic. Biochem. Physiol. (1973) 3, 473.
84. Ruesink, A. W., Plant Physiol. (1971) 47, 192.
85. Constabel, F., in "Plant Tissue Culture Methods," Gamborg, O. L. and Wetter, L. R., eds., p. 11, Prairie Regional Laboratory, Saskatoon, Canada (1975).
86. Cocking, E. C., Annu. Rev. Plant Physiol. (1972) 23, 29.
87. Cocking, E. C., Nature (1960) 187, 962.
88. Farmer, I. and Lee, P. E., Plant Sci. Lett. (1977) 10, 141.
89. Cassells, A. C. and Barlass, M., Physiol. Plant. (1978) 42, 236.
90. Watts, J. W., Motoyoshi, F. and King, J. M., Ann. Bot. (1974) 38, 667.
91. Takebe, I., Otsuki, Y., Honda, Y., Nishio, T. and Matsui, C., Planta (1973) 113, 21.

92.  Gamborg, O. L. and Miller, R. A., Can. J. Bot. (1973) 51, 1795.
93.  Carlson, P. S., Smith, H. H. and Dearing, R. D., Proc. Natl. Acad. Sci. U.S.A. (1972) 69, 2292.
94.  Fuchs, Y. and Galston, A. W., Plant Cell Physiol. (1976) 17, 475.
95.  Rancillac, M., Kaur-Sawhney, R., Staskawicz, B. and Galston, A. W., Plant Cell Physiol. (1976) 17, 987.
96.  Staskawicz, B., Kaur-Sawhney, R., Slaybaugh, R., Adams, W. Jr. and Galston, A. W., Pestic. Biochem. Physiol. (1978) 8, 106.
97.  Boulware, M. A. and Camper, D. N., Physiol. Plant. (1972) 26, 313.

RECEIVED December 20, 1978.

# Xenobiotic Metabolism in Higher Plants: In Vitro Tissue and Cell Culture Techniques

RALPH O. MUMMA and ROBERT H. HAMILTON

Pesticide Research Laboratory and Graduate Study Center and Departments of Entomology and Biology, Pennsylvania State University, University Park, PA 16802

Millions of pounds of xenobiotics have been applied to plants in our environment for the control of pests and plant growth. Some of these chemicals have recognized and well characterized biological effects on animals and plants, while other xenobiotics, such as oils, adjuvants, emulsifiers and inert materials, are applied in even greater quantity, but have been assumed to cause little ecological effect. It is important to understand what happens to all chemicals applied to our environment and to properly interpret the ecological significance of these chemicals and of their degradation products. If we cannot know this in detail, then a general knowledge of persistance and metabolic products is of importance. Since the target organism of these xenobiotics is often plants, it is of the utmost importance to understand the fate of these chemicals in plants. Ultimately, animals and even humans are exposed to these chemicals and/or their subsequent metabolites and degradation products. Most investigations of xenobiotic metabolism in plants have focused on biologically active pest control chemicals. Thus, this review will also focus primarily on plant metabolism of pesticides.

There are many ways to study the metabolism of xenobiotics by plants, but whatever technique is employed, it should predict what would actually happen under field conditions. Metabolism studies have involved whole plants, excised plant parts (meristems, shoots, stems, leaves, roots, leaf disks), plant cell cultures, subcellular particles, and isolated enzymes. Any metabolism study conducted in the laboratory is less than ideal because it is difficult to duplicate many factors that affect the degradation of xenobiotics under field conditions such as weather, light, microsymbionts, soil or method of application. Metabolism of xenobiotics by plant tissue culture offers the obvious advantages of sterility, space, economical use of labeled chemicals, less pigments, etc. These advantages will be discussed in detail later.

The metabolism of xenobiotics by plant tissue culture (1) and the metabolism of endogenous and exogenous chemicals (2) have been reviewed recently. Within the last few years, many new

0-8412-0486-1/79/47-097-035$10.50/0

investigations of xenobiotic metabolism by plant tissue cultures
have been reported.  This review will focus on these more recent
papers with an emphasis on pesticide metabolism.  We will attempt
to evaluate and compare the results obtained with tissue culture
techniques versus those obtained with whole plants and to explore
the many factors (limitations) that affect metabolism studies with
plant tissue culture.

## History and Principles of Plant Tissue Culture

     Plant tissue culture refers to the growth of relatively un-
differentiated plant cells or differentiated organs on solid or
liquid nutrient medium.  The undifferentiated plant tissue growing
on solidified medium is usually referred to as a callus culture
since they are frequently obtained from cut or wounded surfaces
and maintain the appearance of wound callus tissue.  When such
tissues are placed in liquid medium with shaking, many small aggregates of cells and even some single cells may be obtained.
Subcultures of small aggregates or cell clumps in liquid culture
are usually designated as suspension cultures.  The culture of
excised differentiated organs is, of course, organ culture.  Frequently, callus cultures will differentiate with the formation of
xylem elements and sometimes buds and/or roots.  In many callus
cultures with this potential usually a high kinetin/auxin concentration ratio in the medium favors bud formation while the reverse
favors root formation.  In a few cases, by proper manipulation of
the medium, thousands of pseudoembryos can be induced and grown
into normal plants of the same genotype.
     Although the culture of plant tissues was attempted in 1902
(3), success was not achieved until White cultured excised tomato
roots in 1934 and tobacco callus in 1939 (4).  Gautheret and
Nobécourt also described culture of plant callus tissue at about
the same time (5, 6).  White and Gautheret both developed nutrient
media that are used widely today (5, 7).  In addition to essential
salts and sucrose, White added thiamine, nicotinic acid, pyridox-
ine and glycine while Gautheret added thiamine, pantothenic acid,
biotin, inositol and cysteine.  It appears that only thiamine is
essential; but, in some cases, better growth may be obtained by
the addition of other vitamins.  White did not add an auxin for
culture of excised root organ cultures or tobacco tumor tissue,
but Gautheret added naphthaleneacetic acid (NAA).  Van Overbeek
et al. (8) introduced the use of coconut milk and much later
Miller et al. (9) found that kinetin was necessary to culture
tobacco stem pith.  In general, excised root organ cultures,
tumor and some callus cultures (so called habituated) do not
require either auxin or kinetin.  Some tissues do not require
kinetin especially if 2,4-dichlorophenoxyacetic acid (2,4-D) is
used as the auxin (10).  The addition of coconut milk is usually
not essential, and a requirement for gibberellic acid has been
reported rarely.  It is probable that adaptation to the medium

and the selection of tissue that grows well on a particular medium accounts for the wide variation in nutrient requirements for a tissue such as tobacco callus. Other media used widely for plant tissue culture include those of Murashige and Skoog (11), Nitsch and Nitsch (12) and Gamborg (13). In addition, some media formulations are now available from a commercial source (Flow Laboratories, P. O. Box 2226, 1710 Chapman Ave., Rockville, MD 20852).

In theory callus may be derived from any plant tissue containing parenchyma cells. Some species form callus readily and others do not. Tissue sterilization may be accomplished with 70% alcohol (1-2 min dip) and/or a similar treatment with 1 to 5 or 1 to 10 diluted commercial bleach (0.5-1% sodium hypochlorite) containing 0.1% Tween 20. In either case, the tissue is rinsed 2-3 times in sterile water. Seeds are germinated in sterile petri dishes and bits of root or stem tissue are transferred to solidified agar medium containing relatively high auxin levels (0.5-1.0 mg/1 NAA or 2,4-D). Sterilized tissue from bud, leaves or stems may also be used. Formation of enough callus to subculture may vary from 2 weeks to 2 months. Considerable variation in appearance and texture between callus pieces from the same source may be observed. Three to 4 bits of callus (5-7 mm in dia.) are transferred to solidified agar medium (50 ml in a 125 ml Erlenmeyer flask). Difficult tissues may require the addition of 50 ml of autoclaved-filtered coconut liquid and/or 2 g of casein hydrolysate per liter. Growth rates vary, but it is convenient to subculture bits of callus onto fresh medium every 4-6 weeks. Temperature and light requirements may not be critical for most tissues. High temperatures (30°C or more) have caused the loss of kinetin dependence of tobacco callus (14) and inhibited growth. We have maintained cultures under continuous low level fluorescent light at 27°C.

Simple equipment is needed for plant tissue cultures; a temperature controlled incubator or culture room, an autoclave, and a shaker, if suspension cultures are grown. It is also desirable to have a sterile transfer hood.

The genetic and physiological stability of some plant tissue cultures is of concern. Tissue from the same original culture may change in appearance and growth rate over a period of time. It is commonly observed that the ability to regenerate normal plants by the formation of buds and roots is lost with time. It may even be necessary to reisolate callus from the same source, if the callus tissue appears atypical or slow growing. A low growth rate is observed frequently in August or September. Variations in growth rate and tissue appearance may be important factors in metabolism studies and should be examined carefully. A mitotic index at two weeks after transfer may give a good indication of growth rate (15) or fresh weights at the end of 4 or 5 weeks may be used. The source of callus tissue (root, stem, leaf, cotyledons, etc.) also may influence metabolism. The appearance of soybean cotyledon, leaf and root callus was similar and limited

work on 2,4-D metabolism indicated no major qualitative differences (16). Of much more importance was the age or stage of growth of the cultures (15). Most callus cultures exhibit a lag in
growth for 4-7 days after transfer, a log growth phase followed by
a slower growth phase after 4-5 weeks. Cultures 5-9 weeks old are
more active in metabolism of 2,4-D than 3 week old cultures (15).
It should be noted that prolonged pesticide treatment of older
callus in fresh medium may put the tissue into log phase growth
again with probable changes in metabolism.

## Metabolism of Xenobiotics by Plant Tissue Culture

Most investigations with plant tissue cultures and xenobiotics have been concerned with pesticide metabolism. Tables I and
II illustrate the variety of herbicides, insecticides, and plant
tissue cultures that have been used in metabolism studies. The
metabolism of lindane probably represents one of the more extreme
cases where fourteen different plant tissues were used. As is
evident, the source of the plant tissue culture, the type of culture (suspension or nonsuspension) and the media used also varied.
This variation in plant cultures and techniques makes it extremely
difficult to critically compare metabolism studies. As will be
pointed out later, there are also many other factors that affect
metabolism studies with plant tissue cultures.

## HERBICIDES

It is apparent that herbicides exert toxic or physiological
effects on sensitive plant species and that some physiological
effects can be expected on tissue cultures of these species. An
exception may be photosynthetic inhibitors. Due to the sugar in
the plant tissue culture medium, photosynthetic inhibitors should
not be strongly inhibitory unless they have secondary sites of
action. If tolerance is due to metabolism, this might be expected
to lead to qualitative and quantitative differences in metabolism
by plant tissue cultures from susceptible and resistant varieties
or species. Of course, such tissue cultures should also show
differences in actual tolerance.

The metabolism of the herbicide fluorodifen (p-nitrophenyl
$\alpha,\alpha,\alpha$-trifluoro-2-nitro-p-tolyl ether) has been investigated (21)
with tobacco cells in suspension culture (42). The cells were
incubated for 15 days with 1-2 ppm of either $^{14}C_1$- or $^{14}CF_3$-label-
ed fluorodifen. All of the applied fluorodifen was metabolized.
Recovery of added radioactivity varied between 52 and 76%. The
cells contained 60 to 80% of the recovered radioactivity and the
remainder was found in the medium and cell wash. With $^{14}C_1$-label-
ed fluorodifen, 4-nitrophenol (7%) was isolated only from the
medium. Aqueous-soluble conjugated forms of 4-nitrophenol (93%),
primarily the $\beta$-D-glucoside and other acidic conjugates, were present in both the cells and the medium as summarized in Figure 1.

Table I. Metabolism of Herbicides by Plant Tissue Cultures.

| Herbicide | Species | Plant Tissue Culture | | |
| --- | --- | --- | --- | --- |
| | | Source | Medium[a] and Culture Type[b] | Reference |
| Cisanilide | Carrot (Daucus carota L.) Cotton (Gossypium hirsutum L.) | Leaves | B5, S | 17, 18 |
| Diphenimid | Soybean (Glycine max [L.] Merr. 'Wilkin') | Root tips | B5, S | 19 |
| Propanil | Rice (Oryza sativa L. var. Starbonnet) | Root | H, S | 20 |

Table I – page 2

Fluorodifen

Metribuzin

2,4-D

| Plant | Tissue | | Ref. |
|-------|--------|------|------|
| Tobacco (Nicotiana tobacum L. var Xanthi) | | M, S | 21 |
| Soybean (Cultivar Bragg) | Cotyledon | X, S | 22 |
| Soybean (Cultivar Coker 102) | Cotyledon | X, S | |
| Soybean (Glycine max L. var Mandarin) | Root | B5 | 23 |
| Soybean (Glycine max L. var Acme) | Cotyledon | M, C | 24, 25, 26, 27 |
| Jackbean (Canavalia ensiformis) | Pod | M, C | 26, 27 |
| Sweet corn (Zea mays) | Endosperm | M, C | 27 |
| Tobacco (Nicotiana tobacum) | Pith | M, C | 27 |
| Carrot (Daucus carota var Sativa) | Pith | M, C | 27 |
| Sunflower (Helianthus annus) | Pith | M, C | 27 |
| Rice (Oryza sativa var Starbonnet) | Root | M, C | 28 |
| Wheat (Triticum monococcum L.) | | B5, S | 29 |
| Field bindweed (Convolvulus arvenis L.) | Stem | X, C | 30 |

Table I - page 3

2,4,5-T

IAA

| | | | |
|---|---|---|---|
| Soybean (Glycine max L. var Acme) | Cotyledon | M, S | 31 |
| Geranium (Pelagonium hortorum var Nittany Red) | Stem | W, C | 32 |
| Boston ivy (Parthenocissus tricuspidata) | Crown-gall | W, C | 33 |
| Apple (East Malling rootstock 3430) | Bark | W, C | 34, 35 |
| Shamouti orange (Citrus sinensis Osb.) | Ovular | MS, C | 36 |

[a] Basic media:  B5 – Gamborg's; H – Heller's; M – Miller's; MS – Murashige and Skoog's; W – White's; X – Others.

[b] Culture type:  S – Suspension; C – Callus.

Table II.  Metabolism of Insecticides by Plant Tissue Cultures.

| Insecticide | Plant Tissue Culture | | |
|---|---|---|---|
| | Species | Source | Medium[a] and Culture Type[b] | Reference |
| Carbaryl (O-C-NHCH₃ naphthyl structure) | Tobacco (Nicotiana tobacum L. var Xanthi) | | M, S | 37, 38 |
| Lindane (hexachlorocyclohexane structure) | Purple cockle (Agrostemma githago L.) Soybean (Glycine max) Bedstraw (Galium verum) Carrot (Daucus carota) Clover (Meliotus alba) Tobacco (Nicotiana tobacum) Tobacco (Nicotiana glutinosa) Tobacco (Nicotiana sylvestris) Tobacco (Nicotiana glauca) Lettuce (Lactuca sativa) (Beta vulgaris) Parsley (Pstroselinum hortense) Potato (Solanum tuberosum) | | ?, S | 39 |

Table II – page 2

| Compound | Plant | Media/Culture[a][b] | Ref. |
|---|---|---|---|
| Aldrin | Bean (<u>Phaseolus vulgaris</u> var Canadian Wonder) Roots & Shoots | MS, S | 40 |
| | Potato (<u>Solanum tuberosum</u> var Majestic) Tuber | W, S | 40 |
| p,p'–DDT | Parsley (<u>Petroselinum hortense,</u> Hoffm.) Soybean (<u>Glycine max</u> L.) | B5, S | 41 |
| Kelthane (Ascaroside) | Parsley (<u>Petroselinum hortense,</u> Hoffm.) | B5, S | 41 |
| | Soybean (<u>Glycine max</u> L.) | B5, S | 41 |

[a] Basic media:  M – Miller's; W – White's; MS – Murashige and Skoog's; B5 – Gamborg's; X – Other.
[b] Culture type:  S – Suspension; C – Callus.

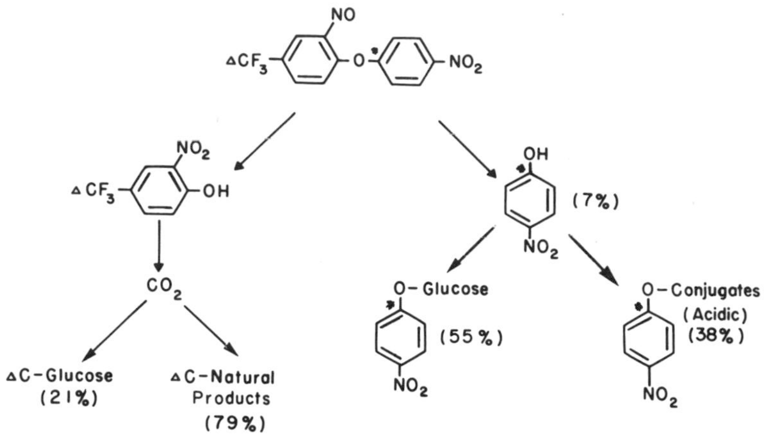

Journal of Agricultural and Food Chemistry

*Figure 1.   Metabolism of fluorodifen by tobacco cell in suspension culture*

These data from plant tissue culture studies are consistant
with results obtained with whole plants where the glucoside of 4-
nitrophenol has been reported as the major product of soybean and
maize seedlings (43, 44).   Whole plant metabolism studies with
fluorodifen (43, 44) suggested that a small percentage of the
applied pesticide may be reduced to 4-aminophenyl 2-amino-4-(trifluoromethyl) phenyl ether, 4-nitrophenyl 2-amino-4-(trifluoromethyl) phenyl ether or 4-aminophenyl 2-nitro-4-(trifluoromethyl)
phenyl ether, but none of these compounds, including 4-amino-
phenyl, was detected in the tobacco tissue  culture studies.

Propanil (3,4-dichloropropionanilide) is an herbicide used to
control weeds in rice.   The resistance of rice to propanil is
attributed to the high levels of an arylacyl amidase (propanil
amidase) that hydrolyzes propanil to 3,4-dichloroaniline and propionic acid.   The enzymatic level of propanil amidase in rice
plants and in rice root suspension cultures has been investigated
(20, 45).   The activity of the enzyme was found to be two to four
times greater in older plants (four leaves) than in younger plants
(less than four leaves).   Propanil amidase was also demonstrated
in the rice suspension culture, but interestingly, the enzymatic
activity could only be demonstrated after the tissue culture had
developed to stationary phase (5.5 days).   This investigation is
important because it documents a change in the biosynthetic
capacity of plant tissue cultures with the age of the culture.
The dependency of several enzymes, including phenylalanine ammonia
lyase, upon illumination of parsley cell cultures also has been
shown (46).

The metabolism of diphenamid (N-N-dimethyl-2,2-diphenylaceta-
mide) by soybean root tip cell suspension cultures has been

investigated (19) at different stages of growth and compared with whole plants. The metabolites found in both plants and suspension cultures were N-hydroxymethyl-N-methyl-2,2-diphenylacetamide (MODA), N-methyl-2,2-diphenylacetamide (MMDA), 2,2-diphenylaceta-mide (DA) and two polar glycosides. One of the glucosides was acidic and was identified as an ester of malonic acid (Figure 2).

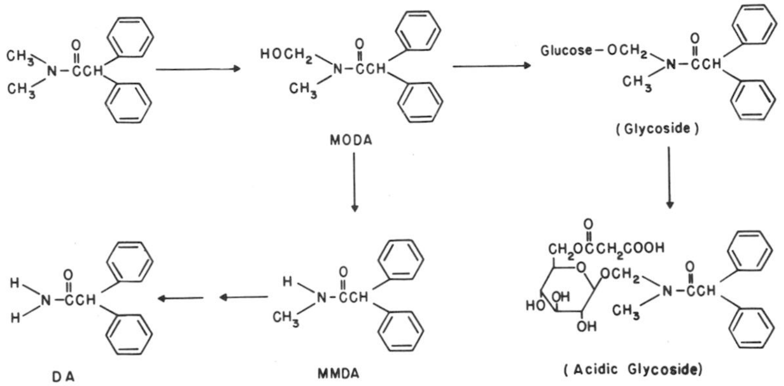

*Figure 2.    Metabolism of diphenamid by soybean root cells in suspension culture*

About 9-22% of the diphenamid was metabolized by the cell cultures at early log (3-7 days) and stationary phases (14-18 days), respectively. However, diphenamid metabolism per gram was about 2 times more rapid by early log phase cells than by stationary cells. Cultures of all ages formed the same metabo-lites with MODA and the dealkylated products predominating. The relative composition of the metabolites is presented in Tables III and IV. The hydroxylated metabolite, MODA, was found almost exclu-sively in the medium 92-99%, and the dealkylated products were found predominantly in the medium (68-94%).

Log phase and stationary phase cells produced larger amounts of the dealkylated metabolites per mg dry weight per day than did early log phase cells. Glycosides consisted of only 6-7% of the total metabolites in cell cultures but were the major metabolites (46-48%) of tomato, pepper and soybean plants.

These cell suspension cultures demonstrate clearly the same metabolic degradation pathways as intact plants, but significant quantitative differences do occur especially in the small amount of glycoside formation by the soybean root suspension cells. No qualitative changes occurred in the metabolism of diphenamid with age of the culture.

The metabolism of cisanilide (cis-2,5-dimethyl-1-pyrrolidine-carboxanilide), a selective preemergence herbicide, has been in-vestigated in excised leaves and cell suspension cultures of

Table III.  Diphenamid Metabolism by Growth Phase of
            Soybean Cell Suspension cultures (19)

| Growth Phase | Diphenamid or Metabolite | nmol per Gram Cells | |
|---|---|---|---|
| | | Cell Extract | Medium |
| Early Log | Diphenamid | 12.8 | 444.8 |
| (3-7 Days) | MODA | 0.1 | 31.6 |
| | Dealkylated | 0.6 | 10.8 |
| | Glucoside | 0.6 | 1.8 |
| Log | Diphenamid | 41.9 | 99.4 |
| (7-14 Days) | MODA | 2.2 | 27.4 |
| | Dealkylated | 10.6 | 27.8 |
| | Glucoside | 1.9 | 1.1 |
| Stationary | Diphenamid | 42.5 | 144.3 |
| (14-18 Days) | MODA | 1.2 | 25.4 |
| | Dealkylated | 6.7 | 14.5 |
| | Glucoside | 0.9 | 1.9 |

Table IV.  Relative Composition of
           Diphenamid or Metabolites
           in Cells and Medium in
           Early Log Phase (19)

| Diphenamid or Metabolite | % | |
|---|---|---|
| | Cell Extract | Medium |
| Diphenamid | 2.8 | 97.2 |
| MODA | 0.3 | 99.7 |
| Dealkylated | 5.5 | 94.5 |
| Glucoside | 25.0 | 75.0 |
| Acidic Glucoside | 100.0 | 0.0 |

carrot and cotton (17, 18).  After 6 days, excised carrot leaves
metabolized ca. 70% of the applied cisanilide, but carrot tissue
cultures metabolized >95% of the applied herbicide in 3 days.
Cotton leaves metabolized cisanilide to a greater extent than
cotton suspension cultures.  The metabolism of cisanilide by carrot and cotton plants is shown in Figure 3 and the relative composition of metabolites in plants and tissue culture is presented
in Table V.

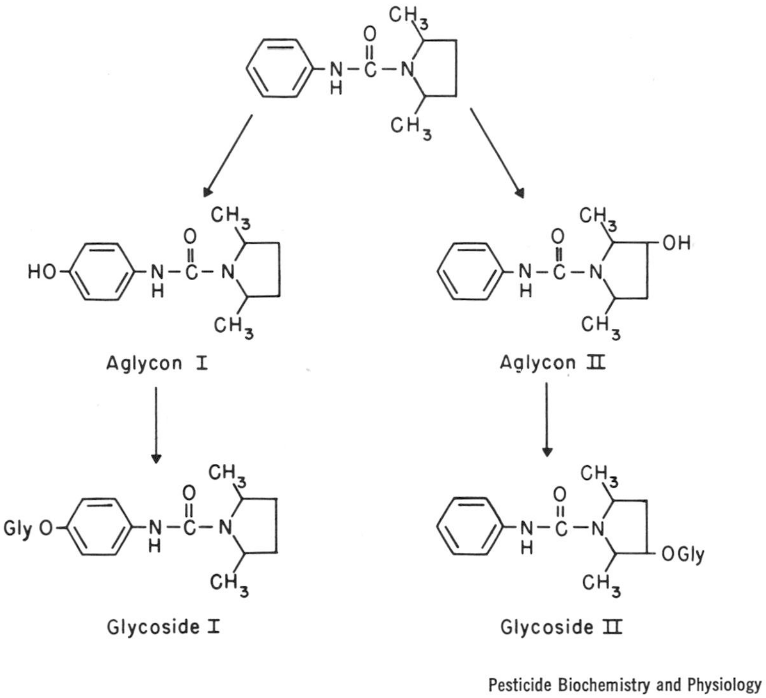

Pesticide Biochemistry and Physiology

*Figure 3.   Metabolism of cisanilide by carrot and cotton plants and cells in culture*

    In the excised plants, glycosides I and II were the major
methanol soluble metabolites and only trace quantities of the
aglycons were detected.  In carrot and cotton cell suspension
cultures, aglycon I or glucoside I was not detected and only
trace amounts of glycoside II were detected.  Aglycon II was a
major metabolite in the medium of the cell suspension cultures.
In the excised plants, less (20-25%) of the $^{14}$C-label was found
in the insoluble residue fraction compared to the cell suspension
cultures (39-40%).

Table V.   Relative Composition of Cisanilide Metabolites (18).

| Fraction | Excised Carrot Leaves (6 Days) % | Carrot Suspension Culture (3 Days)[a] % Cells | % Medium |
|---|---|---|---|
| Total Metabolized | 70 | >95 | |
| Methanol Soluble | 50 (Glycoside I=II) | -- | 40 (Aglycon II) |
| Methanol Soluble (Unknown) | 10 | 20 | -- |
| Insoluble Residue | 20 | 40 | |

| Fraction | Excised Cotton Leaves (2 Days) % | Cotton Suspension Cultures (7 Days) % Cells | % Medium |
|---|---|---|---|
| Total Metabolized | >95 | >76 | |
| Methanol Soluble | 55 (Glycosides I>II) | -- | 24 (Aglycon II) |
| Methanol Soluble (Unknown) | 25 | 13 | -- |
| Insoluble Residue | 18 | 39 | |

[a]Glycoside I was not detected and glycoside II was tentatively identified as a minor component.

At first approximation, it would be easy to conclude that the metabolic degradation pathways were different in the excised plants versus the cell suspensions since aglycon I and glucoside I were not detected in the tissue or the medium. This difference may indicate rapid incorporation of aglycon I into a methanol-insoluble fraction, because when aglycon I was administered to the cell suspension culture, it was rapidly converted to methanol insoluble products. Neither tissue is able to cleave appreciably the urea type structure of cisanilide. This is also the case for the metabolism of other urea herbicides by plants (43). Both tissues possess the ability to form the hydroxyl derivative, aglycon II, but the cell cultures evidently have a reduced capacity to form the glycoside conjugate and consequently aglycon II accumulates in the media. This hydroxylated metabolite is apparently not incorporated into the methanol insoluble product(s). Thus, the metabolic pathways may be somewhat similar except for loss of aglycons into the medium and the increased formation of an insoluble product.

The phytotoxicity and metabolism of the herbicide metribuzin (4-amino-6-t-butyl 3-[methylthio]-as-triazin-5-[4H]-one) has been investigated with dark-grown soybean cotyledon suspension cultures from susceptible ("Coker 102") and resistance ("Bragg") cultivars. Bioassays were based on population changes of viable cells during incubation with metribuzin. Viable cells were classified as cells with structural integrity and cytoplasmic streaming. Differential resistance to metribuzin was demonstrated by the cell suspensions from resistant and susceptible cultivars. Metribuzin had been reported to inhibit photosynthesis, but the demonstrated phytotoxicity toward both cultivars of dark-grown achlorophyllous suspension cultures indicated that phytotoxicity was not restricted to photosynthesis. Detoxification of metribuzin by soybeans has been attributed to formation of an N-glucoside. Enzymatic detoxification of metribuzin did not occur in the susceptible cultivar due to the accumulation of a substance which inhibited the enzyme. The resistant cultivar metabolized the inhibitor to a noninhibitory form. Therefore, metribuzin resistance by the Bragg cultivar was attributed to the ability of this cultivar to metabolize a common enzymatic inhibitor.

Plant tissue culture techniques have been used by numerous investigators (23 - 29) for 2,4-D metabolism studies. In 1968, the metabolism of 2,4-D-2-[14]C by suspension cultures of soybean root grown under continuous light (2000 lux) was examined (23). Most of the [14]C-label in the tissue appeared as two spots on paper chromatography. The faster moving compound has the same Rf as 2,4-D and was assumed to be free 2,4-D. The slower moving spot was a glycoside that yielded glucose and free 2,4-D when treated with emulsin. These investigators assumed that 2,4-D was metabolized only to the β-D glucose ester of 2,4-D. Presumably, the amino acid conjugates, which have been subsequently identified as metabolites of 2,4-D, did not separate from 2,4-D in the

chromatographic solvents used.  The addition of glutamine to the
media increased the uptake of 2,4-D, but did not change the apparent metabolic products when analyzed by their chromatographic solvent systems.  Some 2,4-D was also associated with protein.

Two clones of field bindweed (Convolvulus arrensis L.) that
differed in their susceptibility to 2,4-D under field and green-
house conditions also exhibited similar differences when stem
cells were cultured in liquid and agar media (30).  When amino
acids were added to the culture media, the response to 2,4-D was
altered.  The absorption of 2,4-D was increased with glutamine and
decreased with glutamic acid.  Glutamic acid increased the tolerance of the susceptible clone, but reduced the tolerance of the
resistant clone.  Glutamine increased the susceptibility of the
susceptible clone to a much greater degree than it did the resistant clone.  There was a correlation between 2,4-D susceptibility
and nitrate reductase activity.

When soybean (Glycine max L.) cotyledon callus was incubated
for 32 days with 2,4-D-1-$^{14}$C, metabolites changed qualitatively and
quantatively with time (24).  The water soluble fraction from the
tissue increased in radioactivity.  When it was treated with β-
glucosidase, at least eight aglycons that changed with time were
released (Fig. 4).  4-Hydroxy-2,5-dichlorophenoxyacetic acid (4-
OH-2,5-D) was the most abundant aglycon and 4-hydroxy-2,3-dichlor-
ophenoxyacetic acid (4-OH-2,3-D) was identified as a minor component.  Free 2,4-D also was liberated following enzymatic treatment.
The presumed presence of 2,4-dichlorophenoxyacetyl-β-0-D glucose,
a metabolite reported previously (23), was suggested.

The ether soluble fraction reached a maximum after 2 days and
consisted of seven different regions of components on paper chromatography (Et$_1$-Et$_7$) that varied with time (Fig. 5).  The major
component (Et$_4$) was identified as the glutamic acid conjugate of
2,4-D and its relative composition was maximal after one day.  The
aspartic acid conjugate of 2,4-D (Et$_2$) increased gradually in relative composition.  Surprisingly, free 2,4-D (Et$_7$) did not reach
its maximum until eight days.  These data imply that contrary to
some previous studies, the metabolism of 2,4-D by plant tissue is
quite complex.  Subsequently, five additional amino acid conjugates of 2,4-D have been identified from soybean (27).  These include the alanine, valine, leucine, phenylalanine and tryptophan
conjugates.  A typical distribution of 2,4-D metabolites isolated
from 4-week-old callus tissue is presented in Table VI.

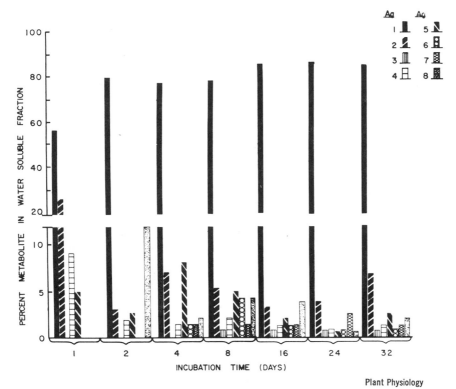

Plant Physiology

*Figure 4.  The relative amounts of the aglycons obtained from the water-soluble fractions of soybean callus tissue incubated with 2,4-D-1-$^{14}$C: (Ag$_1$), primarily 4-OH-2,5-D and 4-OH-2,3-D; (Ag$_7$), 2,4-D.*

Table VI.   Relative Percentage of 2,4-D Metabolites in
            Soybean Callus Tissue[a] (27).

| Ether-Soluble Metabolites | | Aglycons | (emulsin) |
|---|---|---|---|
| Metabolite | % In Tissue | Metabolite | % In Tissue |
| Unk | 1.2 | (4-OH-2,5-D, 4-OH-2,3-D) | 26.3 |
| 2,4-D-Asp | 3.7 | Unk | 2.5 |
| 2,4-D-Gly | 12.9 | Unk | 1.1 |
| Unk | 1.4 | Unk | 1.0 |
| 2,4-D-Ala,-Val) | 5.3 | Unk | 0.8 |
| 2,4-D | 33.7 | Unk | 0.9 |
| 2,4-D-Leu,-Phe -Try) | 4.0 | 2,4-D | 0.8 |
| | | Unk | 0.4 |
| TOTAL | 62.2% | | 33.8% |

[a]Four-week-old callus tissue (10g) incubated for 8 days
with 2,4-D.

Journal of Agricultural and Food Chemistry

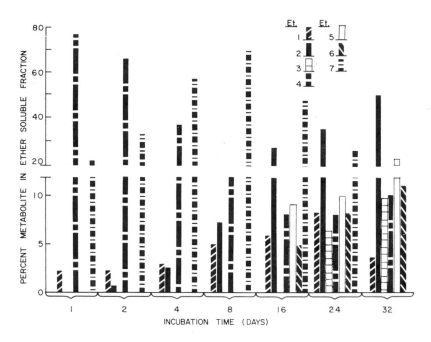

*Figure 5.   Relative amounts of ether solubles isolated from soybean callus tissues incubated with 2,4-D-1-¹⁴C: (Et₂), aspartic acid conjugate; (Et₄), glutamic acid conjugate; and (Et₇), free 2,4-D.*

Additional minor aglycons also have been identified tentatively from corn endosperm callus as 3-hydroxy-2,4-dichlorophenoxyacetic acid (3-OH-2,4-D), 4-hydroxy-2-chlorophenoxyacetic acid (4-OH-2-Cl) (27), and from wheat suspension cultures as 6-hydroxy-2,4-dichlorophenoxyacetic acid (6-OH-2,4-D) and 2-hydroxy-4-chlorophenoxyacetic acid (2-OH-4-Cl) (29). The ethyl ester of 2,4-D has been isolated from the glycoside fraction of rice callus tissue culture following β-glucosidase treatment (28). The ethyl ester was presumed to be an artifact of the isolation procedure probably being derived from the glucose ester that exists in high concentration in this tissue.

The glutamic acid conjugate of 2,4-D is not an end product of 2,4-D metabolism (25). When ¹⁴C-2,4-D-glutamic acid was incubated with soybean callus tissue, free 2,4-D, the aspartic acid conjugate, and other products were found. These data suggest that amino acid conjugates may represent a reservoir of bound 2,4-D

that may be involved in the regulation of 2,4-D levels in the
tissue.

Comparative metabolism studies of 2,4-D in carrot, jackbean,
sunflower, tobacco, corn and rice callus tissue cultures (27, 28)
and a wheat suspension culture (29) are shown in Tables VII and
VIII. All tissues examined, except rice, formed amino acid conjugates and all formed glycosides (phenolic glycosides as well as
glucose esters). The dicots formed a higher relative percentage
of amino acid conjugates while the monocots produced a higher
percentage of glycosides.

The metabolism of 2,4-D in soybean and corn plants has been
compared with 2,4-D metabolism in soybean callus tissue (26).
These data are presented in Tables IX and X. In this experiment,
the 2,4-D-1-$^{14}$C was directly injected into the callus tissue
growing on agar rather than into fresh liquid medium with suspended callus. The callus, therefore did not revert into log phase
growth and its nutrient status was not changed. The metabolites
found in the plants are also present in the callus tissue, but
differ quantitatively. Of particular note is the fact that free
hydroxylated 2,4-D exists in both callus and in plants in contrast
to earlier tissue culture experiments. Free hydroxylated 2,4-D
also has been reported in bean plants (48). These experiments
also suggest that the unknown compounds, Unk$_1$ and Unk$_2$, are amino
acid conjugates of hydroxylated 2,4-D metabolites (primarily the
glutamic acid conjugate of 4-OH-2,5-D) and are common to all tissue examined. A summary of the metabolism of 2,4-D in plants is
presented in Figure 6.

Recently, the metabolism of 2,4-D has been reported in six
intact plants: wheat, timothy, green bean, soybean, sunflower and
strawberry (47). The relative percentage of amino acid conjugates
is low compared to the previously cited work with tissue culture
experiments (Table XI). Of particular notice is the unusually
high percentage of the dichlorophenol glycoside in strawberry.

In contrast to use of true suspension cultures by most other
laboratories, Feung et al. (24-28) usually incubated a fairly
large amount (~10 gms) of small pieces of 4-5 week old callus
taken from solid medium in 25-40 ml liquid medium with shaking
during treatment with 2,4-D-1-$^{14}$C. This technique results in
nearly total uptake of the applied 2,4-D within 48 hours, the
accumulation of significant amounts of glycoside metabolites in
the tissue (phenolic glycosides and glucose ester), insignificant
amounts of primary hydroxylated products and no accumulation of
products in the medium. In cell suspension cultures, absorption
also is rapid but metabolites often accumulate in the medium. In
the study (26) where callus tissue was injected directly with
2,4-D-1-$^{14}$C, additional metabolites were found. Thus, the method
of pesticide administration may be important.

Data with intact plants (Tables IX, X and XI) are consistant
with metabolism data obtained with plant tissue cultures, but significant quantitative differences do occur. The monocots

Table VII.  Relative Percentage of Water-Soluble 2,4-D-1-$^{14}$C Metabolites Isolated from Seven Species of Plant Tissue Cultures as the Aglycons.

| Metabolites | Carrot | Jackbean | Sunflower | Tobacco | Corn | Rice | Wheat |
|---|---|---|---|---|---|---|---|
| | | | | % Total in Tissue[a] | | | |
| (4-OH-2,3-D, 4-OH-2,5-D) | 6.9 | 6.9 | 8.3 | 17.4 | 31.7 | 0.4 | ← |
| Unk | 3.2 | 2.6 | 4.1 | 8.3 | 19.4 | | |
| Unk | 0.7 | 0.4 | 0.8 | 2.0 | 0.5 | | |
| Unk | 0.4 | 0.3 | 0.5 | 1.9 | 1.2 | | 10.2 |
| Unk | 0.1 | 0.3 | 0.8 | 2.3 | | | → |
| Unk | 0.9 | 1.1 | 0.6 | 2.6 | 1.6 | | |
| 2,4-D | 1.0 | 1.2 | 3.2 | 7.7 | 10.2 | 14.9 | 23.9 |
| Ethyl-2,4-D | | | | | | 12.9 | |
| Others | | | | | | 1.5 | |
| TOTAL | 13.2 | 12.8 | 18.3 | 42.2 | 64.6 | 29.7 | |

[a] All were callus tissue cultures (27, 28) except wheat (29).

Table VIII. Relative Percentage of Ether-Soluble 2,4-D-1-$^{14}$ Metabolites Isolated from Seven Species of Plant Tissue Cultures as the Aglycons.

| Metabolites | % Total in Tissue[a] | | | | | | |
|---|---|---|---|---|---|---|---|
| | Carrot | Jackbean | Sunflower | Tobacco | Corn | Rice | Wheat |
| Unk | | | | | 1.9 | | |
| Unk | | | | | 1.7 | | |
| 2,4-D-Asp | 23.8 | 1.2 | | 0.8 | 1.6 | | ← |
| 2,4-D-Glu | 0.8 | 32.5 | 5.0 | 6.7 | 1.3 | | 21.0 |
| Unk | 5.8 | 1.1 | 0.7 | 1.8 | 3.2 | | → |
| Unk | | 5.2 | 5.7 | 5.5 | 0.8 | | |
| 2,4-D | 51.7 | 45.4 | 51.7 | 34.3 | 12.5 | 14.7 | 15.7 |
| Unk | 1.7 | | 15.3 | 4.5 | 2.6 | | |
| Others | | | | | | 1.2 | |
| TOTAL | 83.8 | 85.4 | 78.4 | 53.6 | 25.6 | 15.9 | 36.7 |

[a] All were callus tissue cultures (27, 28) except wheat (29).

Table IX.  Relative Percentage of Water-Soluble 2,4-D-1-$^{14}$C
           Metabolites Isolated from Soybean Callus, Soybean
           Plant, and Corn Plant as the Aglycons (26).

|  | % In Tissue | | |
| Metabolites | Soybean Callus | Soybean Plant | Corn Plant |
|---|---|---|---|
| Unk | 5.18 | 0.39 | 0.94 |
| Unk | 1.67 | | |
| Unk | 1.79 | 0.15 | 0.73 |
| (4-OH-2,3-D* 5-OH-2,4-D) | 8.27 | 1.47 | 2.45 |
| 4-OH-2,5-D | 16.28 | 3.20 | 1.67 |
| 2,4-D | 4.02 | 9.05 | 24.15 |
| Unk | 0.94 | 2.46 | 1.64 |
| Ethyl-2,4-D | | 1.22 | 7.70 |
| TOTAL | 38.15 | 17.94 | 39.28 |

*Major metabolite.

Table X.   Relative Percentage of the Ether-Soluble (at pH 2)
           2,4-D-1-$^{14}$C Metabolites Isolated from Soybean
           Callus, Soybean Plant, and Corn Plant (26).

|  | % In Tissue | | |
| Metabolites | Soybean Callus | Soybean Plant | Corn Plant |
|---|---|---|---|
| Unk | 0.50 | 3.14 | Trace |
| (5-OH-2,4-D 4-OH-2,3-D* 4-OH-2,5-D*) | 1.48 | 3.50 | 7.08 |
| Unk$_1$ | 9.59 | 8.87 | 0.69 |
| Unk$_2$ | 1.49 | 1.94 | 0.25 |
| Asp-2,4-D | 0.62 | Trace | 0.16 |
| (Asp-2,4-D Glu-2,4-D*) | 11.15 | 4.02 | 0.28 |
| Unk | 2.67 | 2.22 | 0.50 |
| Unk | 2.00 | 1.59 | 0.62 |
| Unk | 1.73 | 1.48 | 0.36 |
| (Ala-2,4-D Val-2,4-D*) | 4.07 | 1.37 | 0.86 |
| (Val-2,4-D 2,4-D*) | 11.91 | 43.55 | 29.60 |
| (Phe-2,4-D) Trp-2,4-D Leu-2,4-D*) | 0.51 | 1.63 | 5.60 |
| TOTAL | 47.72 | 73.31 | 46.00 |

*Major metabolite

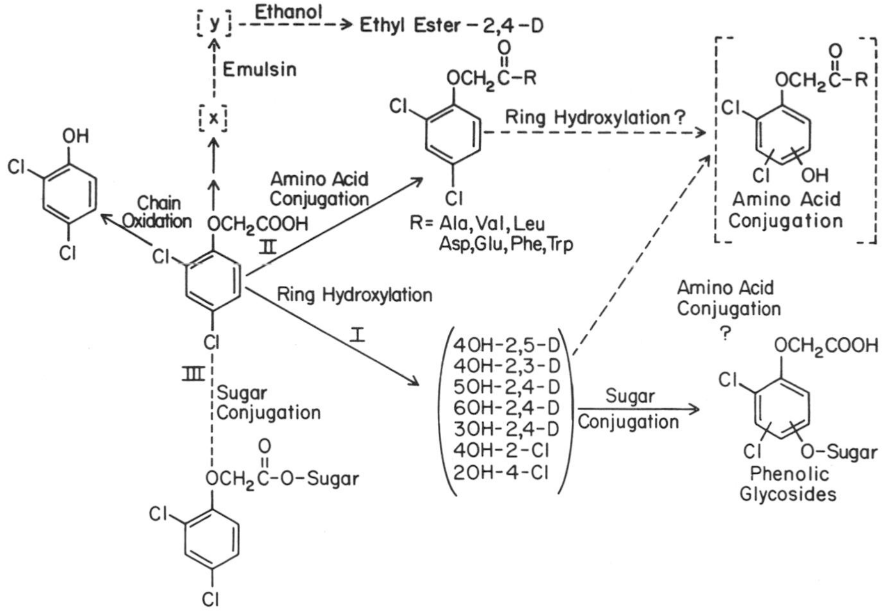

Journal of Agricultural and Food Chemistry

*Figure 6.   Summary of 2,4-D metabolism by plants (26)*

Table XI.   Radioactivity of 2,4-D and its Metabolites, Represented as Percentage of Total $^{14}$C Absorbed, in Plants (47).

| Fraction or Substance | Wheat | Timothy | Bean | Soy-bean | Sun-flower | Straw-berry |
|---|---|---|---|---|---|---|
| 2,4-D | 29.9 | 30.9 | 4.0 | 10.5 | 85.0 | 7.0 |
| 2,4-D-Asp and 2,4-D-Glu | 0 | 0 | 3.2 | 5.6 | 1.5 | 0 |
| 4-OH-2,5-D and 4-OH-2,3-D | 0.8 | 0 | 3.5 | 3.0 | 0 | 0 |
| 2,4-Dichlorophenoxy-acetyl/β-D-glucose | 23.9 | 21.7 | 24.8 | 5.7 | 3.7 | 2.0 |
| Glucosides of 4-OH-2,5-D and 4-OH-2,3-D | 10.2 | 3.3 | 50.1 | 53.0 | 0 | 12.0 |
| Glycoside of 2,4-Di-chlorophenol | 2.2 | 2.4 | — | — | — | 65.0 |
| Unknown 2,4-D Metabolite | 15.0 | 12.6 | 2.5 | 8.0 | 0 | 0 |

consistantly produced large quantities of the glucose ester. Although the amino acid conjugates were present in the dicots, their concentration in intact plants was not as high as in plant tissue cultures.

The lack of substantial amounts of amino acid conjugates in the plants may be explained partially by recent investigations (15). In these studies, it was shown that the age of the callus tissue and the concentration of the applied 2,4-D greatly affected the metabolism of 2,4-D. In young soybean root callus tissue (3 weeks), 2,4-D was metabolized (2 days) to ether soluble metabolites (amino acid conjugates) and to aqueous soluble (ether insoluble) metabolites (glycosides). As the concentration of herbicide increased uptake into the ethanol fraction increased and the amount of free 2,4-D increases proportionately while only a slight increase in metabolites is observed (Fig. 7). In older soybean callus tissue (5-9 weeks), a major biochemical change occurs such that the level of free 2,4-D in the tissue is regulated at ca. 4 nm per gram fresh weight. As the concentration of 2,4-D administered was increased, a greater amount of 2,4-D was converted to amino acid conjugates so the level of free 2,4-D in the tissue was regulated (Fig. 8).

This same phenomena, the regulation of free 2,4-D levels through the formation of amino acid conjugates, was also demonstrated in soybean leaf callus tissue cultures. Although the regulation of the 2,4-D concentration within the tissue is controlled by the formation of the ether soluble metabolites, the aqueous soluble fraction is twice as big in leaf callus as it is in root callus tissue. Differentiated soybean root culture behaves biochemically like old callus tissue. The 2,4-D levels are regulated at ca. 2 nm per gram fresh weight (Fig. 9).

These experiments with 2,4-D have shown the importance of the types of tissue, the age of the tissue, the concentration of the pesticide, and the method of incubation used in plant tissue culture studies. Since each laboratory seems to adopt its own procedures, which may affect results, it is time to standardize some of the procedures used in tissue culture studies. Although the incubation of the pesticide with callus tissue cultures has been used only by a few laboratories (24-28, 31-36, 57), this technique should be examined in more detail with other pesticides to determine whether it may be more representative of whole plant studies.

The metabolism of 2,4,5-T by soybean root callus tissues has been examined recently (31). Studies showed that soybean callus tissue cultures also convert 2,4,5-T into amino acid conjugates (glutamic acid [90%] and aspartic acid [10%]). No glucose ester formation was demonstrated.

Although the metabolism of indoleacetic acid (IAA) by plant tissue cultures has not been studied extensively, the metabolic pathways appear similar to those of intact plants, or excised plant parts. One pathway is the peroxidase-IAA oxidase

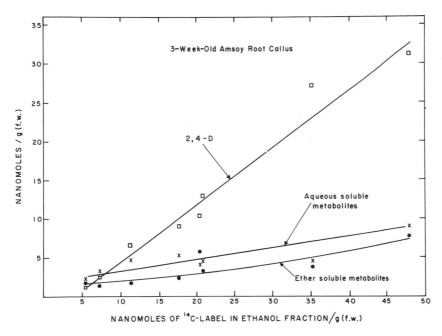

*Figure 7.   Concentration of 2,4-D or 2,4-D metabolites found in various subfractions vs. total concentration in the ethanol extract of 3-week-old soybean root callus tissue following incubation for 48 hr with various levels of 2,4-D-1-$^{14}$C (1.8 × 10$^{-6}$ to 1.1 × 10$^{-5}$M). The free 2,4-D content was subtracted from the total ether-soluble metabolites (mostly amino acid conjugates).*

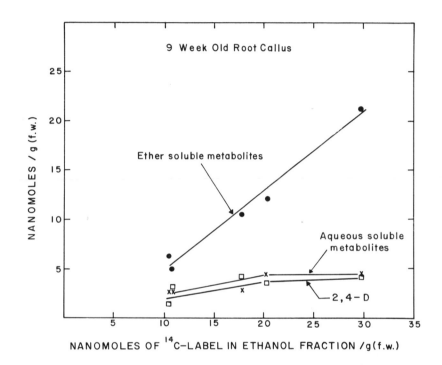

*Figure 8.    Concentration of 2,4-D or 2,4-D metabolites found in various subfractions vs. total concentration in the ethanol extract of 9-week-old soybean root callus tissue following incubation for 48 hr with various levels of 2,4-D-1-14C (1.8 × 10⁻⁶ to 1.1 × 10⁻⁵M). The free 2,4-D content was subtracted from the total ether-soluble metabolites (mostly amino acid conjugates).*

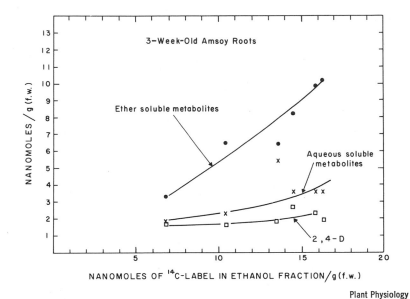

Plant Physiology

*Figure 9.   Concentration of 2,4-D or 2,4-D metabolites found in various subfractions vs. total concentration in the ethanol extract of 3-week-old differentiated soybean roots following incubation for 48 hr with various levels of 2,4-D-1-¹⁴C (9 × 10⁻⁷ to 2.3 × 10⁻⁶M). The free 2,4-D content was subtracted from the total ether-soluble metabolites (mostly amino acid conjugates).*

oxidation of IAA in the presence of $Mn^{+2}$ and phenolic cofactors.
The second pathway (in common with 2,4-D) is the conjugation of
IAA with amino acids or sugars.

It now appears that peroxidases are as widely distributed in
plant tissue cultures as they are in intact plants (49). These
so-called isozymes that are observed on gel electrophoresis often
change with the stage of development or hormonal treatment (49,
50, 51) of plants. Since genetic information is not available
(52) and peroxidase contains carbohydrate (53), the term isozyme
is probably a misnomer. These "isozymes" have varying activities
on peroxidase substances or act as an IAA oxidase.

An IAA oxidase has been found in Picea glauca callus cultures
(54) and the first extra-cellular IAA oxidase was detected in
Parthenocissus tricuspidata crown gall cultures (55). An extra-
cellular IAA oxidase and the products of an intracellular IAA
oxidase from this tissue have also been characterized (56, 57).
Although the enzymatic products were 3-hydroxymethyloxindole and
ultimately its dehydration product 3-methyleneoxindole, neither
metabolite was found in the tissue (57). However, small amounts
of 3-methyloxindole were found in the medium in confirmation of
its reported occurrence in pea seedlings (58). Extensive decarboxylation of IAA-1-$^{14}$C supplied to this tissue (50% in 24 hours)
suggests the degradation of IAA by IAA oxidase and conversion of
the oxindole to unidentified products. In 12 week old apple callus, 90% decarboxylation of IAA-1-$^{14}$C was found in 4 hours compared to 20% decarboxylation in 4 hours by 6 week old apple callus
(35). Six week old apple callus accumulated elevated IAA levels
in the tissue, and two metabolites, thought to be oxindoles, were
detected in 12 week and 6 week old apple callus (34).

The conjugation of IAA to aspartic acid has been reported in
geranium stem callus (32) and in embryogenic habituated ovular
callus of orange (36) where it is suggested to maintain levels
favorable to embryogenesis. The major conjugates found in Parthenocissus tricuspidata crown gall callus were the glycine,  alanine, and valine conjugates (33). Minor amounts of the aspartic
and glutamic acid conjugates also were found. Chromatographic
separation of the glycine conjugate from IAA as well as the aspartic conjugate from the glutamic conjugate is difficult (59). Thus,
the glutamic and glycine conjugates may have remained undetected
in intact plants or excised tissue.

The glucose ester of IAA has been detected in many plant
tissues (60, 61, 62, 63, 64), but does not appear to have been
identified in plant tissue cultures.

INSECTICIDES

The metabolism of carbaryl (1-naphthyl methylcarbamate) by
tobacco cells in suspension culture has been reported (37, 38).
The first report (37) indicated that up to 16% of the total metabolites of carbaryl might be conjugates of N-hydroxycarbaryl

(1-naphthyl N-hydroxy-N-methyl carbamate) a potential mutagen. In
a more thorough investigation (38) no N-hydroxy carbaryl or derivatives could be detected. In these later studies, [14]C-labeled
$C_1$-naphthyl, carbonyl and N-methyl carbaryl (9 ppm) were incubated
in the dark with tobacco cell suspensions for 14 days. The cells
metabolized 36% of the carbaryl of which 7.9% represented nine
metabolites. The only metabolite found in the medium was $N-CH_2OH-$
carbaryl. It represented 18.38% of the metabolites. Free N-
$CH_2OH-$carbaryl and its glycoside were found in the cells, but in
very low concentrations. The major tissue metabolite was the β-D-
glucoside of α-naphthol. This metabolite was found present only
in trace amounts in intact bean plants (65). Small amounts of
conjugated 4-OH-(0.3%), 5-OH-(0.3%) and 7-OH-(0.82%) carbaryl were
also identified in the suspension cultures. These conjugates were
the major metabolites in intact bean plants (65). Of considerable
interest was the tentative identification of two new metabolites
of carbaryl, 1,4-dihydro-1,4-epiperoxynaphthalene (0.39%) and 0-1-
naphthylcholesterol (3.0%), the latter metabolite being a unique
ether. A summary of the metabolism of carbaryl by tobacco suspension culture is presented in Figure 10. The relative composition
of metabolites in tobacco cell in suspension culture (38) and
intact bean plants (65) are compared in Table XII.

Metabolites that have been identified in whole plants are
also found in the tobacco tissue culture, but there is a large
quantitative difference between bean plants and tobacco suspension
cultures. A more detailed study of the metabolites found in intact plants of the same species should be made to see if any of
the newly discovered metabolites found in tobacco cell suspension
cultures also exist in intact tobacco plants. In bean plants, the
glycosides of 4-OH, 5-OH and $N-CH_2OH-$carbaryl predominate. The
primary hydroxylated product $N-CH_2OH-$carbaryl is perhaps excreted
into the suspension culture media before the glycoside is formed.
Strangely, the α-naphthol was found only as the glycoside in tobacco suspension culture cells. In contrast, the glycoside of N-
$CH_2OH-$carbaryl was present in the cells in only minor amounts.

The metabolism of [35]Cl-labeled lindane (α-hexachlorocyclohex-
ane) by various plant cell cultures has been compared to its metabolism in intact plants (39). With intact plants (28 day incubation), very little [35]Cl was liberated, but plant suspension
cultures (12-28 days incubation) metabolized from 0% (soybean) to
6.8% (wild carrot) of the applied lindane. Trace quantities of
1,2,4-trichlorobenzene (1%) were identified in tobacco cultures,
but were not detected in the other cultures. The main metabolite
of carrot suspension cultures had not been reported previously in
plants and was tentatively identified as a glucoside of
trichlorophenol.

Tissue cultures showed a higher uptake and metabolic rate for
lindane than intact plants. No degradation to $CO_2$ was detected,
and lettuce plants were not able to metabolize lindane to penta-
chlorophenol as has been reported (66). These studies also showed

Table XII.  Percentage of $^{14}$C-Carbaryl Metabolites Isolated from Bean Plants and Tobacco Suspension Cultures.

| | Percentage of $^{14}$C-Labeled Compound | | | |
| | Bean Plants[a] | | Tobacco Suspension Culture[b] | |
| Carbaryl or Metabolite | Ether Soluble | Conjugated (Aglycons) | Ether Soluble (Medium) | Conjugated (Aglycons) (Cell) |
|---|---|---|---|---|
| Carbaryl | + | 1.0 | 64.72 | 0. |
| 1-Naphthol | 0 | Trace | 0 | 5.72 |
| 4-Hydroxy Carbaryl | 0 | 33.0 | 0 | 0.02 |
| 5-Hydroxy Carbaryl | 0 | 25.0 | 0 | 0.02 |
| 7-Hydroxy Carbaryl | 0 | 0 | 0 | 0.06 |
| N-Hydroxymethyl Carbaryl | 0 | 18.1 | 1.47 | 0.20 |
| Dihydrodihydroxy Carbaryl | 0 | 15.6 | | |

[a]Data taken from (65)
[b]Data taken from (38)

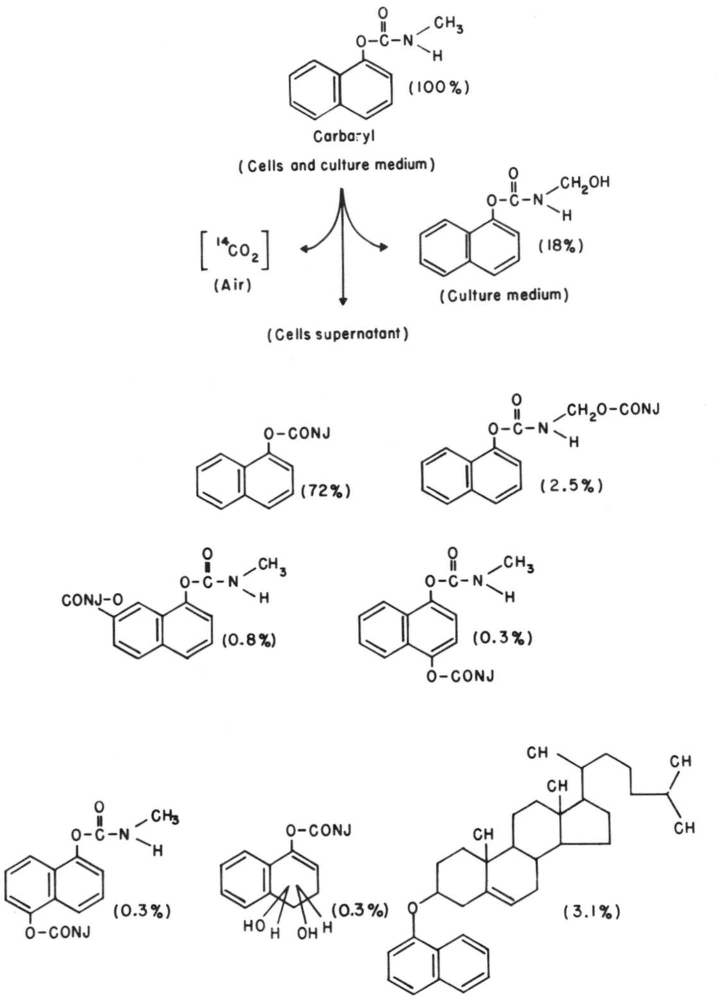


Archives of Environmental Contamination and Toxicology

*Figure 10. The metabolism of carbaryl by tobacco cell suspension cultures*

that intact plants were contaminated with epiphytic microorganisms
that could metabolize lindane.

The metabolism of aldrin has been investigated in suspension
cultures from bean roots, bean shoots and potato tubers (40). The
effect of media variations on metabolism also were studied. In
intact plants, aldrin was converted to dieldrin, photodieldrin,
dihydrochlorodene dicarboxylic acid and aldrin trans-diol (Fig.
11). Aldrin (40%) was metabolized mainly to dieldrin by the plant
suspension cultures (28 days). The dieldrin was located primarily
in the cells. Aldrin trans-diol was also isolated in small
amounts, but only in the bean shoot and potato tuber cultures.

Small quantities of photodieldrin were detected when larger
quantities of aldrin (10 mg) were added to bean root cultures.
Conversion of aldrin to photodieldrin was only found in mixed bean
root and shoot cultures although it was formed from dieldrin in
all cultures. These data support the direct formation of photodieldrin by plants in the dark rather than by a light induced
photochemical reaction or microorganisms.

The metabolism of aldrin by plant tissue cultures is in good
qualitative agreement with similar intact plant experiments, except that the dicarboxylic acid isolated in low levels from intact
plants grown under field conditions was not detected in plant suspension cultures. Variation in the culture media affected the
quantitative distribution of metabolites. Differences also ex-
isted between bean root and shoot cultures and between potato
tuber cultures. Aldrin trans-diol was only found in cultures
incubated with aldrin, never with dieldrin, and suggest that
aldrin trans-diol is directly formed from aldrin.

The metabolism of DDT and Kelthane has been examined in cell
suspension cultures of parsley and soybean (41). After 44-48 hr
incubation, only 0.6 to 2.2% of the applied DDT was metabolized.
DDE (1,1-dichloro-2,2-bis-[4-chlorophenyl]-ethylene) was identified as the major metabolite of DDT. Other metabolites were detected but were not identified. Parsley suspension cultures
converted Kelthane to a nonpolar (0.1%) and a polar (0.3%)
metabolite.

## Phytotoxicity and Bioassays

A number of investigators (22, 67-74) have used plant tissue
cultures as a means of studying phytotoxicity. These investigations usually have not focused on the metabolism of the xenobiotic
directly but have concentrated on the physiological affect of the
xenobiotic on the plant tissue. Indirectly, these investigators
may be measuring the ability of the tissue culture to metabolize
the xenobiotic to nontoxic substances. An important example is
the prior mentioned investigation (22) of metribuzin phytotoxicity
in soybean suspension cultures where the principle of resistance
was the ability to metabolize an inhibitor of an enzyme that
metabolized metribuzin to a nontoxic form.

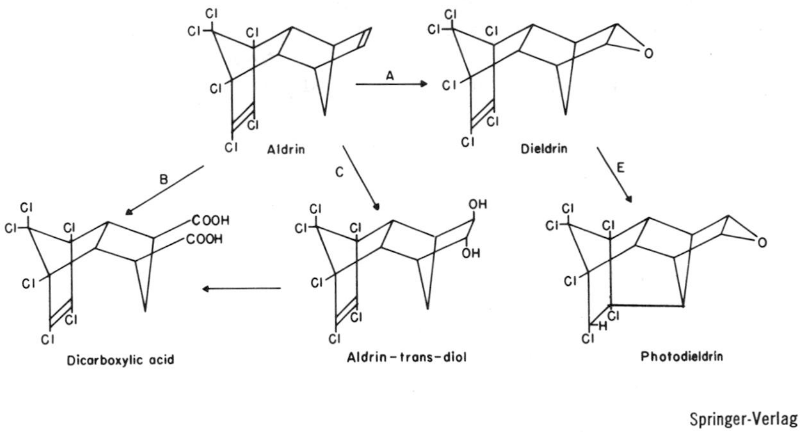

Springer-Verlag

Figure 11.    Metabolism of aldrin and dieldrin. The dicarboxylic acid metabolite
could not be detected in plant cell suspension cultures.

The effects of organic solvents on growth and ultrastructure of plant cell suspensions have been studied recently (75). These studies have bearing on most metabolism studies. The phytotoxic effects of solvents increased in the following order: chloroform, dimethyl sulfoxide, methanol, acetone, isopropanol, and ethanol. At concentrations of 0.25%, chloroform had no apparent affect on cell growth, however, ethanol inhibited growth at concentrations as low as 0.05%. These data suggest that small amounts of organic solvents, often used to introduce the xenobiotic to the plant tissue culture, must be carefully considered.

Plant tissue culture techniques have been used to evaluate the biological activity of growth stimulating herbicides and their metatolites or potential metabolites. Amino acid conjugates of 2,4-D (76), 2,4,5-T (77), and IAA (78) were added to culture media ($10^{-4}$-$10^{-8}$ M) of soybean callus tissue and evaluated for their ability to stimulate cell division and growth as measured by increase in weight. Amino acid conjugates of 2,4-D and IAA stimulated the growth of callus tissue and some conjugates of 2,4-D stimulated growth even better than 2,4-D itself. Surprisingly, the amino acid conjugates of 2,4,5-T did not stimulate growth of soybean root callus.

## Production of Secondary Substances

Plant tissue cultures have been evaluated as a potential means of production of plant products sometimes referred to as secondary products. Plant products of potential commercial use such as steroids, alkaloids, glycosides, vitamins and others have received some attention of investigators, especially those of medicinal importance (79-83). The metabolism of three alkaloids, vindoline, catharanthine HCl, and vincaleukoblastine sulfate have been examined with suspension cultures of Catharanthus roseus (L.) (84). Vindoline formed two metabolites, desacetylvindoline and dihydrovindoline. No metabolites of catharanthine HCl were detected. Vincaleukoblastine sulfate formed three metabolites.

The biosynthesis of alkaloids by suspension cultures may be enhanced greatly by incubation of the plant tissue with selected intermediates (85). In this way, the cell media would be supplemented with key intermediates that would be metabolized further to the desired alkaloid.

The biosynthesis of edulinine and furoquinoline alkaloids from selective quinoline derivatives by Ruta graveolens cell suspension cultures has been studied (86). The biogenetic synthesis of the alkaloids in the tissue culture experiments were consistant with pathways discovered in rutaceous plants. The metabolic intermediates differed quantitatively from intact plants and varied with the age of the culture and with different culture isolates.

Berberine and plamatine, two medicinally important alkaloids, are produced by plant tissue cultures of Coptis japonica (79). The production of ginseng glycosides has been studied in plant

tissue cultures of <u>Panax ginseng</u> (<u>79</u>).  Nitroquanidine and X-ray
treatments were used to obtain mutants that had higher titers of
saponins.  These genetic mutation techniques may also be useful
in the selection of resistant and nonresistant cultivars by altering their metabolism of xenobiotics.  So far, large scale commercial drug production using plant tissue cultures has not been
achieved.

It has been suggested (<u>87</u>) that through proper selection of
plant species, tissue culture techniques may be useful for the
preparation of metabolites of xenobiotics in quantities needed for
standards and for structural characterization.  For example, the
glucose ester of 2,4-D can be mass produced with rice callus tissue (<u>28</u>) and amino acid conjugates of 2,4-D can be mass produced
from soybean callus tissue when culture conditions are selected
for optimization of amino acid conjugates (<u>15</u>).

## Advantages and Disadvantages

In general, all studies indicate that the same metabolic
pathways of degradation appear to be operating in intact plants
and plant tissue cultures.  Thus, xenobiotic metabolism by plant
tissue cultures is a desirable model for estimating metabolic
pathways in the intact plant.  However, at the present time, work
with intact plants (or parts) is also necessary to confirm and
evaluate the quantitative aspects of xenobiotic metabolism.  Plant
tissue cultures are sterile, homogenous, rapidly growing and do
not require extensive facilities.  Because of ease of standardization of conditions, reproducibility should be achieved more readily, data are amenable to statistical analysis and results could
be compared directly in different laboratories.  Use of tissue
cultures obviates the difficulties of poor penetration, translocation, and perhaps there is less compartmentation of metabolic pools
than encountered with intact plants.  Plant tissue cultures permit
the use of lower levels of radiolabeled material and the isolation
of metabolites that are free of many interfering substances so
troublesome with intact plants.  Metabolism by different plant
species or by different tissues of the same plant can be compared
readily.  However, it is not at all clear that callus started from
different tissues will show major differences in metabolism.  However, one would expect organ culture to exhibit clear differences
in the metabolism of xenobiotics.  Plant tissue cultures are also
useful for studying the mode of action of phyto-active xenobiotics
because of ease of controlling the various parameters of growth.
Cultures have been used as a technique for the bioassay of chemicals that cause physiological changes such as growth stimulation,
cell division and phytotoxicity.  In addition, plant tissue culture techniques offer great potential in the mass production of
metabolites as well as medicinally important chemicals.

Obvious disadvantages do exist in the use of plant tissue
cultures.  The technique does not show the importance of cuticular

penetration, of root absorption, of microorganisms associated with
the intact plant, or of vascular transport. Tissue cultures
would not indicate the importance of environmental factors such
as wind, nutrition, disease, water stress, temperature or sunlight
on metabolic products and pool sizes. In tissue cultures, the
photosynthetic apparatus is often absent or only marginal. If
photosynthesis is important for the metabolism of the xenobiotic,
then tissue culture technqiues might be undesirable. Experiments
with tissue cultures have shown the importance of culture age and
the method of xenobiotic administration in determining metabolite
levels. These conditions would be different with intact plants.

## Conclusions

Xenobiotic metabolites isolated from plant tissue cultures are
qualitatively the same as metabolites found in whole plants, but
with quantitative differences. Therefore, metabolic pathways
operating in whole plants also seem to be operating plant tissue
cultures. With some metabolites, such as glycosides and aglycons,
there may be a large quantitative difference between the two techniques. This is especially true with plant suspension culture
technqiues which often produce quantitatively lower amounts of
glycosides and higher amounts of aglycons than studies with intact
plants. Apparently the aglycons can be excreted from the cells
before the glycosides are formed. Perhaps the level of carbohy-
drates in the media affects glycoside synthesis.

Common reactions found in plant tissue cultures are oxidations
at both aliphatic and aromatic carbons, dealkylations, hydrolytic
enzymes such as amidases, and esterases, dehydrochlorinations,
dechlorinations, hydrogenations and conjugations with sugars,
amino acids and acids. Plant tissue cultures can reflect the tolerance of the parent plant, e.g., cultivars showing resistance to
phytotoxic xenobiotics also exhibit resistance in tissue culture.

Many factors affect xenobiotic metabolism by plant tissue
cultures. The source of the tissue is important. Different tissues from the same plant show minor variations, and tissue from
different species (or even varieties) of plants show greater
variations (e.g., monocot and dicot plant tissue cultures may exhibit major differences in metabolism). The tissue culture method
is also very important. Suspension cultures may give rise to sig-
nigicant amounts of metabolites in the medium and low relative
proportions of glycosides. In the few cases reported, incubations
with callus tissue results in rapid absorption of the xenobiotic,
no significant metabolites in the medium and accumulation of gly-
goside conjugates similar to that found in intact plants. The
method of administrating the xenobiotic to the culture may also
be important. Direct injection of 2,4-D into the callus tissue
seemingly gave different results from callus tissue incubated in
solution with 2,4-D (26). Another factor, of some importance, is
the composition of the medium (40). In intact plants, illumination

has been shown to stimulate the formation of the glucose ester (60) and enzymes such as phenylalanine ammonia lyase (46). This parameter has not been examined thoroughly in plant tissue cultures and needs further study. The physiological stage or age of the tissue culture has been demonstrated to show a significant effect on metabolism (15). In some cases only older tissues demonstrated enzymatic activity (20) and controlled metabolism (15). In spite of these limitations, investigations of the metabolism of xenobiotics by plant tissue cultures provides a reasonable approximation of the metabolism expected with intact plants.

With so many factors affecting metabolism and each research laboratory using different tissues and culture conditions, there is a need for the standardization of some tissue culture parameters. Perhaps certain well studied plant tissues should be used by all laboratories as a base of comparison. Selected plant tissues should include some important dicot and monocot plants. Tobacco tissue has been suggested as at least one possibility for routine use (38). Perhaps a plant tissue bank, similar to those established for microorganisms, could be established for laboratories working with plant tissue cultures.

Additional research is needed to determine which of the many factors affecting metabolism in plant tissue cultures are most important before we can suggest standardization of these factors. Really, only a few xenobiotics and pesticides have been examined, e.g., few compounds from the important organophosphate or triazine pesticides have been examined. Fungicides appear to have been neglected. Therefore, additional investigations with other pesticides and xenobiotics are desirable before we can properly evaluate the relative merits of studying metabolism with plant tissue cultures and the extrapolation of these results to intact plants.

## ABSTRACT

Xenobiotic metabolism by plant tissue cultures are reviewed
with an emphasis on pesticide metabolism.  The results obtained
with tissue culture techniques are evaluated and compared with
results using whole plants.  Some factors affecting metabolism
studies with plant tissue culture techniques are also considered.

Some advantages of the plant tissue culture techniques
include:  sterility, a rapidly growing homogenous tissue with
low pigment content, moderate cost and space requirements, ease
of duplication of treatment conditions, rapid uptake and metabolism of xenobiotics, and ease of isolation of metabolites.  It
offers the opportunity to mass produce desired metabolites as
well as evaluate phytotoxicity or physiological changes of the
plant tissue.  Obvious disadvantages of this technique are its
failure to evaluate such factors as:  penetration, absorption,
microorganisms, vascular transport and environmental influences.
Other factors affecting xenobiotic metabolism by plant tissue
cultures are:  culture method, source of the tissue, method of
treatment and concentration of xenobiotic, composition of medium
and physiological age of tissue.

Although quantitative and perhaps qualitative differences
may be found, it is concluded that xenobiotic metabolism by
plant tissue culture provides a useful approximation of metabolic
pathways in intact plants.

## Literature Cited

1. Sandermann, H., Diesperger, H., Scheel, D., In "Plant Tissue Culture and Its Bio-Technological Application," Barz, W., Reinhard, E., Zenk, M. H., Eds., Springer-Verlag, Berlin, Heidelberg, New York, (1977), pp. 178-196.
2. Barz, W., In "Plant Tissue Culture and Its Bio-Technological Application," Barz, W., Reinhard, E., Zenk, M. H., Eds. Springer-Verlag, Berlin, Heidelberg, New York, (1977), pp. 153-177.
3. Haberlandt, G., Sitzungsber. Acad. Wiss. Wien, Math.-naturw. Kl. (1902), 111, 69.
4. White, P. R., Amer. J. Bot. (1939) 26, 59.
5. Gautheret, R. J., C.r. Acad. Sci., Paris (1939) 208, 118.
6. Nobécourt, P., C.r. Soc. Biol., Paris (1939) 130, 1270.
7. White, P. R., The Cultivation of Animal and Plant Cells, The Ronald Press, New York, NY (1954).
8. Van Overbeek, J., Conklin, M. E., Blakeslee, A. F., Sci. (1941) 94, 350.
9. Miller, C. O., Skoog, F., Okumura, S., Von Sultza, H., Strong, F. H., J. Am. Chem. Soc. (1955) 77, 2662.
10. Miller, C. O., In Paech, K. and Tracey, M. V. Eds., Modern Methods of Plant Analysis, Springer-Verlag, Berlin (1963) 6, 194.
11. Murashige, T., Skoog, F., Physiol. Plant (1962) 15, 473.
12. Nitsch, J. P., Nitsch, C., Science (1969) 163, 85.
13. Gamborg, O. L., In "Plant Tissue Culture Methods," Gamborg, O. L., Wetter, L. R., Eds., Natl. Res. Council (Canada) Ottawa, Canada (1975), p. 1.
14. Meins, F., In "Tissue Culture and Plant Science," Street, H. E., Ed., Acad. Press (1974), p. 233.
15. Davidonis, G. H., Hamilton, R. H., Mumma, R. O., Plant Physiol. (1978) 62, 80.
16. Unpublished data.
17. Frear, D. S., Swanson, H. R., Davison, K. L., 170th Nat. Meet. of the Am. Chem. Soc., Aug. 24-29 (1975).
18. Frear, D. S., Swanson, H. R., Pest. Biochem. and Physiol. (1975) 5, 73.
19. Davis, D. G., Hodgson, R. H. Dusbabek, K. E., Hoffer, B. L., Physiologia plantarum (1970) 44, 87.
20. Ray, T. B., Still, C. C., Pest. Biochem. Physiol. (1975) 5, 171.
21. Locke, R. K., Baron, R. L., J. Agric. Food Chem. (1972) 20, 861.
22. Oswald, T. H., Smith, A. E., Phillips, D. V., Pest. Biochem. Physiol. (1978) 8, 73.
23. Ojima, K., Gamborg, O. L., Proc. Sixth Int. Conf. Plant Growth Subst. (1968) p. 857.
24. Feung, C.-S., Hamilton, R. H., Witham, F. H., Mumma, R. O., Plant Physiol. (1972) 50, 80.

25. Feung, C.-S., Hamilton, R. H., Mumma, R. O., J. Agric. Food Chem. (1973) 21, 637.
26. Feung, C.-S., Loerch, S. L., Hamilton, R. H., Mumma, R. O., J. Agric. Food Chem. (1978) 26, 1064.
27. Feung, C.-S., Hamilton, R. H., Mumma, R. O., J. Agric. Food Chem. (1975) 23, 373.
28. Feung, C.-S., Hamilton, R. H., Mumma, R. O., J. Agric. Food Chem. (1976) 24, 1013.
29. Bristol, D. W., Ghanuni, A. M., Oleson, A. E., J. Agric. Food Chem. (1977) 25, 1308.
30. Harvey, R. G., Muzik, T. J., Weed Sci. (1973) 21, 135.
31. Arjmand, M., Hamilton, R. H., Mumma, R. O., J. Agric. Food Chem. (1978) 26, 1125.
32. Troxler, R. F., Hamilton, R. H., Plant Physiol. (1965) 40, 400.
33. Feung, C.-S., Hamilton, R. H., Mumma, R. O., Plant Physiol. (1976) 58, 666.
34. Epstein, E., Klein, I., Lavee, S., Plant and Cell Physiol. (1975) 16, 305.
35. Epstein, E., Lavee, S., Plant and Cell Physiol. (1975) 16, 553.
36. Epstein, E., Kochba, J., Neumann, H., Z. Pflanzenphysiol. (1977) 88, 263.
37. Locke, R. K., Bastone, V. B., Baron, R. L., J. Agric. Food Chem. (1971) 19, 1205.
38. Locke, R. K., Chen, J. T., Damico, J. N., Dusold, L. R., Sphon, J. A., Arch. of Environ. Contam. and Toxicol. (1976) 4, 60.
39. Stöckigt, J., Ries, B., In "Plant Tissue Culture and Its Bio-technological Applications," Barz, W., Reinhard, E., Zenk, M. H., Eds., Springer-Verlag, Berlin, Heidelberg, New York (1977), pp. 204-210.
40. Brain, K. R., Lines, D. S., In "Plant Tissue Culture and Its Bio-technological Applications," Barz, W., Reinhard, E., Zenk, M. H., Eds., Springer-Verlag, Berlin, Heidelberg, New York, (1977) pp. 197-203.
41. Scheel, D., Sandermann, H., Planta (1977) 133, 315.
42. Filner, P., Exp. Cell Res. (1965) 39, 33.
43. Geissbühler, H., Bannock, I., Gross, D., "Radioisotope and Chromatographic Techniques for Tracing the Fate of Herbicides in Plants and Soils," IUPAC Symposium, Johannesburg (1969).
44. Rogers, R. L., J. Agric. Food Chem. (1971) 19, 32.
45. Lieb, H. B., Ray, T. B., Still, C. C., Plant Physiol. (1973) 51, 1140.
46. Hahlbrock, K., In "Plant Tissue Culture and Its Bio-technological Applications," Barz, W., Reinhard, E., Zenk, M. H., Eds., Springer-Verlag, Berlin, Heidelberg, New York (1977) pp. 95-111.

47. Chkanikov, D. I., Makeyev, A. M., Pavlova, N. N., Grygoryeva, L. V., Dubovoi, V. P., Klimov, O. V., Arch. Environ. Contam. Toxicol. (1976) 5, 97.

48. Hamilton, R. H., Hurter, J., Hall, J. K., Ercegovich, C. D., J. Agric. Food Chem. (1971) 19, 480.

49. Schneider, E. A., Wightman, F., Ann. Rev. Plant Physiol. (1974) 25, 487.

50. Lee, T. T., Plant Physiol. (1971) 48, 56.

51. Lavee, S., Galston, A. W., Am. J. Bot. (1968) 55, 890.

52. Scandalios, J. G., Ann. Rev. Plant Physiol. (1974) 25, 225.

53. Shannon, L. M., Kay, E., Lew, J. Y., J. Biol. Chem. (1966) 241, 2166.

54. Reinert, J., Schraudolf, H., Tazawa, M., Naturwiss (1957) 44, 588.

55. Lipetz, J., Galston, A. W., Am. J. Bot. (1959) 46, 193.

56. Witham, F. H., Gentile, A. C., J. Exp. Bot. (1961) 12, 188.

57. Hamilton, R. H., Meyer, H. E., Burke, R. E., Feung, C.-S., Mumma, R. O., Plant Physiol. (1976) 58, 77.

58. Tuli, V., Moyed, H. S., Plant Physiol. (1967) 42, 425.

59. Feung, C.-S., Hamilton, R. H., Mumma, R. O., J. Agric. Food Chem. (1975) 23, 1120.

60. Bandurski, R. S., Schulze, A., Cohen, J. D., Biochem. Biophys. Res. Comm. (1977) 79, 1219.

61. Davies, P. J., Physiol. Plant (1972) 27, 262.

62. Patrick, J. W., Wolley, D. J., J. Exp. Bot. (1973) 24, 949.

63. Zenk, M. H., In "Régulateurs Naturels de la Croissance Végétale," C.N.R.S. Paris, (1964) pp. 241-249.

64. Zenk, M. H., Nature (1961) 191, 493.

65. Kuhr, R. J., Casida, J. E., J. Agric. Food Chem. (1967) 15, 814.

66. Kohli, J., Weisgerber, I., Klein, W., Pest. Biochem. Physiol. (1976) 6, 91.

67. Diaz-Colon, J. D., Bovey, R. W., Davis, F. S., Baur, J. R., Physiol. Plant (1972) 27, 60.

68. Bovey, R. W., Baur, J. R., Diaz-Colon, J. D., Weed Sci. (1974) 22, 191.

69. Zilkah, S., Gressel, J., Plant Cell Physiol. (1977) 18, 815.

70. Davis, F. S., Villarreal, A., Baur, J. R. Goldstein, I. S., Weed Sci. (1972) 20, 185.

71. Zilkah, S., Gressel, J., Plant Cell Physiol. (1977) 18, 641.

72. Barg, R., Umiel, N., Z. Pflanzenphysiol. (1977) 83, 437.

73. Zilkah, S., Bocion, P. F., Gressel, J., Plant Cell Physiol. (1977) 18, 657.

74. Davis, D. G., Hoerauf, R. A., Dusbabek, K. E., Dougall, D. K., Physiol. Plant (1977) 40, 15.

75. Davis, D. G., Wergin, W. P., Dusababek, K. E., Pest. Biochem. Physiol. (1978) 8, 84.

76. Feung, C.-S., Mumma, R. O., Hamilton, R. H., J. Agric. Food Chem. (1974) 22, 307.

77. Arjmand, M., Hamilton, R. H., Davidonis, G. H., Mumma, R. O.,
    J. Agric. Food Chem. (1979) (in press).
78. Feung, C.-S., Hamilton, R. H., Mumma, R. O., Plant Physiol.
    (1977) 59, 91.
79. Misawa, M., In "Plant Tissue Culture and Its Bio-technologi-
    cal Application," Barz, W., Reinhard, E., Zenk, M. H., Eds.,
    Springer-Verlag, Berlin, Heidelberg, New York (1977) pp.
    17-26.
80. Muhle, E., Hoesel, W., Barz, W., Phytochem. (Oxf.) (1976)
    15, 1669.
81. Heeger, V., Leienbach, K.-W., Barz, W., Hoppe-Seyler's Z.
    Physiol. Chem. (1976) 357, 1081.
82. Leienbach, K.-W., Barz, W., Hoppe-Seyler's Z. Physiol. Chem.
    (1976) 357, 1069.
83. Koop, W., Barz, W., Phytochem. (Oxf.) (1976 15, 1581.
84. Carew, D. P., Drueger, R. J., Phytochem. (1977) 16, 1461.
85. Strek, W., In "Plant Tissue Culture Methods," Gamborg,
    O. L., Wetter, L. R., Eds., Natl. Res. Council (Canada)
    Ottawa, Canada (1975), p. 83.
86. Boulanger, D., Bailey, B. K., Steck, N., Phytochem. (1973)
    12, 2399
87. Mumma, R. O., Hamilton, R. H., In "Bound and Conjugated
    Pesticide Residues," Kaufman, D. D., Still, C. C., Paulson,
    G. D., Bandal, S. K., Eds., ACS Symposium Series No. 29,
    Am. Chem. Soc. (1976), pp. 68-85.

RECEIVED December 20, 1978.

# Pesticide Metabolism in Higher Plants: In Vitro Enzyme Studies[1]

G. L. LAMOUREUX and D. S. FREAR

Metabolism and Radiation Research Laboratory, Agricultural Research, Science and Education Administration, U. S. Department of Agriculture, Fargo, ND 58105

The study of xenobiotic metabolism in plants has developed primarily as a result of the use of pesticides to protect plant crops from damage by weeds, insects and other pests. Great stimulus for research in this field was experienced in the early 1960's when increased concern was raised over the possible hazards of pesticide residues to man and his environment.

The complexity of xenobiotic metabolism studies is a continuum with in vivo studies conducted in the natural environment at one end, and the use of isolated enzymes to study molecular reactions at the other. Each technique in this continuum has its own particular limitations, but can be used to great advantage under the proper conditions. In the previous two reports, the use of cell cultures, tissue cultures, isolated cells and isolated plant organs were considered.

This report will examine the use of isolated plant enzyme systems in xenobiotic metabolism studies. The primary topic will be a discussion of the enzymes involved in the four basic metabolic reactions of xenobiotics in plants: oxidation, reduction, hydrolysis and conjugation. The literature regarding key enzymes within these classes will be reviewed. Specific examples of in vitro plant enzyme systems used to study xenobiotic metabolism will be presented. A detailed discussion of various techniques will not be attempted.

## OXIDATION REACTIONS:

Oxidations are among the most important reactions in the metabolism of pesticides because they are frequently the primary

[1] Mention of a trademark or proprietary product does not constitute a guarantee or warranty of the product by the U. S. Department of Agriculture and does not imply its approval to the exclusion of other products that may also be suitable.

reaction that results in detoxication or activation of a pesticide.  In mammals and insects, oxidation reactions have been the
subject of many in vitro studies.  It is now evident that mixed
function oxidases are responsible for many of the oxidation
reactions in these organisms.  Although plants have mixed
function oxidase systems, their role in pesticide metabolism has
not been widely demonstrated.  In addition to mixed function
oxidases, peroxidases, lacasses and polyphenol oxidases are
found universally in the plant kingdom and some of these enzymes
may also play a role in oxidative pesticide metabolism.  At the
present, our knowledge of the enzyme systems involved in many of
the pesticide oxidation reactions that occur in plants is limited
and there is great need for more research.

   Peroxidases:

     The plant peroxidases catalyze two general types of oxi-
dation reactions, the classical peroxidative reaction that
requires hydrogen peroxide and the oxidative reaction that
utilizes molecular oxygen.  The horseradish peroxidase (HRP)
peroxidative reaction normally proceeds by the following
mechanism (1, 2):

   $HRP + H_2O_2 \rightarrow HRP-I$
   $HRP-I + AH_2 \rightarrow HRP-II + AH\cdot$
   $HRP-II + AH_2 \rightarrow HRP + AH\cdot$
   $2 AH\cdot \rightarrow Products$

The oxidative reactions are not as well understood as the
peroxidative reactions.  In $Mn^{++}$ inhibited reactions, the
oxidative hydroxylation of several substrates can be catalyzed by
peroxidase in the presence of dihydroxyfumaric acid (3).  Other
oxidative reactions require an aromatic co-factor such as 2,4-
dichlorophenol and $Mn^{++}$ (4).  In some oxidative reactions, a
catalytic amount of hydrogen peroxide is needed as an initiator,
but oxygen is used in stoichiometric amounts (5).
     Plant peroxidases catalyze the oxidation of a large and
diverse class of endogenous and exogenous substrates such as
phenols, aromatic amines, enediols, ascorbate, ferrocyanide,
cytochrome C, indole-3-acetic acid, and the leuco form of many
dyes.  Phenols and aromatic amines are among the most commonly
used substrates and the reaction catalyzed is generally an
oxidative condensation of the substrate (6).  In addition to
oxidative condensations, decarboxylations, sulfur oxidations, N-
demethylations, ring hydroxylations, carbon-halogen bond
clevages, and oxidation of aromatic methyl groups have all been
attributed to peroxidases (3) (Figure 1).  Peroxidases are
ubiquitous in the plant kingdom (3).  They occur throughout the
plant cell and have been found in the cytoplasm, cell wall,
membranes, nuclei, mitochondria and ribosomes (7).  Peroxidase
isozymes have been demonstrated in horseradish (4, 8-11) and
several other species (4, 8-13).  Striking differences have been

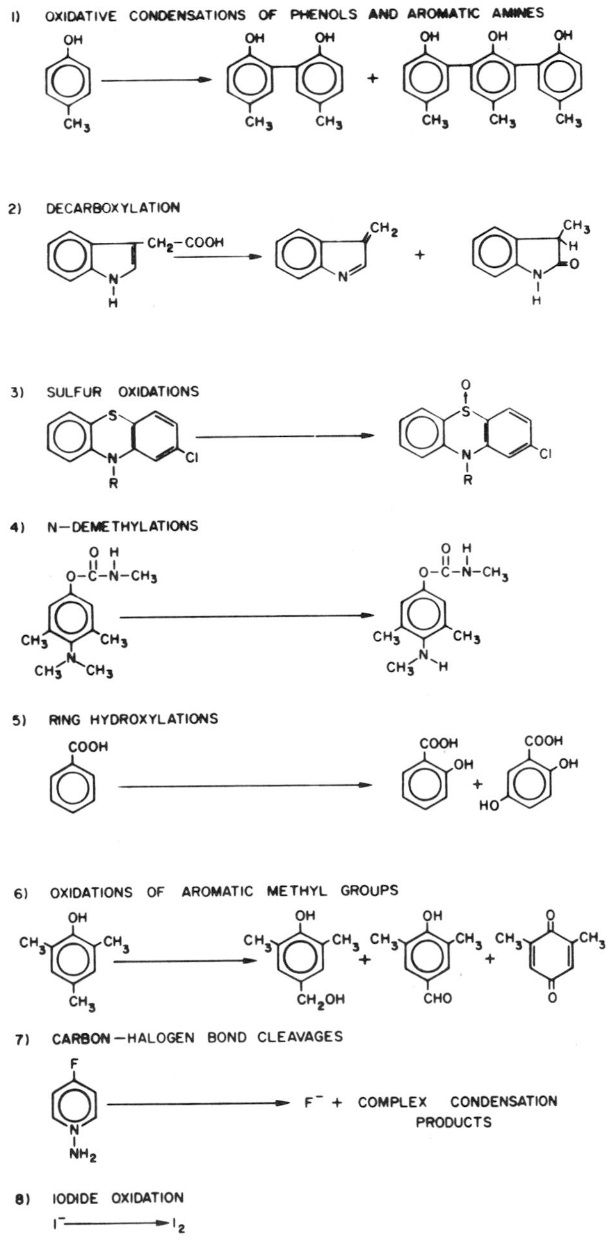

Figure 1. Types of reactions attributed to plant peroxidases (3, 22, 188, 189, 190)

noted in the substrate specificity of several HRP isozymes (14).

In spite of their widespread occurrence, the physiological role of peroxidases is uncertain. Their ability to utilize indole-3-acetic acid (15-18) and flavonoids (19) as substrates suggests that peroxidases may be important in the metabolic regulation of these endogenous substrates. Peroxidases are also thought to be involved in the lignification process (20). The high concentration of peroxidase activity associated with the cell wall (12) is consistent with this theory.

Several reports have associated peroxidase activity with pesticide metabolism. The oxidation of parathion to paraoxon and the hydrolysis of both parathion and paraoxon can be catalyzed by HRP (21) (Figure 2). The reaction occurs under both oxidative and peroxidative conditions. A peroxidase was also isolated from bean hypocotyl that was approximately 50% as active as HRP in the oxidation and hydrolysis of parathion (21). This enzyme was equal to HRP in the oxidation of guiacol. The in vitro reaction of ten [$^{14}$C-carbonyl]carbamate insecticides with hydrogen peroxide in the presence of HRP has been examined (22). Conversion to ether-soluble products that could be differentiated from the reactants by TLC or conversion to water-soluble products were used as the criteria for a reaction. Of the ten substrates tested (banol, baygon, carbaryl, HRS-1422, isolan, mesurol, UC-10854, matacil and zectran), only matacil and zectran reacted. The highest percentage of radioactivity was in the form of unidentified water-soluble products; however, several ether-soluble products were identified (Figure 3). The ether-soluble products represented various stages of N-dealkylation. This may suggest a minor role for peroxidases in N-dealkylation. Mesurol, a carbamate insecticide that contains an arylmethylsulfide, and cysteine, thioglycolic acid, mercaptoethanol, thiourea and thiouracil were not substrates for HRP (22, 23); however, chloropromazine, a heterocyclic sulfide, was a substrate (3). The precise role of peroxidases in sulfur oxidation is thus uncertain.

Anilines are known degradation products of phenylcarbamates, phenylureas, and acyl anilide herbicides; therefore, the fate of anilines in the environment is an important consideration. A number of workers have shown that various anilines are converted to azobenzenes and other products by the action of HRP and hydrogen peroxide (3). However, it is of particular note that the chloroanilines that formed azobenzenes in vitro as the result of HRP and hydrogen peroxide were the same as those that formed azobenzenes in the soil as a result of microbial action (24) (Figure 4). The HRP system served as a model to predict the likelihood of azobenzene formation in the soil. In these studies, no effort was made to identify products other than the azobenzene analogs or to quantitate the reaction; therefore, the full scope of products produced and the yields are not known.

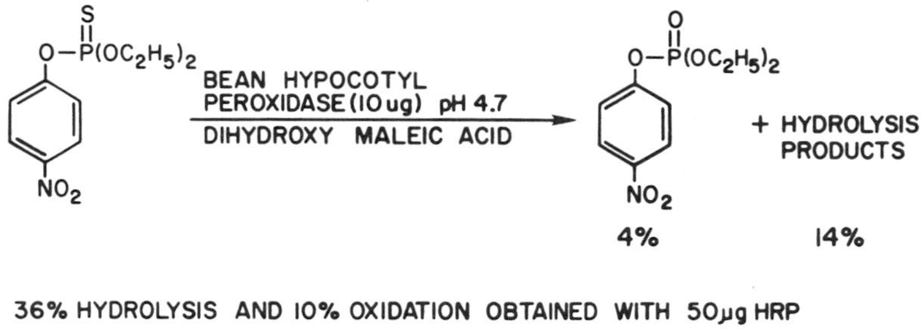

36% HYDROLYSIS AND 10% OXIDATION OBTAINED WITH 50μg HRP

Figure 2.   *Oxidation and hydrolysis of parathion by plant peroxidases (21)*

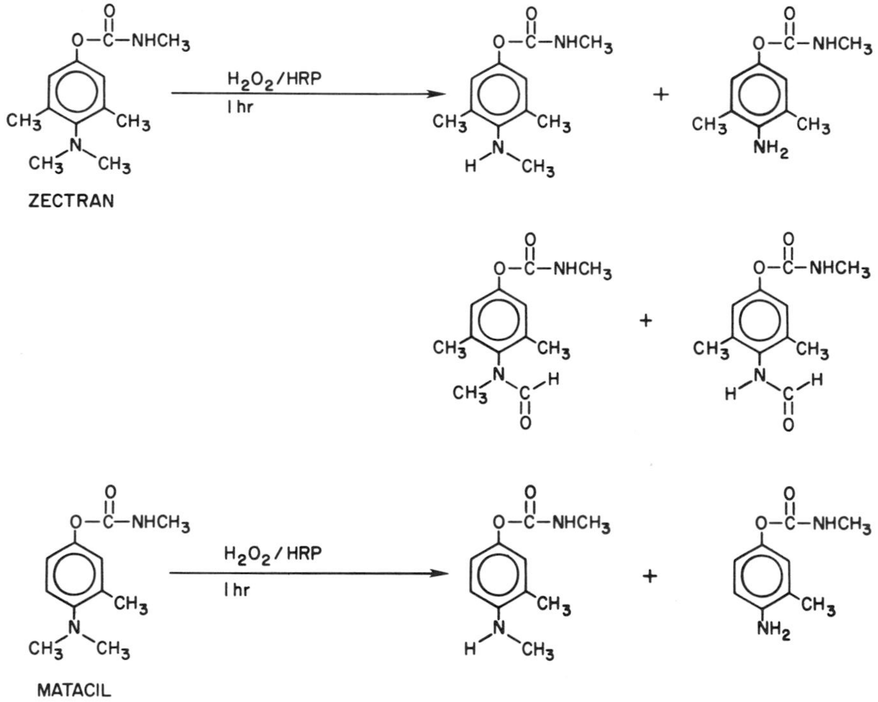

Figure 3.  N-*Demethylation of substituted phenylcarbamate insecticides by horse-radish peroxidase (22)*

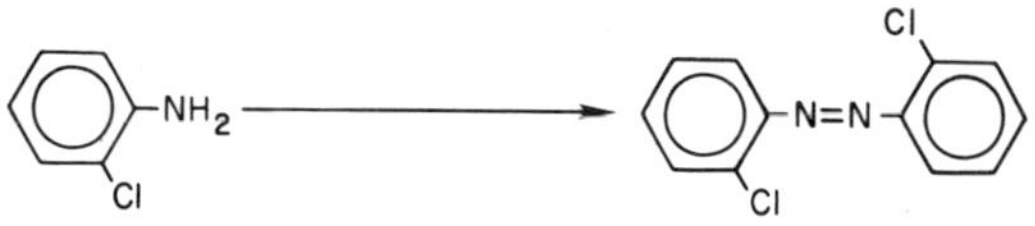

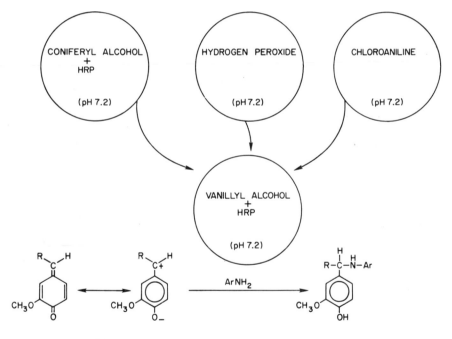

Figure 4.   HRP catalyzed formation of azobenzenes from various chloroanilines
(3, 24)

Figure 5.   Model system for incorporation of chloroanilines into synthetic lignin
(26)

Although azobenzenes do not appear to be metabolites of chloroanilines in higher plants, chloroanilines may be incorporated into lignin or converted to lignin-like products (25). In an effort to determine the chemical nature of the chloroaniline residue in the lignin fraction, a model system was developed that uses HRP to catalyze the free radical formation of a synthetic lignin-like material (26). In this system, the [14]C-labeled pesticide metabolite, 3-chloroaniline or 3,4-dichloroaniline, was co-polymerized with coniferyl alcohol, a building block of natural lignin (Figure 5). The polymerization was accomplished by simultaneously pumping solutions of (a) coniferyl alcohol and HRP in pH 7.2 buffer, (b) hydrogen peroxide in pH 7.2 buffer, and (c) the [14]C-labeled chloroaniline in pH 7.2 buffer into a buffered solution of vanillyl alcohol and HRP. After 10 hr in the dark, the insoluble [14]C-labeled polymeric product was removed by centrifugation, washed and subjected to gel permeation chromatography. Based upon an average molecular weight of 1,000, 1.19 residues of 3-chloroaniline or 1.68 residues of 3,4-dichloroaniline were incorporated per molecule of polymer formed. In vivo incorporation into rice lignin was also greater for 3,4-dichloroaniline than for 3-chloroaniline. When acetylated anilines were used in the model HRP system, the incorporation rate was reduced by over 50%. This may indicate the involvement of the aniline nitrogen in the co-polymerization reaction.

A number of techniques were used for the analysis of the synthetic lignin. The most successful method was pyrolytic GC/MS. Pyrolysis released over 80% of the radioactivity in a volatile form. Over 60% of the released [14]C was 3-chloroaniline or 3,4-dichloroaniline. Similar results were obtained with natural lignin isolated from chloroaniline-treated rice, but with much lower yields. It was concluded that a high percentage of the chloroaniline in the lignin-like material was covalently bonded between the aniline nitrogen and the α-carbon of the polymer (Figure 5).

HRP was also used to study the metabolism of botran (27). Botran was not a direct substrate for HRP, but its reduction product (2,6-dichlorophenylenediamine) was readily converted to at least 8 products upon treatment with HRP (Figure 6). One of the most abundant products was identical to a soil metabolite of botran. High resolution mass spectrometry of the soil metabolite indicated a molecular formula of $C_{12}H_6N_4Cl_6$. A botran metabolite, N-(4-amino-3,5-dichlorophenyl)malonamic acid, was found in soybean plants and in soybean callus cultures (28). The presumed intermediate of this metabolite (2,6-dichlorophenylenediamine) was not detected; however, plants contain a system that is capable of reducing arylnitro groups (29). The diamine of botran could thus be formed in the plant and serve as a substrate for a malonyl transfer reaction, a peroxidase-catalyzed oxidation or lignin incorporation.

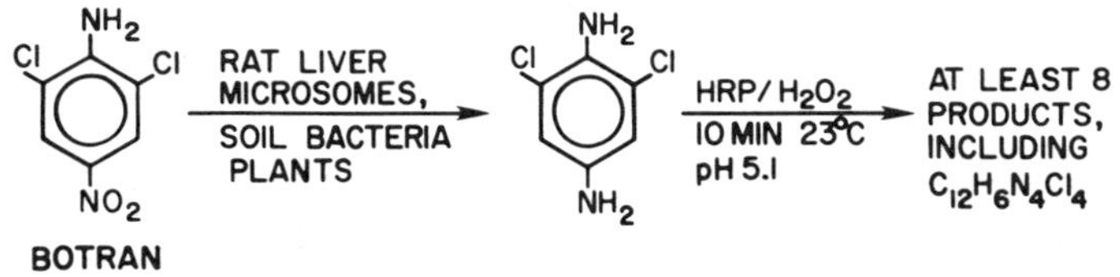

*Figure 6.   A possible role for peroxidases in botran metabolism (27, 28, 29)*

Table I.   Relationship between resistance to iodide and absence of peroxidase
           capable of oxidizing iodide.*

| Species | Peroxidase Activity | | Iodide accumulation (mg/g dry weight) | Resistance |
|---|---|---|---|---|
| | Guaiacol donor (units/mg protein) | Iodide donor (units/mg protein) | | |
| tomato | 2.6 | 0 | 70 | short term |
| buttercup | 2.0 | 9 | 13 | resistant |
| cabbage | 6.7 | 26 | 4 | resistant |
| bean | 12.7 | 28 | 15 | susceptible |
| mettle | 15.3 | 75 | 5 | susceptible |
| pea | 82 | 123 | 8 | susceptible |

*Adapted from (32).

The finding that ioxynil liberated iodide when exposed to ultraviolet light or when subjected to plant or animal metabolism resulted in an examination of the herbicidal properties of iodide. Subsequently, iodide was shown to possess some selectivity as a herbicide (30). The ability of plant peroxidases to oxidize iodide to iodine (31) varied greatly with the plant species (32) and this ability was related to resistance to iodide toxicity (Table I). Iodine was shown to be $10^5$ times more powerful than iodide as an inhibitor of the Hill reaction (33). This suggested that iodide toxicity was due, in part, to intracellular oxidation of iodide to iodine. When 30 iodo-benzoic acids were assayed for herbicidal activity, only those that liberated iodide in vivo were toxic to Phaseolus vulgaris seedlings. It was suggested that liberation of iodide might be one factor in the herbicidal activity of these compounds (30).

In addition to in vitro studies that suggested an active role for peroxidases in pesticide metabolism, several studies have indicated that certain pesticides may increase the level of peroxidases in plants. EPTC was reported to increase peroxidase activity and lignification in corn seedlings; these increases could be alleviated by treatment with a protectant, N,N-diallyl-2,2-dichloroacetamide (9). Stimulation of peroxidase activity was also observed when Phaseolus radiatus seedlings were treated with sodium diethyldithiocarbamate (34).

A microsomal hydroperoxide-dependent oxidizing system (hydroperoxidase) was recently isolated from pea seeds (35, 36) (Figure 7). This enzyme hydroxylated indole, phenol, α-naphthol, and aniline to indoxyl, hydroquinone, α-napthylhydroquinone, and N-hydroxyaniline, respectively. Hydrogen peroxide, tert-butyl hydroperoxide, cumene hydroperoxide, or linoleic acid hydroperoxide served as sources of oxidizing power. A well-defined pH optimum at pH 7.2 was observed with linoleic acid hydroperoxide, but a broad pH optimum around 8.7 was observed with the other hydroperoxides. An allosteric effect was noted with linoleic acid hydroperoxide, but not with the other hydroperoxides. It was speculated that the natural hydroperoxides for this system were produced by the action of lipoxygenases ón substrates such as linoleic acid. Studies with $O^{18}$-labeled linoleic acid hydroperoxide indicated a direct oxygen transfer from the hydroperoxide to the hydroxylated substrate. No participation of molecular oxygen was observed. Pre-treatment with p-chloromercuriobenzoate resulted in a slight promotion of the hydroperoxidase reaction, indicating no involvement of P450. Other properties of this system also indicated that activity was distinct from that of P450.

Although none of the in vitro peroxidase studies discussed proves that these enzymes play an important role in pesticide metabolism in plants, it is clear that the spectrum of substrates utilized by these enzymes does encompass many pesticides or pesticide metabolites. The apparent universal occurrence of

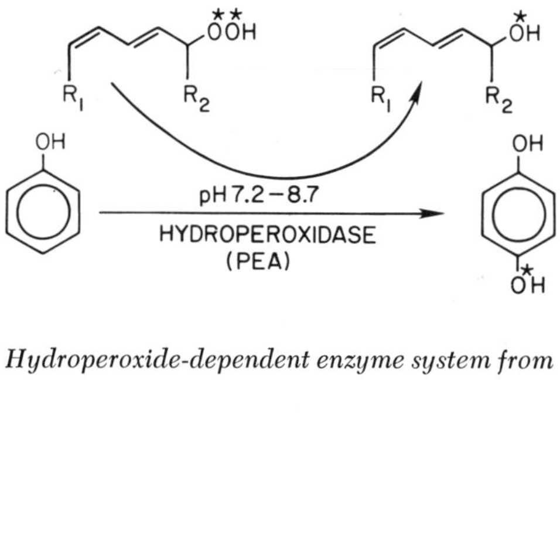

*Figure 7.   Hydroperoxide-dependent enzyme system from pea (35, 36)*

peroxidases in the plant kingdom and throughout the cell
contributes greatly to the possible involvement of these enzymes
in pesticide metabolism.  A number of possible roles for peroxidases in the metabolism of specific pesticides or classes of
pesticides have been pointed out.  The utility of HRP in model
systems to produce metabolites found in the soil and to aid in
the study of the pesticide residues found in the plant lignin
fraction have been clearly demonstrated.

### Mixed Function Oxidases:

Extensive research over the last 28 years has shown that
mixed function oxidases are of great importance in xenobiotic
metabolism in insects and animals (37).  The presence of mixed
function oxidases in higher plants has been established in the
last 10 years by experiments conducted with both endogenous
substrates (38-42) and xenobiotics (43-48).  Based upon light
reversible CO inhibition (39, 44) and spectral properties (49),
several mixed function oxidase (mfo) systems in plants appear to
resemble the cytochrome P450 mfo systems found in animals and
insects.  Other plant mfo systems, however, appear to be quite
different (38, 40).

Based upon our knowledge of insect and mammalian mfo systems
and our knowledge of metabolites produced in plants, a number of
reactions in plants should be considered as possible mixed
function oxidase-catalyzed reactions.  Some of these are N-dealkylation, O-dealkylation, aromatic hydroxylation, alkyl oxidation, epoxidation, desulfuration, sulfur oxidation, ester
hydrolysis, and nitrogen oxidation (Figure 8).  The demonstrated
mfo reactions in plants are more limited.

There are several examples of mfo-catalyzed N-dealkylations
in plants.  A mfo system from cotton that catalyzes the N-demethylation of phenylurea herbicides (47, 48, 50) and mfo
systems from castor beans (51) and avocado pear (46) that
catalyze the N-demethylation of p-chloro-N-methylaniline have
been reported.  The O-demethylation of p-nitroanisole has been
detected with an in vitro system from avocado pear (46).  A
similar mfo-catalyzed dealkylation might explain the presence of
the phenol of 2,4-D that has been reported as a metabolite in
certain plant systems.  The formation of the phenol of 2,4-D does
not seem to involve an initial decarboxylation (52).  The
reported in vivo alkyl oxidation of the plant growth regulator
flurenol butyl ester might also be explained by a mfo (53).
Several mixed function oxidase systems that catalyze aromatic
ring hydroxylations have been studied in vitro with both
xenobiotic (44-46) and endogenous substrates (38-41, 45, 54-57).
Because of the large number of potential substrates, this reaction
is of particular interest.  The epoxidation aldrin has been
demonstrated by in vitro systems isolated from pea and bean
(43, 58-62).  The aldrin epoxidase systems have not been clearly

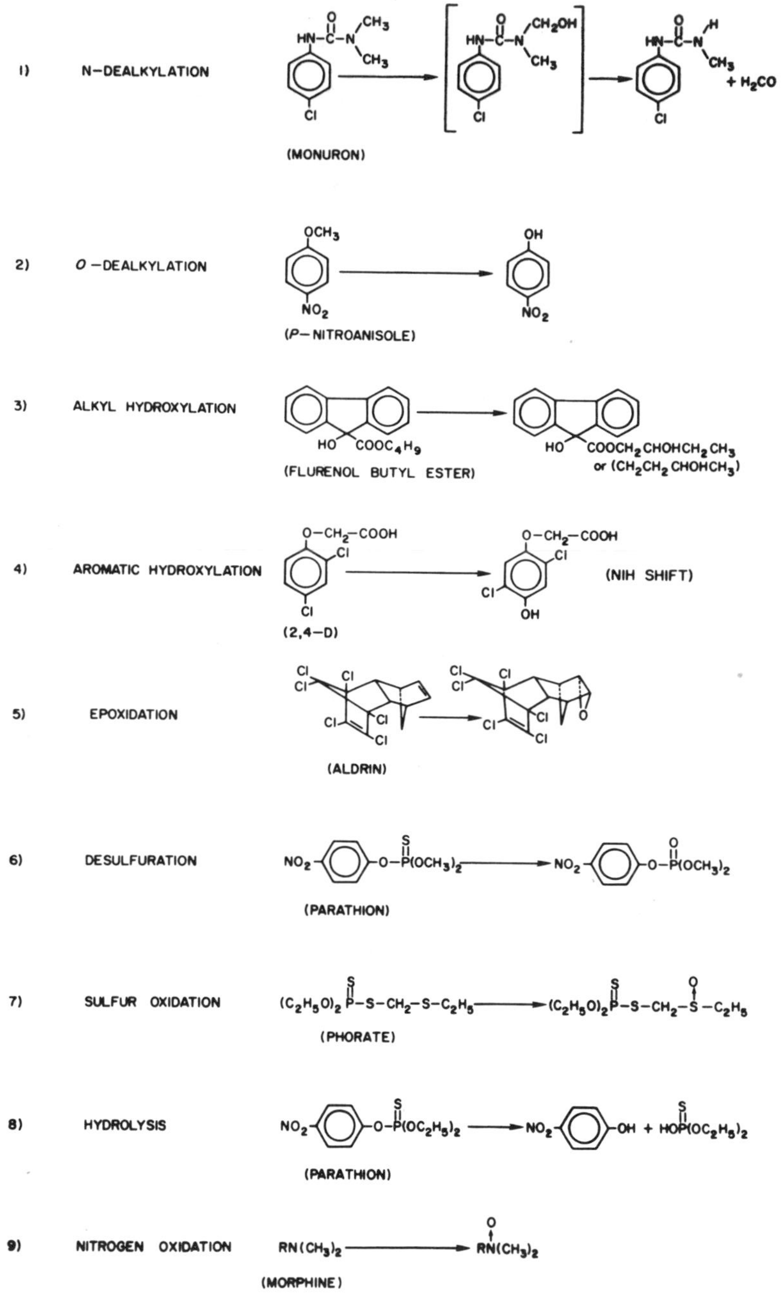

*Figure 8.  Reactions for which a mfo mechanism is known or might be expected*

demonstrated to be mfo systems.  The conversion of organophos-
phorothioates to phosphates in plants has been well established.
This conversion involves mixed function oxidases in animals and
insects (63).  Mixed function oxidases may also catalyze this
reaction in plants, but the possibility that other enzyme
systems may be involved should be considered (21).  The oxidation of a number of thio-ethers to sulfoxides and sulfones has
been reported in plant metabolism studies; again, the enzymes
responsible for these reactions have not been well characterized.
An enzyme that catalyzes the sulfoxidation of phorate has been
isolated from soybean root (64).  Additional studies are needed
to characterize this system.  In animals, organophosphate ester
hydrolysis can be catalyzed by both mixed function oxidases and
glutathione S-transferases (63).  In plants, this reaction may be
catalyzed by esterases or peroxidases (21, 65, 66), but the
reaction mechanism needs further study at the in vitro level.
In plants, N-oxide formation does not appear to be a common
reaction in pesticide metabolism.  However, an enzyme that
catalyzes the formation of the N-oxide of morphine has been
detected in Papaver somniferum latex (67).  Since peroxidases
and polyphenol oxidases are found in high concentrations in plant
latex, the possibility that this reaction may be catalyzed by one
of these enzymes should also be considered.

The N-demethylase from cotton (47) and the cinnamic acid
hydroxylase from cucumber (44) are two mfo systems that have
been shown to utilize pesticides as substrates.  The N-demethylase system appears to have limited substrate specificity, only
N-methyl substituted phenylureas were found to be active substrates.  The N-demethylation reaction was strongly and competitively inhibited by carbamate insecticides that had high electron density at the position ortho to the carbamate group (50,
68).  Inhibition by substituted phenylureas was also demonstrated.  This inhibition was dependent upon the presence of a
proton on the aniline nitrogen atom (50).  Field observations
(69, 70) and an in vitro study (71) indicated an antagonistic
interaction of carbamates with dimethylphenylurea herbicides.
A positive correlation between resistance to phenylurea
herbicides and the presence of an active N-demethylase system
was supported by in vitro determinations of N-demethylase
activity in 12 plant species.  In cotton, the specific activity
of the mfo system varied over a 10-fold range, depending upon
the age of the plant and the specific tissue.

A recent study has shown that 2,4-D is hydroxylated by an
in vitro mfo system from cucumber leaves (44).  This appears to
be the first reported ring-hydroxylation of a pesticide
catalyzed by an isolated plant mfo system.  Cinnamic acid was
also hydroxylated by this system.  Hydroxylase activity was
increased 2- to 3-fold by spraying the cucumber leaves with
2,4-D before enzyme isolation.  Other studies have shown that
certain plant mfo systems were induced or stimulated by light

(39, 72).  The NIH shift was observed in the hydroxylation of
2,4-D.  The primary product was 4-hydroxy-2,5-dichlorophenoxy-
acetic acid.  The NIH shift was also demonstrated in the 4-
hydroxylation of cinnamic acid by a mfo system from pea (73).
These studies suggest that additional investigations on the
induction of plant mfo systems may be warranted.  They also
suggest the need to conduct kinetic studies on the cinnamic acid
4-hydroxylase reaction with 2,4-D and related pesticides as
possible inhibitors.  Since microsomal mixed function oxidases
play an important role in the metabolic pathway of some
endogenous substrates (39, 41), the induction or inhibition of
these reactions by pesticides could have important implications.

In animals, the microsomal fraction has typically displayed
a broad specificity range (37) that can be explained by the
presence of a series of P450 cytochromes (74).  In contrast,
mixed function oxidases from plants appear to have a fairly
narrow substrate specificity range with some tissue specificity.
The mfo system from castor bean (51) displayed 4-hydroxylase
activity for cinnamic acid and N-demethylase activity for p-
chloro-N-methylaniline, N-methylaniline, and N,N-dimethylaniline,
but displayed no activity for 15 other compounds that contained
N-, O-, or S-methyl groups.  The system from avocado pear may
have one of the broadest specificity ranges of the isolated
plant systems.  It apparently has hydroxylase activity for
biphenyl and aniline, O-demethylase activity for p-nitroanisole,
and N-demethylase activity for p-chloro-N-methylaniline (46).

Mixed function oxidase systems isolated from plants
typically display very low levels of activity.  Specific
activities are frequently in the range of 1- to 10-nmol product/mg
protein/hr.  This low level of activity can be explained by the
report that P450 concentrations in plants range from 0.007 to
0.02 nmol P450/mg microsomal protein as compared to 0.9 to 1.2
nmol P450/mg microsomal protein in rat liver (49). Because of
the low levels of mfo activity in plant tissues, the use of
radioactive substrates in assays is often necessary.

The properties of isolated plant mfo systems are highly
variable (Table II).  Some mfo systems are microsomal, undergo
light reversible CO-inhibition, require NADPH as a co-factor and
behave much like mammalian P450 mfo systems (39).  Others require
illuminated chloroplasts as a co-factor and may be soluble (38).
Some systems require only one co-factor (47), but other systems
require several (40).  Ascorbic acid, NADH, NADPH, dithionite,
illuminated chloroplasts, and an unidentified natural product
(probably a pteridine) have all been utilized in various in vitro
plant mfo studies (38, 39, 40, 47).  The response of these
systems to various inhibitors is also quite variable.  Mercaptoethanol was an inhibitor of phenylalanine hydroxylase (40) and
gibberellin A1 hydroxylase (41), but it was necessary to
demonstrate 4-hydroxylase activity with cinnamic acid (39).
Chelating agents inhibited an N-demethylase (47) and a

Table II.   Properties of plant enzymes with mfo type activity.

| Enzyme | Co-factors | Activators or factors used to demonstrate activity | Inhibitors | Reference |
|---|---|---|---|---|
| N-demethylase | NADH or NADPH | NaCN, isoascorbate, poly-clar AT | CO, ionic detergents sulfhydryl reagents, chelating agents and electron acceptors. | 47 |
| aldrin epoxidase | NADPH (activity present at reduced level without) | chelating agents and detergents | electron acceptors, CN, phenols, aniline. | 43 |
| 2,4-D hydroxylase and cinnamic acid hydroxylase | NADPH | mercaptoethanol | CO-light reversible. | 44 |
| biphenyl hydroxylase (microsomal) | NADPH | safrole and 3,4-benzopyrene are stimulatory to 2-hydroxylation. | weak with CO, SKF 525A, $Cu^{++}$, NADH. | 45,46 |
| pyroloxygenase | illuminated chloroplasts, or dithionite | | chelating agents, dithiothreitol and mercaptoethanol. | 38 |
| phenylalanine hydroxylase | NADPH or NADH, and an unidentified product or THFA | ascorbate | aminopteridine, sulfhydryl-containing compounds; i.e., mercaptoethanol. | 40 |
| gibberellin A1 hydroxylase | NADPH, ascorbate $Fe^{++}$ | | mercaptoethanol, EDTA | 41 |
| cinnamic acid hydroxylase | NADPH | mercaptoethanol | CO-light reversible, azide. | 39 |
| cinnamic acid, hydroxylase and N-demethylase | NADPH (or NADH with 2nd substrate) | EDTA | CO lipases, menadione, 1,4-napthoquinone, riboflavin. | 51 |

pyroloxygenase (38), but slightly stimulated an aldrin epoxidase
(43). Safrole and 3,4-benzopyrene stimulated a biphenyl 2-
hydroxylase from avocado, but other mfo activities were unaffected (46). Castor bean N-demethylase was strongly inhibited by
Kp$_i$ buffer and was assayed with tricine buffer (51). In sharp
contrast, N-demethylase from cotton was inhibited by tricine, but
not by Kp$_i$ (47). Based on differences in co-factor requirements,
responses to different inhibitors and responses to different
buffers, it would appear that a variety of different plant mfo
systems exist.

    Although most mfo systems in plants are associated with
particulate (microsomal) fractions, a gibberellin A$_1$ hydroxylase
(41) and a biphenyl hydroxylase (45, 46) are soluble systems.
The nature of several other mfo systems (38, 40) is uncertain.
The solubilization of Swede root cinnamic acid 4-hydroxylase with
Triton X-100 has been reported (75) and both soluble and particulate aldrin epoxidase (60, 61) and biphenyl hydroxylase (45,
46) have been isolated from the same tissues. It appears that
isolated active fractions may not always be a true indication of
the nature and location of the enzyme in the native state, but
may also be a function of the combination of techniques and
tissue used.

    A number of different procedures and special precautions were
used to isolate mfo activity from plant sources (Table III). In
the isolation of N-demethylase activity from cotton, the tissue
was ground under liquid nitrogen (47, 48) and in the isolation of
aldrin epoxidase from pea (43), totally anaerobic conditions were
used. Most extraction and isolation procedures utilized pH 7.5
buffers that contained either polyvinyl pyrrolidine or polyclar
AT. The buffer used to extract N-demethylase activity from
cotton contained isoascorbate, polyclar AT and sodium cyanide.
Mercaptoethanol, chelating agents, sucrose, and bovine serum
albumin have also been used with varying frequency to help
protect mfo systems during isolation. Differential centrifugation
has been the most commonly used fractionation method, but DEAE
chromatography, sephadex chromatography, ammonium sulfate
fractionation and density gradient centrifugation have also been
employed.

    Based on this brief survey, it is apparent that the number
of xenobiotics shown to be metabolized by in vitro plant mixed
function oxidases is very limited. Some of these oxidative
systems have not been well defined. Considerable effort is needed
to isolate and characterize these systems. The methods used for
enzyme isolation have been highly variable. Because of the
extremely low levels of enzyme activity associated with many of
the mfo systems, they are frequently difficult to study and
special methods are often needed to measure reaction rates. This
is further complicated by the presence of endogenous inhibitors
and the instability of many of these systems.

Table III.  Methods used to isolate mixed function oxidase-like activity from higher plants.

| Enzyme | Tissue Source | General Isolation Procedure | Special Precautions | Reference |
|---|---|---|---|---|
| N-demethylase (microsomal) | *cotton leaves | pulverized in liquid N2, extract (pH 7.5), filter, differential and density gradient centrifug. | NaCN, polyclar AT, isoascorbate | 47 |
| aldrin epoxidase (microsomal) | pea root | extract (pH 7.5), filter, Sephadex G-100 and differential centrifug. | anaerobic isolation, polyclar AT | 43 |
| 2,4-D and cinnamic A. hydroxylase (microsomal) | *cucumber leaves | extract (pH 7.5), filter, diff-erential centrifug. | PVP | 44 |
| biphenyl hydroxy-lase (microsomal and soluble) | avocado pear | extract (pH 7.4), filter, diff-erential centrifug. | none apparent | 45,46 |
| pyroloxygenase | *wheat germ | water-extract, $(NH_4)_2SO_4$ frac-tionation, DEAE and Sephadex G-100 | remove high m.w. inhibitor | 38 |
| phenylalanine hydroxylase | spinach leaves | pulverize frozen tissue, water-extract, filter, acetone fraction-ation, DEAE-cellulose and calcium phosphate gel adsorption. | none apparent | 40 |
| gibberellin A1 hydroxylase | snap bean | homogenize decoated imbibed seeds (pH 6.5), differential centrifug. | sucrose, PVP | 41 |
| cinnamic acid hydroxylase (microsomal) | castor bean | pulverize in pH 7.5 buffer, filter, differential centrifug. or density gradient centrifug. | EDTA, sucrose | 51 |
| cinnamic acid hydroxylase (microsomal) | aged Swede root | homogenize in pH 7.5 buffer, filter, differential centrifug. | EDTA, sucrose, mercaptoethanol | 75 |
| cinnamic acid hydroxylase (microsomal) | wounded Jerusalem artichoke tuber | homogenize in pH 7.5 buffer, filter, differential centrifug. and density gradient centrifug. | mercaptoethanol, EDTA, serum albumin, poly-clar AT, mannitol. | 76 |

*Also isolated from other sources.

REDUCTION REACTIONS:

Although reductive reactions have not been demonstrated to
play a major role in xenobiotic metabolism in higher plants,
several investigators have reported the reduction of aromatic
nitro groups in plants (77-82) and callus culture (82).  A
reductive dehalogenation (83) and the reduction of a sulfoxide
to a sulfide (84) have also been reported.  The reported arylnitro reductions of pentachloronitrobenzene (PCNB) (77) and
fluorodifen (p-nitrophenyl-α,α,α-trifluoro-2-nitrophenyl-p-tolyl
ether) (79, 80, 85, 86) were in competition with glutathione
conjugation.  In studies with fluorodifen, arylnitro reduction
was a minor metabolic pathway.  However, in studies with pentachloronitrobenzene, about 28% of the pesticide was converted to
pentachloroaniline.
    The only reductive reactions involving pesticides that
appear to have been studied in detail in plants are those
catalyzed by aryl nitroreductases.  Aryl nitroreductase activity
has been isolated from peanut (77) and pea (78).  The soluble
arylnitroreductase system from peanut was isolated in conjunction
with studies on GSH S-transferase activity.  Magnesium chloride
was used in the isolation procedure to precipitate the microsomal
fraction (87) and to avoid high speed centrifugation.  With PCNB
as the substrate, reductase activity was detected with enzyme
preparations from roots and hypocotyls of 7-day-old etiolated
peanut seedings.  Aryl nitroreductase activity was detected only
when the reaction was run under a nitrogen atmosphere in the
presence of both FAD and NADPH.  The aryl nitroreductase isolated
from soybean seedling roots catalyzed the reduction of dinoben
(2,5-dichloro-3-nitrobenzoic acid) when the system was incubated
under nitrogen at pH 8.2 with either NADPH or NADH (78).  When
this enzyme system was purified further, FAD or FMN was required
in addition to NADH or NADPH.  The fact that in vitro reduction
could be demonstrated only under a nitrogen atmosphere suggests
that these reactions may become more important in vivo under
conditions of low oxygen tension.
    In many cases in which reduction reactions have been
reported, plants have been grown and treated in such a manner that
microbial action could have accounted for the reaction.  This
possibility should be considered in any study in which reductive
reactions are reported in xenobiotic metabolism in plants.  The
reduction of the aryl nitro groups of PCNB and dinoben with in
vitro enzyme systems isolated from plants and the apparent
reduction of the aryl nitro group of 2,6-dichloro-4-nitroaniline
in soybean callus culture suggests, however, that aryl nitro
reductions may result from plant metabolism.

HYDROLYTIC REACTIONS:

Aryl Acylamidases:

Aryl acylamidases that hydrolyze the herbicide propanil
(3',4'-dichloropropionanilide) have been isolated from bacteria
(88), fungi (89), birds (90), mammals (91, 92) and plants (93–
110) (Figure 9). Of the hydrolytic enzymes that play important
roles in the metabolism of pesticides in plants, the aryl acylamidases appear to be the most thoroughly studied. Studies with
homogenates of rice plants (101, 105, 106) established the
enzymatic nature of propanil hydrolysis. Hydrolytic activity was
associated with a particulate fraction (93, 94). The enzyme was
stable, required no co-factors, and had a pH optimum of 7.5–7.9.
A comparison of the enzyme activity in rice and barnyard grass
showed a 60-fold higher level of enzyme activity in rice (94).
This suggested that propanil resistance was based on the presence
of the aryl acylamidase in sufficient concentration to detoxify
the herbicide before sensitive sites could be attacked. Enzyme
activity in rice seedlings was a function of the developmental
stage of the plant and maximum activity was reached at the fourth
leaf stage. In field studies, however, seedlings in the third
and fourth leaf stages were more sensitive to propanil than were
younger seedlings (98). Aryl acylamidase activity was also
reported in rice root callus suspension cultures (98), but in
vitro activity was demonstrated only in cultures that were at
least 120 hr old. This did not correspond with the much earlier
appearance of 3,4-dichloroaniline in propanil-treated cultures.

Inhibitor studies showed that carbamate insecticides were
powerful competitive inhibitors of the aryl acylamidase from
rice (94). The phosphorothioate insecticides, parathion and
sumithion were much weaker inhibitors of the enzyme, but their
oxidized analogs, paraoxon and sumioxon, were respectively 100X
and 200X more effective as inhibitors (95). Phosphorothioate
insecticides are partially converted to their oxygen analogs in
plants (103). The strength of paraoxon as an inhibitor of the
hydrolysis reaction in vitro was correlated with its synergistic
effect in reducing the fresh weight of propanil-treated rice
seedlings (95). The synergistic effect between propanil and the
organophosphorthioate and carbamate insecticides (101, 107) can
thus be explained on the basis of competitive inhibition of the
aryl acylamidase enzyme necessary for the detoxication of
propanil.

A particulate aryl acylamidase enzyme has also been isolated
from red rice (108) and soluble aryl acylamidases have been
isolated from tulip (99) and dandelion (109). Substrate specificities of these enzymes are shown in Tables IV and V. Significant and potentially useful differences exist in the substrate
preferences of these enzymes for different halogenated propion-
anilides. 2',3'-Dichloropropionanilide was the preferred substrate
for the amidase from cultivated rice, but it was the poorest
substrate for red rice. In contrast, propanil was the best
substrate for red rice, but had a relative rate of metabolism of
only 42% in cultivated rice. Substrate preferences for

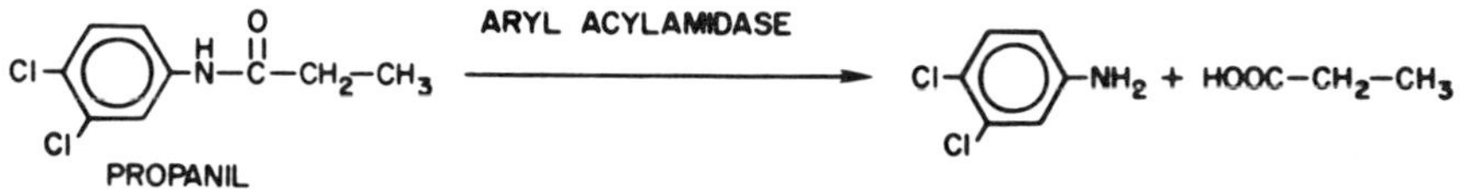

*Figure 9. Hydrolysis of 3',4'-dichloropropionanilide (propanil) by an aryl acyl-amidase*

different alkyl side chains were similar for these enzymes, each had a marked preference for the propionic side chain. These aryl acylamidases were not capable of hydrolyzing carbamate or urea herbicides. Some differences were found in the response of these enzymes to inhibitors (Table VI). These differences between the aryl acylamidases suggest that substrate specificity tests might be used to develop more selective compounds or compounds with more desirable biological stability. Differences in response to sulfhydryl inhibitors suggests that inhibitor studies with isolated enzyme systems could provide an effective means for the development of selective pesticide synergists.

Table IV.   Substrate specificity of aryl acylamidase from red rice (108), rice (94), tulip (99) and dandelion (109): the effect of chlorine ring substitution.

| | Relative Activity (%) | | | |
| Substrate | Red Rice | Rice | Tulip | Dandelion |
| --- | --- | --- | --- | --- |
| 2',3'-dichloropropionanilide | 29 | 100 | 41 | 14 |
| 2',4'-dichloropropionanilide | 47 | 84 | 100 | 49 |
| 2'-chloropropionanilide | 29 | 60 | 66 | 37 |
| 3'-chloropropionanilide | 73 | 42 | 27 | 51 |
| 3',4'-dichloropropionanilide | 100 | 42 | 100 | 100 |
| 3',5'-dichloropropionanilide | 33 | 30 | -- | -- |
| 2',5'-dichloropropionanilide | 27 | 27 | -- | -- |
| 4'-chloropropionanilide | 38 | 21 | 99 | 54 |
| 2',6'-dichloropropionanilide | -- | 1 | 2 | 0 |
| propionanilide | 58 | -- | -- | -- |

Table V.    Substrate specificity of aryl acylamidases from red
            rice (<u>108</u>), rice (<u>94</u>), tulip (<u>99</u>) and dandelion (<u>109</u>):
            the effect of various 3',4'-dichloroanilide alkyl
            analogs.

| Substrate | Relative Activity (%) | | | |
|---|---|---|---|---|
| | Red Rice | Rice | Tulip | Dandelion |
| 3',4'-dichloroacetanilide | 82 | 59 | 49 | 49 |
| 3',4'-dichloropropionanilide | 100 | 100 | 100 | 100 |
| 3',4'-dichlorobutyranilide | 18 | 32 | 18 | 37 |
| 3',4'-dichlorovaleranilide | 40 | 39 | 3 | 12 |
| 3',4'-dichloro-2-methyl propionanilide | -- | 2 | -- | -- |
| 3',4'-dichloro-2-methyl acrylanilide | 0 | 0 | 2 | 8 |
| 3',4'-dichloro-3-methyl butyranilide | -- | 0 | -- | -- |

Thirty-eight different horticultural and agronomic crop
species representing 10 different plant families were assayed
for aryl acylamidase activity with propanil as the substrate (<u>96</u>).
Enzyme activity was reported in over half of the species.  Only
one family, leguminosae, was devoid of activity.  A similar study
was conducted with 19 genera of weeds.  Enzyme activity was
assayed with propanil, 1,1-dimethyl-3-phenylurea (fenuron), and
isopropylcarbanilate (propham) (<u>97</u>).  Propanil was hydrolyzed at
widely varying rates by approximately 70% of the species.  Fenuron
and propham, however, were hydrolyzed by the enzyme preparation
from only one species, wild cucumber.  The distribution of aryl
acylamidases in other members of the plant kingdom has also been
reported (<u>100</u>, <u>110</u>).

Extensive studies with aryl acylamidases have shown that
these enzymes are widely distributed in the plant kingdom.
Activity varies widely within different plant tissues and among
different plant species.  Resistance to propanil is dependent
upon the presence of these enzymes.  Detailed substrate
specificity studies with four aryl acylamidases revealed subtle
differences in substrate specificity and response to inhibitors.
Inhibitor studies with carbamate and organophosphate insecticides
have clearly shown that these compounds are strong competitive
inhibitors of the aryl acylamidases from rice.  Interactions
observed in the field between propanil and these insecticides
can be attributed to the inhibition of aryl acylamidases.

Table VI. Inhibition of aryl acylamidases from red rice (108), rice (94), tulip (99) and dandelion (109).

|  | Source of Enzyme | | | | | | | |
|  | Red Rice | | Rice | | Tulip | | Dandelion | |
| Inhibitor | Conc. | % Inhib. | Conc. | % Inhib. | Conc. | % Inhib. | Conc. | % Inhib. |
| o-iodosobenzoate | -- | -- | 0.5mM | 74 | 0.25mM | 5 | 0.25mM | 27 |
| Na$_2$AsO$_2$ | -- | -- | 1.0mM | 74 | -- | -- | -- | -- |
| HgCl$_2$ | -- | -- | 0.1mM | 74 | 0.25mM | 100 | 0.5mM | 89 |
| CuSO$_4$ | 0.2mM | 60 | 0.2mM | 59 | 0.25mM | 16 | 0.5mM* | 86 |
| p-chloromercuribenzoate | 0.2mM | 4 | 0.5mM | 50 | -- | -- | 0.25mM | 61 |
| p-benzoquinone | 0.2mM | 35 | 0.5mM | 47 | -- | -- | 0.50mM | 50 |
| N-ethylmaleimide | 0.2mM | 6 | 0.5mM | 44 | 0.50mM | 9 | 1.0mM | 23 |
| iodoacetate | 0.2mM | 6 | 0.5mM | 18 | 0.50mM | 2 | 1.0mM | 2 |
| 2,4-dichlorophenoxyacetic | 0.2mM | 2 | -- | -- | -- | -- | -- | -- |
| pyrocatecol | 0.2mM | 29 | -- | -- | -- | -- | 0.5mM** | 73 |
| CoCl$_2$ | -- | -- | -- | -- | 0.50mM | 1 | 1.0mM | 16 |
| FeCl$_3$ | -- | -- | -- | -- | 0.50mM | 0 | 1.0mM | 6 |

*CuCl$_2$ used instead of CuSO$_4$

**Catechol used instead of pyrocatechol.

Esterases:

Many carboxylic acid ester pesticides are readily hydrolyzed
to free acids in vitro. In most cases, the free acid form of the
pesticide is presumed or known to be the active agent. Esterases
that hydrolyze carboxylic acid ester pesticides are important,
not only because they play a role in the degradation of the
pesticide, but also because they may be involved in activation,
selectivity or detoxication. Some esterases may be inducible
(111). Common inhibitors of these enzymes include a number of
the organophosphate and carbamate insecticides (112-114). The
possibility of pesticide interaction between carboxylic acid
ester herbicides and certain insecticides exists. Research on
the induction, activation, inhibition, and substrate specificity
of esterases should have important and direct application to the
improvement and better use of pesticides.

Esterases are probably ubiquitous and have been isolated
from many plant species. The stability of plant esterase preparations varies with the source and may be related to the
presence of phenol oxidases and polyphenols. Gel electrophoresis
has been a valuable tool in studying plant esterases and has shown
that these enzymes are a complex family of isozymes with
differences in substrate preference and susceptibility to
inhibitors (115-118). Polyacrylamide-gel electrophoresis
separated 7 esterases from pea and 14 esterases from green bean
(114). Separated isozymes responded differently to the assay
substrates, α-naphtylacetate, α-naphthylbutyrate, and α-naphthyl-
propionate. Differential response to inhibitors such as
parathion, paraoxon and diisopropylphosphorofluoridate was also
observed. Gel electrophoresis of enzyme preparations from
cabbage indicated the presence of 6 esterases (113). With 2-
naphthylacetate as the substrate, inhibition was demonstrated
with carbofuran, eserine and several other compounds. The
partially purified esterase from cabbage had a pH optimum of
approximately 7, and an estimated molecular weight of 69,000.
This enzyme lost 50% of the original activity when it was stored
for 22 days at -22°.

A few studies have reported the hydrolysis of pesticides by
in vitro esterase systems (Figure 10). Recent studies showed
that apple and cucumber leaves contain esterases that hydrolyze
fungicidal nitrophenyl esters (115). Esterase activity was
detected with 18 different substrates. Hydrolysis rates varied
100-fold, depending upon the substrate. Selective inhibition with
paraoxon and several other compounds was also demonstrated.
Eserine and EDTA were not inhibitory. Differences in isozyme
patterns were observed between the two species.

The carboxylic acid ester herbicide chlorfenprop-methyl
(methyl 2-chloro-3-(4-chlorophenyl)propionate) is hydrolyzed in
vivo and in vitro to an active herbicide (119). Active esterases
were isolated from 2 cultivars of oat, wild oat, wheat and beet

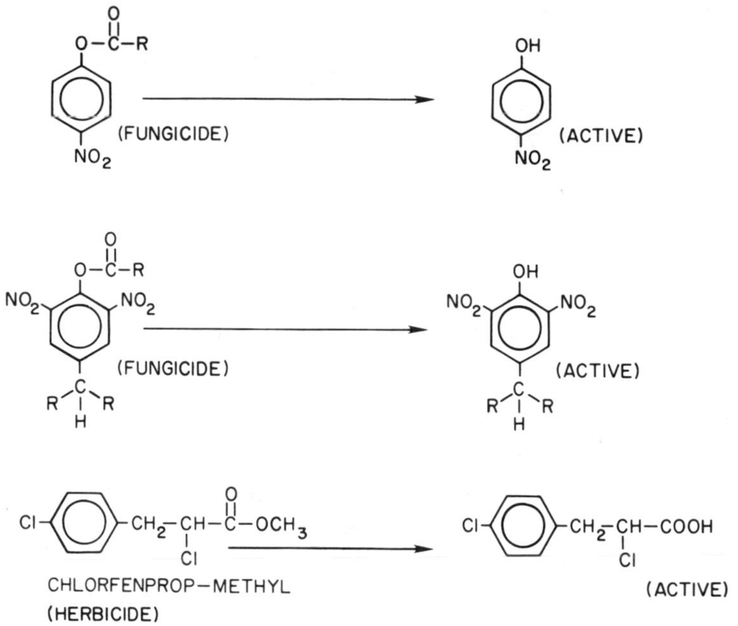

Figure 10.  Hydrolysis of fungicides and herbicides by plant esterases (115, 119)

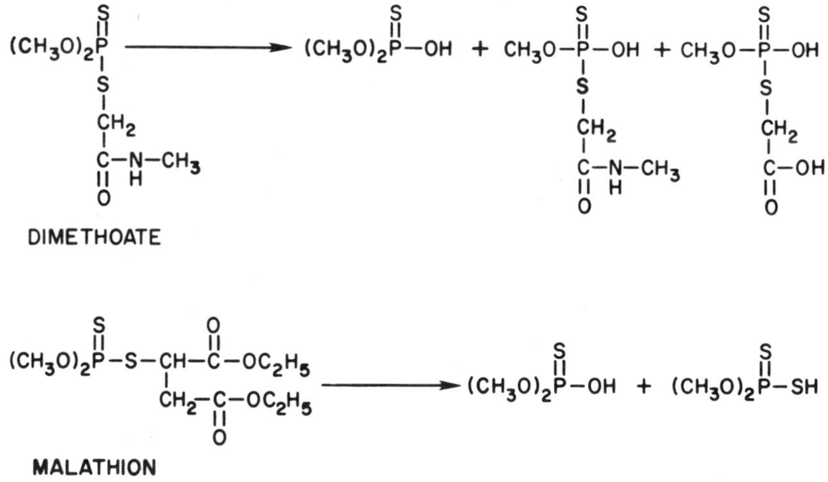

Figure 11.  Hydrolysis of organophosphorus insecticides by plant esterases (127, 128)

(119). Estimates of in vivo rates of hydrolysis based upon in vitro data indicated that herbicide selectivity was not related to esterase activity. Two related herbicides, flamprop-isopropyl [(±)-N-benzoyl-N-(3-chloro-4-fluorophenyl)alanine isopropyl ester] and benzoylprop-ethyl [(±)-N-benzoyl-N-(3,4-dichlorophenyl) alanine ethyl ester] are also hydrolyzed to active herbicides, presumably by plant esterases (120, 121). Very low levels of activity have been reported for the in vitro hydrolysis of bifenox [methyl 5-(2,4-dichlorophenoxy)-2-nitrobenzoate] in homogenates of velvetgrass (122).

These in vitro and in vivo studies have shown that plant esterases can catalyze the hydrolysis of a number of pesticides. These studies do not, however, answer important questions regarding the localization of the enzymes within the cell or the distribution of the enzymes in various tissues of the plant. In the case of herbicides, these factors may play an important role in selectivity.

A number of organophosphorous compounds are metabolized in higher plants to products that are consistent with the involvement of hydrolytic enzymes (123-129). In vivo and in vitro studies showed that wheat and sorghum grains rapidly degrade dimethoate [O,O-dimethyl-S-(N-methylcarbamoylmethyl)phosphoro-thiolothionate] to a number of products including O,O-dimethyl-phosphorothionate, mono-O-methyl S-N-methyl-carbamoylmethylphos-phorothiolothionate and mono-O-methyl-S-carboxymethyl-phosphoro-thiolothionate (127) (Figure 11). The apparent hydrolysis of malathion (O,O-dimethyl-S-bis(carboethoxy)ethyl phosphorodi-thioate) to dimethylphosphorothionate and dimethylphosphorothiol-thionate with crude extracts from wheat germ was also demonstrated (128). Unfortunately, these studies do not establish the significance of esterases or phosphohydrolyases in the hydrolysis of organophosphorous pesticides. In animals and insects, glutathione S-transferases and mixed function oxidases play important roles in the metabolism of organophosphorus compounds (126). These enzymes may form some of the same products produced by esterases. Unless experiments are conducted properly, it may not be possible to discern whether GSH S-transferase, esterase or mixed function oxidase-related reactions are responsible for ester hydrolysis. In addition, plant peroxidases may also catalyze the cleavage of organophosphorous compounds (21).

In vivo and in vitro studies have shown that chloramben (3-amino-2-5-dichlorobenzoate) is rapidly metabolized to a stable N-glucoside in resistant plant species (130). In addition to the N-glucoside, susceptible species also form the chloramben glucose ester (130, 131). The glucose ester was not stable in vivo and appeared to act as a chloramben reservoir (Figure 12). Crude homogenates from cucumber and barley tissues hydrolyzed the chloramben glucose ester quite rapidly. Since other benzoic acid or phenoxy herbicides may form glucose ester conjugates, these hydrolytic enzymes could play an important role in regulating

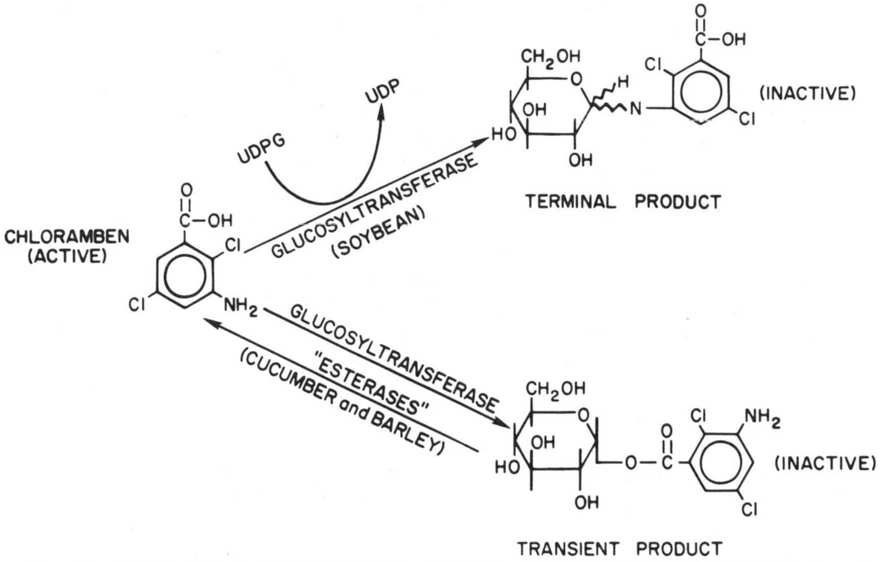

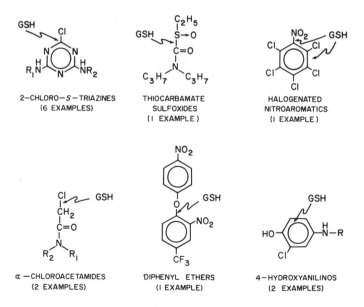

Figure 12.   Chloramben conjugation and hydrolysis (130, 131)

Figure 13.   Agricultural chemicals known to be enzymatically conjugated to GSH
in plants

the levels of these herbicides in vivo.

CONJUGATION:

### Glutathione S-Transferase:

In animals, glutathione (GSH) conjugation is an important reaction in the metabolism of a wide range of xenobiotics and has been the subject of a number of reviews (132-136).

$$
R-X \;+\; \underset{\text{GSH}}{\underset{\text{Substrate}}{
\begin{array}{l}
HN-CH_2-COOH \\
\quad | \\
\quad C=0 \\
\quad | \\
CH_2-CH \\
|\quad | \\
SH\;\; HN-C=0 \qquad COOH \\
\qquad\quad | \qquad\qquad\quad | \\
\qquad CH_2-CH_2-CH \\
\qquad\qquad\qquad | \\
\qquad\qquad\qquad NH_2
\end{array}}}
\;\;\xrightarrow{\text{GSH S-transferase}}\;\;
\underset{\text{GSH Conjugate}}{
\begin{array}{l}
HN-CH_2-COOH \\
\quad | \\
\quad C=0 \\
\quad | \\
CH_2-CH \\
|\quad | \\
S\;\; HN-C=0 \qquad COOH \\
|\qquad\quad | \qquad\qquad\quad | \\
R\qquad CH_2-CH_2-CH \\
\qquad\qquad\qquad | \\
\qquad\qquad\qquad NH_2
\end{array}}
\;+\; HX
$$

Recent findings (137-146) have established that GSH conjugation is also important in plants. Although the range of xenobiotic compounds that have been demonstrated to undergo GSH conjugation in plants is limited (Figure 13), it can be assumed that GSH conjugation of additional classes of compounds will be shown as more studies are conducted. Glutathione conjugation should be considered as a possible metabolic reaction with any xenobiotic that possesses an electrophilic center and an appropriate leaving group, or with xenobiotics that can be activated by oxidation or by some other means to afford an active substrate. Glutathione conjugation is of particular importance in plants (a) because of the wide range of potential substrates, (b) because it may determine the nature of the terminal residues in the plant, and (c) because it may be a major factor in pesticide detoxication or herbicide selectivity.

Glutathione S-transferases have been found in 21 plant species (Table VII) and appear to be widespread in the plant kingdom. Glutathione S-transferases from animals (133) and plants (140, 142, 143, 145, 146) appear to be soluble enzymes. Glutathione S-transferase activity may not be detected in crude enzyme preparations until after gel chromatography (140) or may have limited stability when partially purified (142).

Table VII.  Species which have been examined in vitro for GSH S-transferase activity and cysteine S-transferase activity.

| Plant | Substrate Used to Assay for Activity | | | | |
| | Atrazine (143) | Fluorodifen (142) | PCNB (146) | EPTC (144) | 4-hydroxy chlorpropham (191) |
|---|---|---|---|---|---|
| barley | N. D. | | | | |
| corn | H | H | H | H | L |
| cotton | | H | H | | |
| crabgrass | | | H | | |
| foxtail | | | H | | |
| lambsquarter | | | H | | |
| johnsongrass | H | | | | |
| oat | N. D. | | | L | H |
| okra | | H | | | |
| pea | N. D. | H | H | | |
| peanut | | H | H | | |
| pigweed | N. D. | | H | | |
| soybean | | H | H | | L |
| sorghum | H | | | | |
| sudangrass | H | | | | |
| sugarcane | H | | | | |
| squash | | L | | | |
| tomato | | L | | | |
| wheat | N. D. | | H | | |
| cucumber | | L | | | L |
| rice | | | | | L |

The first demonstrated GSH conjugation of a pesticide in plants was reported in sorghum (137). Atrazine (2-chloro-4-ethylamino-6-isopropylamino-s-triazine) was isolated as a GSH conjugate. The conjugation reaction was enzymatic (143) and active enzyme systems were subsequently isolated from atrazine-resistant corn, sorghum, johnsongrass, sudangrass and sugarcane. Atrazine-susceptible species (pea, oats, wheat, barley and pigweed) contained no detectable enzyme activity. The finding that GSH S-transferase activity was easily isolated from resistant species, but not from susceptible species, indicated that resistance to atrazine was based on the presence of this enzyme. Subsequent studies with an inbred corn line showed that GSH S-transferase activity was present in high concentrations in the resistant line, but not in the susceptible line. This was correlated to the production of the atrazine-GSH conjugate and lack of photosynthetic inhibition in the resistant line (147) (Table VIII). It was further shown that a number of resistant corn lines contained high concentrations of GSH S-transferase activity. These studies confirmed the importance of GSH S-transferase activity in the selectivity of atrazine.

In the tolerant species, corn and sorghum, GSH S-transferase activity was concentrated in the foliar tissue. Partially purified enzyme preparations from corn leaves were stable and could be stored with little loss in activity. Unfortunately, attempts to further purify the enzyme were not successful (148). Substrate specificity studies with several 2-chloro-s-triazine, 2-methoxy-s-triazine, and 2-methylmercapto-s-triazine herbicides showed that the 2-chloro-s-triazines were the only effective substrates. A later study showed that the sulfoxide of a 2-methylmercapto-s-triazine was a good substrate for GSH conjugation (149). The isolated corn enzyme was specific for GSH. Dithiothreitol, mercaptoethanol, 2,3-dimercaptopropanol or L-cysteine did not function as sulfhydryl substrates. Results from substrate specificity studies with the corn enzyme were comparable to those obtained with excised sorghum leaves (Table IX). Although in vitro studies indicated that 2-chloro-4-amino-6-isopropyl-amino-s-triazine was a poor substrate for GSH S-transferase in corn, in vivo studies with sorghum (150) showed that this substrate was conjugated with GSH. This difference may be attributed to differences in the substrate specificity of the GSH S-transferases from sorghum and corn.

The GSH S-transferase mediated cleavage of fluorodifen (p-nitrophenyl α,α,α-trifluoro-2-nitro-p-tolyl ether) to S-(4-trifluoro-2-nitrophenyl)glutathione and 4-nitrophenol appears to be the first demonstrated cleavage of a diphenylether by a GSH transferase system (142). When S-(4-trifluoromethyl-2-nitro-phenyl)glutathione was first detected in vivo, the nature of this metabolite was not understood. A crude enzyme that produced the same product in the presence of GSH was isolated from pea epicotyl tissue. Subsequent large-scale enzyme incubations

Table VIII.    Relationship between GSH-transferase activity, formation of GSH conjugates,
               and inhibition of photosynthesis in atrazine resistant and susceptible corn. **

| Corn line | Response to atrazine | GSH transferase* activity in vitro | % GSH conjugate in leaf disc after 5 hours | % Inhibition of photosynthesis in leaf discs after 2 hours |
|---|---|---|---|---|
| GT112RfRf | resistant | 1.63 | 43.1 | 8.6 |
| GT112 | susceptible | 0.03 | 0.4 | 64.9 |
| 6 other resistant lines | resistant | 2.62 ± 1.0 | --- | --- |

*nmoles/mg protein/hour.
** adapted from (147).

produced $\underline{S}$-(4-trifluoromethyl-2-nitrophenyl)glutathione in good
yield and greatly facilitated the development of analytical
techniques that were used in the isolation and identification of
the $\underline{\text{in vivo}}$ metabolite ($\underline{141}$, $\underline{142}$).

Table IX.    Comparison of the relative substrate specificity of
excised sorghum leaves ($\underline{138}$, $\underline{150}$) with the substrate
specificity of the glutathione $\underline{S}$-transferase from
corn ($\underline{143}$).

| Substrate | Relative activity in vitro (corn) | Relative activity in vivo (sorghum) |
|---|---|---|
| atrazine | 0.68 | 1.00 |
| GS-13529 | 1.00 | 0.93 |
| cyprazine | 0.52 | 0.92 |
| propazine | 0.42 | 0.90 |
| simazine | 0.05 | 0.62 |
| 2-chloro-4-amino-6-isopropylamino-$\underline{s}$-triazine | 0.01 | active* |
| 2-hydroxy-4-ethylamino 6-isopropylamino-$\underline{s}$-triazine | 0.01 | -- |

*Glutathione-related conjugates were the primary
products produced, but experimental conditions
were different from those used with the other
$\underline{S}$-triazines.

   The isolated GSH $\underline{S}$-transferase from pea was stable, but
crude enzyme preparations from corn, peanut and cotton underwent
irreversible inhibition when stored for several hours at 4°.
Enzyme activity was detected in higher concentrations in
resistant species (cotton, corn, peanut, pea, soybean and okra)
than in susceptible species (cucumber, tomato and squash).
Fluorodifen selectivity appeared to be based on enzyme distribution and concentration. A broad substrate specificity study was
not conducted with this enzyme, but two other diphenylether
herbicides were tested and found to be inactive. It was hypothesized that only diphenylethers that were highly activated at
the C-1 position would act as substrates. Mercaptoethanol,
2,3-dimercaptopropanol, dithiothreitol and cysteine would not
function as the sulfhdryl substrate with the enzyme from pea.
   Recent studies have shown that the fungicide PCNB (pentachloronitrobenzene) is also converted to GSH conjugates with an
enzyme system isolated from pea ($\underline{145}$). Additional studies will
be needed to determine if the same enzyme is involved in the
metabolism of both PCNB and fluorodifen. A unique feature of the

PCNB GSH S-transferase assay system was the inclusion of tert-
butanol to increase PCNB solubility and enzymatic activity
(Figure 14). The use of tert-butanol in enzyme systems has been
previously reported (151). This system has not been completely
studied with respect to the PCNB-GSH conjugation reaction.

Detailed inhibitor studies were conducted with the GSH S-
transferases isolated from both corn and pea (Table X). Both
enzymes gave similar responses to sulfhydryl compounds and to the
classical inhibitors of mammalian GSH S-transferase activity,
sulfobromophthalein and 1,2-dichloronitrobenzene. Inhibition by
sulfobromophthalein was competitive in mammalian systems and also
appeared to be competitive in both plant systems. Propachlor
(2-chloro-N-isopropylacetanilide) and barban (4-chloro-2-butynyl-
m-chlorocarbanilate) were inhibitors of the enzymatic reactions
with atrazine and fluorodifen. Inhibition by alkylating agents
was also observed. The fact that sulfobromophthalein was a
competitive inhibitor of both enzymes suggested some commonality
of the active site(s). On the other hand, the fact that atrazine
was neither a substrate nor an inhibitor of the pea enzyme
suggested important differences. Inhibition of the pea enzyme by
other diphenylether compounds, phenylureas and acetamide
herbicides suggested the possibility of pesticide interactions
with these compounds. A number of s-triazines were tested as
inhibitors of the corn enzyme. These studies suggested that the
bis(alkylamino)-methoxy-s-triazines and the methylmercapto
analogs were probably competitive inhibitors capable of binding
at the active site, but incapable of undergoing reaction. Hydro-
xytriazines and the dealkylated triazines were not effective
inhibitors. It is of particular interest to note that a known
synergist of atrazine, 2,3,6-trichlorophenylacetic acid, was an
inhibitor of the GSH S-transferase from corn.

EPTC (S-ethyl dipropylthiocarbamate) does not appear to be a
GSH S-transferase substrate. However, after oxidation to the
sulfoxide, it readily undergoes conjugation in the presence of
GSH S-transferases isolated from rat liver (152) or corn root
(144).

$$C_2H_5-S-\overset{\overset{O}{\|}}{C}-N(C_3H_7)_2 \longrightarrow C_2H_5-S-\overset{\overset{O}{\uparrow}\overset{O}{\|}}{C}-N(C_3H_7)_2$$

EPTC                                  EPTC Sulfoxide

$$C_2H_5-\overset{\overset{O}{\uparrow}\overset{O}{\|}}{S}-C-N(C_3H_7)_2 \xrightarrow[\text{GSH-transferase}]{\text{GSH}} GS-\overset{\overset{O}{\|}}{C}-N(C_3H_7)_2$$

EPTC Sulfoxide                        S-Carbamyl-GSH

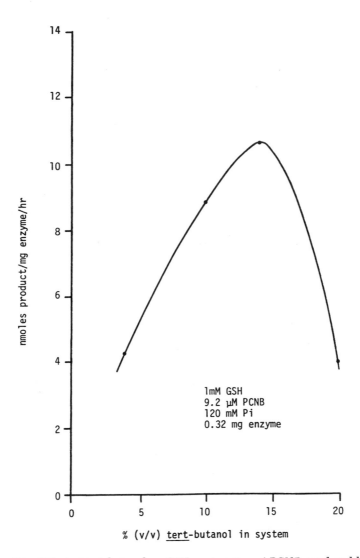

Figure 14.   *Effect of* tert-*butanol on GSH conjugation of PCNB catalyzed by an enzyme system isolated from pea* (192)

Table X.  Inhibitor studies with the glutathione S-transferases isolated from corn (143) and pea (142).

| Inhibitor | Inhibitor concentration (mM) | % Inhibition of GSH-transferase (pea) | % Inhibition of GSH-transferase (corn) |
|---|---|---|---|
| dithiothreitol | 1 | 14 | 40 |
| S-methyl glutathione | 1 | 6 | 11 |
| 2,3-dimercaptopropanol | 1 | 86 | 72 |
| cysteine | 1 | 0 | 0 |
| atrazine | 0.1 | 3 | N.A. |
| 2,4-bis(isopropylamino-6-methyl-mercapto-s-triazine* | 0.06 | -- | 61 |
| 2,3,6-trichlorophenyl acetic acid | 0.1 | -- | 29 |
| propachlor | 0.1 | 28 | 29 |
| barban | 0.1 | 60 | 34 |
| sulfobromophthalein | 0.1 | 88 | 41 |
| 1,2-dichloro-4-nitrobenzene | 1 | 79 | 54 |
| nitrofen* | 0.03 | 55 | -- |
| diuron* | 0.1 | 57 | -- |
| propanil | 0.1 | 68 | -- |
| 1-chloro-3-tosylamido-7-amino-L-2 heptane-HCl* (alkylating agents) | 1.0 | 58 | -- |

*Related compounds were tested with similar results.

This is comparable to a previous observation that a methylmercapto-s-triazine would not undergo conjugation until after
oxidation to the sulfoxide (149). Recent studies have also shown
that chlorpropham (isopropyl m-chlorocarbanilate) is not a
substrate for GSH S-transferase activity in oat, but its
oxidation product, 4-hydroxychlorpropham, readily undergoes an
enzymatic reaction with cysteine or GSH (139, 140). These
observations illustrate the need to consider the possible role
of activating reactions in GSH conjugation.

When corn is treated with N,N-diallyl-2,2-dichloroacetamide
(R-25788), herbicidal injury due to EPTC is greatly reduced (153).
Glutathione S-transferase activity and the concentration of GSH
were increased 2- to 3-fold by treatment with 0.3 to 30 ppm of
R-25788. It was concluded that decreased herbicidal injury was
due to an increased rate of GSH conjugation brought about by the
elevated levels of GSH and GSH S-transferase activity (152). In
EPTC-susceptible oat seedlings, the levels of GSH and GSH S-
transferase did not increase in response to R-25788. The action
of R-25788 appears to be selective. No increase in activity was
noted when the isolated corn system was treated with R-25788;
therefore, R-25788 does not appear to be a simple activator.
Increased levels of GSH S-transferase activity were observed in
both crude and partially purified enzyme preparations after
treatment with R-25788. Although it was not proven, the results
suggest that enzyme induction or possible removal of endogenous
inhibitors may be responsible for the observed increases in
enzyme activity. Twenty-eight compounds were compared to
R-25788 for their effectiveness in increasing GSH S-transferase
activity and GSH content in corn seedling roots. Although
significant exceptions were noted, the effectiveness of these
compounds as antidotes generally correlated with increased GSH
and GSH S-transferase levels.

Chlorpropham (isopropyl m-chlorocarbanilate) and cisanilide
(cis-2,N-phenyl-1-pyrrolidinecarboxanilide) are metabolized to
hydroxylated derivatives in certain plant species (139, 154).
Recent evidence indicates that the 4-hydroxylated derivatives of
chlorpropham and cisanilide are converted to GSH and cysteine
conjugates in oat shoot sections (139, 140) (Figure 15). The
soluble enzyme complex that catalyzes conjugate formation was
isolated from oat. When cysteine and 4-hydroxychlorpropham were
incubated with the enzyme, a polar metabolite was formed. When
GSH was substituted for cysteine, a more polar product was formed.
The in vitro enzyme system was used to produce sufficient
metabolite from the reaction with cysteine and 4-hydroxychlor-
propham to allow isolation and partial characterization of the
product (139). Because of the low yield of this product in the
in vivo system and difficulties encountered in its isolation, the
use of an in vitro system for product formation greatly
facilitated the characterization of this product. In the
characterization of the cysteine conjugate, cysteine C-S lyase

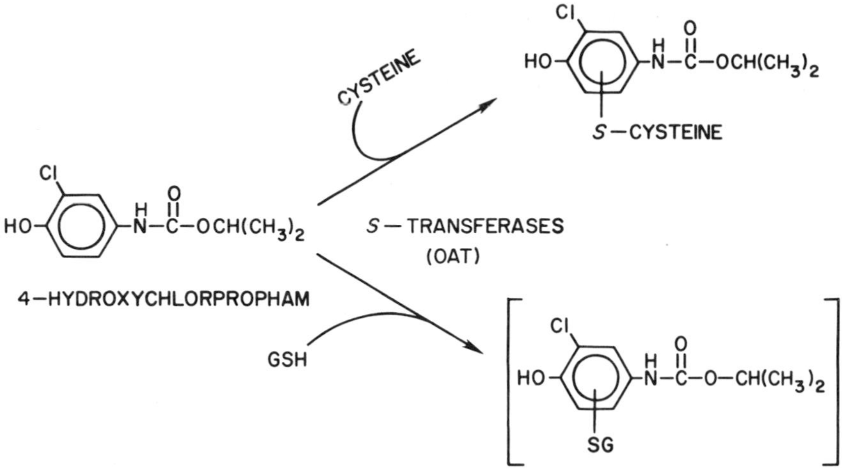

Figure 15.  Reactions thought to be catalyzed by a GSH/cysteine S-transferase
from oat (139, 140)

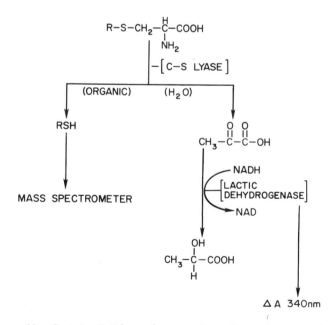

Figure 16.  Cysteine C–S lyase cleavage of cysteine conjugates (139, 150)

was used to cleave the cysteine moiety from the aryl group to yield pyruvic acid and a thiophenol (Figure 16). The reaction was quantitative and the liberated pyruvic acid was measured by coupling the cysteine C-S lyase reaction to a lactic acid dehydrogenase reaction. These coupled reactions were previously used in the characterization of a GSH-related conjugate of atrazine (150).

Glutathione S-transferase activity with GSH and 4-hydroxychlorpropham was not demonstrated until the crude enzyme was partially purified by Sephadex gel chromatography. This behavior suggested the presence of endogenous inhibitors. Detailed inhibitor studies showed that several naturally occurring aromatic compounds and 3-chloro-4-hydroxyaniline were powerful inhibitors of the cysteine S-transferase activity (155). It was suggested that these enzyme systems may use naturally occurring hydroxylated aromatic compounds or aryl hydroxylated xenobiotics as substrates. Two transferase enzyme systems were apparently present in oat shoots. One exhibited nearly comparable activity with either cysteine or GSH and the other displayed much greater activity with cysteine. The latter enzyme also functioned as a GSH S-transferase when the ethylester of cysteine was added to the reaction mixture (140). The nature and the significance of this activation is not understood.

These are the first studies to suggest that cysteine may be utilized as a substrate much like GSH in a transferase reaction (139, 140, 155). This system should be studied in greater detail to better evaluate its significance to xenobiotic metabolism.

Glutathione S-transferase activity was recently isolated from 10 agriculturally important plant species and screened for activity with 8 different pesticide substrates (146). Of the substrates examined, GSH S-transferase activity was demonstrated in all species with PCNB, propachlor and CDAA (N,N-diallyl-chloroacetamide). The results suggested that certain types of GSH S-transferase activity may be widely distributed in higher plants.

These limited studies have clearly shown that GSH S-transferases play an important role in xenobiotic metabolism in plants. Some GSH S-transferases appear to be widely distributed in the plant kingdom, but others appear to be more limited in their distribution. Glutathione S-transferase enzymes play an important role in the selectivity of certain herbicides, such as the 2-chloro-s-triazines, fluorodifen and EPTC sulfoxide, but their role in the selectivity of herbicides such as the α-chloro-acetamides is uncertain. The possibility that herbicidal selectivity may be increased by selectivity stimulating or inducing GSH S-transferase levels has been raised. Additional studies are needed to determine the distribution of GSH S-transferases in higher plants and to better determine the properties of the individual transferases.

Glucose Conjugation:

The reports that ethylenechlorohydrin was converted to a
β-O-D-glucoside and a gentiobioside in wheat (156) and tomato
(157) were among the first indications that plants had the
ability to convert certain xenobiotics to glucosides. It was
later shown that most higher plants (158, 159) had the ability to
convert exogenous phenols to β-O-D-glucosides. This ability was
apparently lacking in algae, fungi and certain aquatic plants
(158). The formation of O-, N-, and S-glucosides, acylated
glucosides, gentiobiosides, and glucose esters have all been
demonstrated either in vitro or in vivo with xenobiotics or
natural substrates (160). The formation of glucosides is
extremely important in pesticide biochemistry for the following
reasons: there is a wide range of potential substrates for
conjugation, glucoside formation may affect the nature of
terminal residue, and glucosylation may play a role in pesticide
selectivity or detoxication. The most common types of glycoside
reactions encountered in pesticide metabolism appear to involve
an initial UDPG-dependent glucosyl transfer reaction (Figure 17).
The formation of simple O-glucosides from polyhydroxylated
phenols was demonstrated with an in vitro system from wheat germ
(161). Substrate specificity tests showed that the wheat germ
glucosyltransferase could use a number of polyhydroxy phenols
as substrates, but was not active with simple phenols. After
purification of this enzyme, activity for certain substrates
was lost; thus, the presence of more than one transferase was
indicated. The in vitro synthesis of 14 phenolic glucosides by
crude enzymes from wheat germ and bean was compared with the
in vivo synthesis in bean (162). The only products detected
in vitro were generally the primary products formed in vivo.
The enzyme systems from wheat germ and bean could not utilize
simple mono-hydroxylated phenols as substrates; it is, therefore,
questionable whether these enzymes are involved in the formation
of β-O-D-glucosides from pesticides or pesticide metabolites.
A number of UDPG:sterol glucosyltransferases have been isolated
from various plant sources (163-166). These enzymes are usually
associated with the particulate fraction (164). For some
phenolic xenobiotics, the possibility should be considered that
UDPG:glucosyltransferase activity may be membrane bound.
A UDPG-dependent enzyme that catalyzes the formation of
β-O-D-glucosides with a variety of phenols, alkyl alcohols and
other substrates has been isolated from germinating mung bean
(167). Attempts to demonstrate the presence of this enzyme in
seedlings were not successful. The ammonium sulfate fractionated
enzyme from germinating mung beans could be stored in liquid
nitrogen with little loss in activity, but the more highly
purified enzyme lost all activity upon freezing. This enzyme
utilized UDPG as the glucosyl donor, had an estimated M.W. of
62,000 and had a pH optimum of approximately 10. The pH optimum

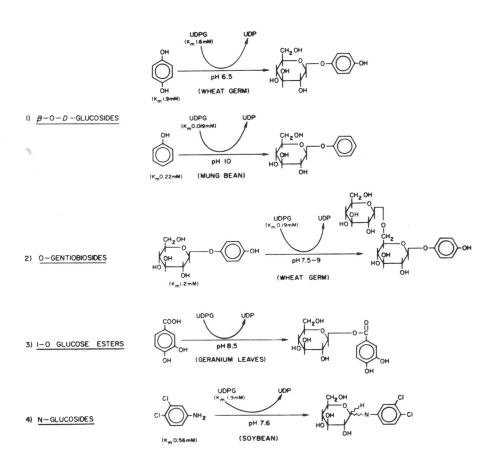

*Figure 17.   Glucosyl transferase systems that use UDPG as the glucosyl donor*

for most other glucosyl transferases is between 6.5 and 9.
Detailed substrate studies showed that reaction rates with the
mung bean enzyme were primarily dependent upon the size of the
acceptor substrate.  n-Butanol was the most active alkyl acceptor
and phenol was the most active aryl acceptor.  The $K_m$ values
observed with a number of low molecular weight substrates
suggested that this enzyme was non-specific and could play an
important role in the metabolism of pesticides and other
xenobiotics.

A crude enzyme system from wheat germ was shown to contain
an enzyme that utilized arbutin as a substrate in the formation
of the corresponding gentiobioside (168).  This enzyme was
separated from UDPG:polyhydroxyphenol glucosyl transferase
activity and was partially purified.  A broad range of phenolic
β-glucosides were substrates for this enzyme, but it was not
active with free phenols.  This type of enzyme may be involved
in the formation of pesticide gentiobioside conjugates such as
diphenamid (169).  A similar enzyme that catalyzes the formation
of an O-α-L-rhamnosyl-(1-O)-β-D-glucosyl conjugate of quercetin
has been isolated from mung beans (170).  Pesticide conjugates
of this type have not been reported.

The in vitro formation of the 1-O-glucose ester of anthran-
ilic acid was demonstrated with a UDPG-dependent transferase from
lentils (171, 172).  The formation of 1-O-glucose esters of
several 4-hydroxy cinnamic acid derivatives (p-coumaric, caffeic,
ferulic, and sinapic acids) and several hydroxybenzoic acids
(vanillic, isovanillic and syringic acid) was demonstrated with
an acetone powder from geranium leaves (173).  The crude enzyme
system from geranium leaves required UDPG for activity, had a pH
optimum of approximately 8.5 for ester formation, and was also
capable of forming β-O-glucosides with phenols at pH 7.4.  The
1-O-glucose esters of both chloramben (131) and naphthelene-
acetic acid (174) have been reported in plants.  These products
may also be formed by UDPG-dependent systems such as those from
lentils or geranium leaves.  The formation of 1-O-glucose ester
conjugates of herbicides may not be a permanent detoxication
mechanism since these products are readily hydrolyzed in vivo
and in vitro as previously discussed.

The formation of 2-O, 4-O and 6-O glucose esters of
carboxylic acid appears to involve a different mechanism
(Figure 18).  A soluble enzyme from sweet corn kernels was shown
to catalyze the formation of 2-0, 4-0 and 6-0 glucose esters of
indole-3-acetic acid in the presence of ATP, CoA, and $Mg^{++}$ (175).
Products such as these may also be important in pesticide
metabolism in higher plants (160).

The in vitro formation of substituted aniline N-glucosides
was demonstrated with enzyme systems from soybean (176, 177) and
pea (178) (Figure 17).  The UDPG:arylamine glucosyltransferase
from soybean utilized UDPG or TDPG as the glucosyl donor for 15
different arylamine acceptors (176).  During the isolation of this

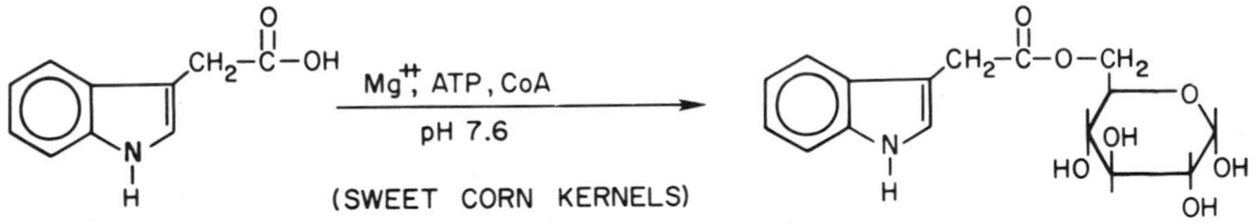

*Figure 18.   Formation of 2–0, 4–0, and 6–0 glucose ester conjugates (175)*

enzyme, activity was demonstrated with arylamines and hydro-
quinones; however, the ratio of these activities changed
dramatically during purification.  It appears that more than one
transferase was originally present.

In vivo studies indicated a direct relationship between
chloramben N-glucoside formation and resistance (179).  Several
arylamine herbicides are metabolized directly to N-glucosides in
plants and a number of other herbicides have been reported to be
metabolized to arylamines by plants (160).  These metabolites
might also be expected to form N-glucosides.  Based upon our
knowledge of the metabolism of herbicides to aniline derivatives
and the broad specificity of the UDPG:arylamine glucosyltransferase from soybean, it would appear that this enzyme plays an
important role in xenobiotic metabolism.

The formation of 6-O-malonyl-β-D-glucosides of endogenous
substrates (180-182) as well as the pesticides fluorodifen (183)
and flamprop (184) have been reported.  The reaction, with flavone
glycosides as substrates, has been studied in vitro with an
enzyme isolated from illuminated cell suspension cultures of
parsley (185).  The enzyme is a malonyl coenzyme A:flavone
glycoside malonyl-transferase.  The enzyme did not appear to be
specific for the few glycoside substrates tested and no cofactors other than malonyl coenzyme A were required.

In addition to the UDPG-dependent glucosyl transferase
systems, an enzyme that utilizes an endogenous glucoside, iso-
succinimide β-glucoside, as the glucosyl donor has been characterized from pea (186) (Figure 19).  This soluble enzyme has a pH
optimum of 5.5 and converts ethanol and isopropanol to their
corresponding β-O-D-glucosides.  Isotope studies showed that the
reaction was essentially irreversible.  Various phenolic
glucosides also functioned as glucosyl donors, but at a reduced
rate.  UDPG, glucose-1-P and related compounds did not function
in this capacity.  A high $K_m$ for ethanol, 0.5 M, suggested that
ethanol and isopropanol were probably not the natural substrates
for this enzyme.

A similar or identical system from pea was recently shown to
utilize polyethoxylated alkylphenol detergents as substrates
(187).  An unidentified endogenous glucoside and several
exogenous phenolic glucosides functioned as glucosyl donors.
Additional studies on the substrate specificity, distribution,
and kinetics of this enzyme are needed to properly evaluate its
importance in the metabolism of detergents and other xenobiotics.

SUMMARY:

Based on the enzyme studies considered in this report, it
can be concluded that in vitro enzyme techniques can be used to
great advantage to study pesticide metabolism in plants.
Important advantages that may be offered by these techniques
are as follows:

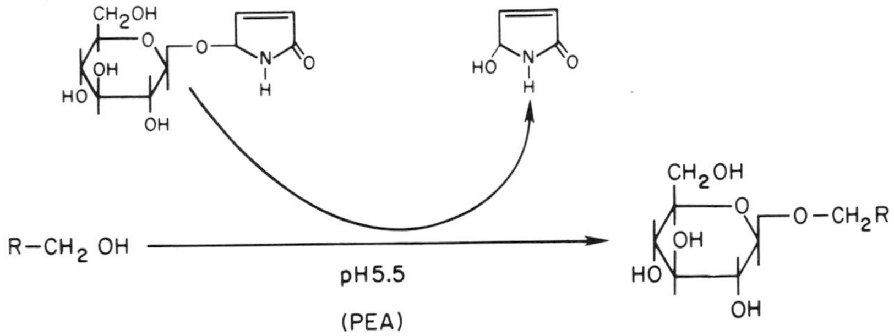

*Figure 19.  Non-UDPG-dependent glycosyl transferase system from pea (186, 187)*

Advantages:

(1) Specific metabolic reactions can be isolated from competing reactions and studied in a simplified system. Details of the reaction mechanism can be examined. Transitory or unstable intermediates can be detected or isolated.

(2) Extensive inhibitor and activator studies can be efficiently conducted. Possible pesticide interactions may be identified and nonpesticidal agents can be screened for use in combinations with pesticides to change their selectivity or improve their efficacy.

(3) Broad structure-activity studies can be conducted easily to determine the structural requirements for a specific metabolic reaction.

(4) Screening studies can be conducted with enzymes isolated from many different plant species and varieties to obtain basic information on genetic differences in metabolism or the mechanism of herbicide resistance.

(5) Enzyme induction studies can help in the development of protectants and other useful chemicals that function by stimulating the formation of key enzymes involved in metabolism.

(6) Isolated enzymes may be used effectively for the biosynthesis of specific metabolites in quantities that simplify their isolation and identification.

(7) Specific enzymes can be used to characterize and degrade more complex metabolites.

(8) Model enzyme systems can be developed to help solve difficult problems such as those associated with the bound residues of pesticides.

(9) Certain metabolic reactions may be studied in vitro without the need for radioactive substrates.

(10) Enzyme concentrations as a function of age or tissue type can be studied.

(11) Enzyme kinetic studies can be used to determine reaction mechanisms and to evaluate the importance of competing metabolic reactions.

The use of isolated enzymes to study xenobiotic metabolism is not without certain disadvantages. In addition to specific problems associated with the isolation of enzymes from plants, such as low levels of enzyme activity within the plant and the presence of phenolics and their oxidative enzymes that can result in enzyme inactivation or degradation during extraction and isolation, there are a number of disadvantages or problems associated with in vitro enzyme techniques in general. Those most relevant to xenobiotic metabolism are as follows:

Disadvantages:

(1) Results of isolated enzyme studies must usually be verified by in vivo studies.

(2) The enzyme may be extremely difficult to isolate in an active form or may be labile and require reisolation for each study.

(3) The nature of the enzyme system may be unknown and it may be difficult to determine the proper co-factors.

(4) If the desired enzyme activity is found in several fractions, the researcher must decide whether to study only one fraction, study each fraction separately, or study the crude system.

(5) Endogenous inhibitors may be present. If not properly handled, they can yield misleading results.

(6) The system may be susceptible to substrate or product inhibition or the kinetics may be dependent upon the substrate concentration.

(7) The solubility of the substrate may be too low to obtain reliable kinetic data and it may be necessary to use detergents or solvents to solubilize the substrate. These agents may alter the kinetics or inhibit the enzyme.

(8) The methods necessary to isolate a specific enzyme activity from different plant species may vary sufficiently to make it difficult to conduct broad screening studies.

(9) It may be difficult to obtain the enzyme in sufficiently pure form to conduct meaningful kinetic studies.

(10) Low enzymatic activity generally makes necessary the use of radioactive substrates or other more sensitive assay methods.

This brief survey has documented the role played by various isolated enzyme studies in answering important questions related to pesticide metabolism in plants. It has shown that when proper consideration is given, in vitro techniques can be used to great advantage. Currently, our ability to use isolated enzymes to study certain areas of pesticide metabolism is limited by our basic knowledge of the enzymes involved. As this knowledge becomes available, our ability to use in vitro enzyme techniques to study additional areas of pesticide metabolism will be increased.

## Abstract

The four basic biochemical reactions commonly involved in pesticide metabolism in higher plants (oxidation, reduction, hydrolysis and conjugation) are discussed in relation to the enzyme systems capable of catalyzing these reactions. The literature regarding the use of enzymes from these classes to study pesticide metabolism is reviewed. The following enzymes are considered: peroxidases, mixed function oxidases, hydroperoxidases, aryl nitroreductases, aryl acylamidases, esterases, glutathione S-transferases, cysteine S-transferases and various glucose-conjugating enzyme systems. The advantages and disadvantages of in vitro enzyme techniques as they related to pesticide metabolism studies are also discussed.

Literature Cited:

1.  Chance, B., _Arch. Biochem. Biophys._ (1952) <u>41</u>, 416.
2.  George, P., _Nature_ (1952) <u>169</u>, 612.
3.  Saunders, B. C., Homes-Siedle, A. G. and Stark, B. P., _In_: "Peroxidase," Butterworths, Washington (1964).
4.  Kay, E., Shannon, L. M. and Yew, J. W., _J. Biol. Chem._ (1967) <u>242</u>, 2470.
5.  Wilson, J. M. and Wong, E., _Phytochem._ (1976) <u>15</u>, 1333.
6.  Westerfeld, W. W. and Lowe, C., _J. Biol. Chem._ (1942) <u>145</u>, 463.
7.  Lee, T. T., _Physiol. Plant._ (1973) <u>29</u>, 198.
8.  Gove, J. P. and Hoyle, M. C., _Plant Physiol_. (1975) <u>56</u>, 684.
9.  Harvey, B. M. R., Chang, F. Y. and Flecher, R. A., _Can. J. Bot._ (1975) <u>53</u>, 225.
10. Delincee, H. and Radola, B. J., _Europ. J. Biochem._ (1975) <u>52</u>, 321.
11. Iordachescu, D., Dumitry, I. F. and Niculesau, S., _Experientia_ (1973) 1215.
12. Gardiner, M. G. and Cleland, R., _Phytochem._ (1974) <u>13</u>, 1707.
13. Frenkel, C. and Hess, C. E., _Can. J. Bot._ (1974) <u>52</u>, 295.
14. Chlielnicka, J., Ohlsson, P. I., Paul, K. G. and Stigbrand, T., _FEBS Letters_ (1971) <u>17</u>, 181.
15. Ockerse, R. and Mumford, L. M., _Can. J. Bot._ (1973) <u>51</u>, 2237.
16. Raa, J., _Physiol. Plant._ (1973) <u>29</u>, 247.
17. Loh, J. W. C. and Severson, J. G. Jr., _Phytochem._ (1975) <u>14</u>, 1265.
18. Machackova, I., Ganceva, K. and Zmrhal, Z., _Phytochem._ (1975) <u>14</u>, 1251.
19. Schreiber, W., _FEBS Letters_ (1974) <u>41</u>, 50.
20. Sarkanen, K. V., _In_: "Lignins: Occurrence, Formation, Structure and Reactions," pp. 95-163 (Edited by Sarkanen, K. V. and Ludwig, C. H.), John Wiley and Sons, New York (1971).
21. Knaak, J. B., Stahmann, M. A. and Casida, J. E., _J. Agric. Food Chem._ (1962) <u>10</u>, 154.
22. Kuhr, R. J. and Casida, J. E., _J. Agric. Food Chem._ (1967) <u>15</u>, 814.
23. Sorbo, B. and Ljunggren, C., _Acta Chem. Scand._ (1958) <u>12</u>, 470.
24. Bartha, R., Linke, H. A. B. and Pramer, D., _Science_ (1968) <u>161</u>, 582.
25. Balba, H. M., Still, G. G. and Mansager, E. R. (1977) 174th National ACS Meeting, Aug. 29-Sept. 2, Chicago, Ill.
26. Still, G. G., Balba, H. M. and Mansager, E. R. (1978), In preparation.
27. Van Alfan, N. K. and Kosuge, T., _J. Agric. Food Chem._ (1976) <u>24</u>, 584.
28. Kadunce, R. E., Stolzenberg, G. E. and Davis, D. G. (1974) National ACS Meeting, Sept. 8-13, Atlantic City, N.J.

29. Lamoureux, G. L. and Rusness, D. G. (1976) 172nd National ACS Meeting, Aug. 29–Sept. 3, San Francisco, Calif.

30. Wain, R. L. and Smith, M. S., In: "Herbicides, Physiology, Biochemistry and Ecology," (Edited by Audus, L. J.), 2nd Ed., Vol. 2, Academic Press (1976).

31. Morrison, M. and Schonbaum, G. R., Ann. Rev. Biochem. (1976) 45, 861.

32. Mynett, M. and Wain, R. L., Pestic. Sci. (1971) 2, 238.

33. Mynett, M. and Wain, R. L., Weed Res. (1973) 13, 101.

34. Ram, C., Balasimha, D. and Tewari, M. N., Plant Biochem. J. (1975) 2, 61.

35. Ishimaru, A. and Yamazaki, I., J. Biol. Chem. (1977) 252, 6118.

36. Ishimaru, A. and Yamazaki, I., J. Biol. Chem. (1977) 252, 199.

37. Hodgson, E. (Ed.) In: "Enzymatic Oxidations of Toxicants," N. Car. State Univ., Raleigh, N. C. (1968).

38. Frydman, R. B., Tomaro, M. L. and Frydman, B., Biochim. Biophys. Acta (1972) 284, 63.

39. Russell, D. W., J. Biol. Chem. (1971) 246, 3870.

40. Nair, P. M. and Vining, L. C., Phytochem. (1965) 4, 401.

41. Patterson, R. and Rappaport, L., Phytochem. (1975) 14, 363.

42. Russell, D. W. and Conn, E. E., Arch. Biochem. Biophys. (1967) 122, 256.

43. Earl, J. W. and Kennedy, I. R., Phytochem. (1975) 14, 1507.

44. Makeev, A. M., Makoveichuk, A. I. U. and Chkanikov, D. C., Dokl. Acad. Nauk. S.S.S.R. (1977) 233, 1222.

45. McPherson, F. J., Markham, A., Bridges, J. W., Hartman, G. C., and Parke, D. V., Biochem. Soc. Trans. (1975) 3, 281.

46. McPherson, F. J., Markham, A., Bridges, J. W., Hartman, G. C. and Parke, D. V., Biochem. Soc. Trans. (1975) 3, 283.

47. Frear, D. S., Swanson, H. R. and Tanaka, F. S., Phytochem. (1966) 8, 2157.

48. Frear, D. S., Science (1968) 162, 674.

49. Markham, A., Hartman, G. C. and Parke, D. V., Biochem. J. (1972) 130, 90.

50. Tanaka, F. S., Swanson, H. R. and Frear, D. S., Phytochem. (1972) 11, 2709.

51. Young, O. and Beevers, H., Phytochem. (1976) 15, 379.

52. Fleeker, J. R., Phytochem. (1973) 12, 757.

53. Wotschokowsky, M., Weed Res. (1972) 12, 80.

54. Madyastha, K. M. and Coscia, C. J., Fed. Proc. (1975) 34, 2163.

55. Potts, J. R. M., Weklych, R. and Conn, E. E., J. Biol. Chem. (1974) 249, 5019.

56. Murphy, P. J. and West, C. A., Arch. Biochem. Biophys. (1969) 133, 395.

57. Meehan, T. D. and Coscia, C. J., Biochem. Biophys. Res. Commun. (1973) 53, 1043.

58. Oloffs, P. C., Pestic. Sci. (1970) 1, 228.
59. McKinney, J. D. and Mehendale, H. M., J. Agric. Food Chem. (1973) 21, 1079.
60. Lichtenstein, E. P. and Corbett, J. R., J. Agric. Food Chem. (1969) 17, 589.
61. Mehendale, H. M., Skrentny, R. F. and Dorough, H. W., J. Agric. Food Chem. (1972) 20, 398.
62. Yu, S. J., Kiigemagi, U. and Terriere, L. C., J. Agric. Food Chem. (1971) 19, 509.
63. Eto, M., In: "Organophosphorus Pesticides: Organic and Biological Chemistry," CRC Press Inc., Cleveland, Ohio (1974).
64. Krueger, H. R., Pest. Biochem. Physiol. (1975) 5, 396.
65. Main, A. R. and Braid, P. E., Biochem. J. (1962) 84, 255.
66. Rowlands, D. G., Residue Rev. (1967) 17, 105.
67. Fairbairn, J. W., Handa, S. S. and Phillipson, J. D., Phytochem. (1978) 17, 261.
68. Frear, D. S., Swanson, H. R. and Tanaka, F. S., In: "Symposia of the Phytochemical Society of North America," (Edited by Runeckles, V. C.), Academic Press, New York (1972).
69. Bowling, C. C. and Hudgins, H. R., Weeds (1966) 14, 94.
70. Hacskaylo, J. K., Walker, J. K. Jr., and Pires, E. G., Weeds (1964) 12, 288.
71. Swanson, C. R. and Swanson, H. R., Weed Sci. (1968) 16, 481.
72. Benveniste, K., Salaun, J. P. and Durst, F., Phytochem. (1978) 17, 359.
73. Russell, D. W., Conn, E. E., Sutter, A. and Grisebach, H., Biochim. Biophys. Acta. (1968) 170, 210.
74. Werringloer, J. and Estabrook, R. W., Arch. Biochem. Biophys. (1975) 167, 270.
75. Hill, C. A. and Rhodes, M. J., Phytochem. (1975) 14, 2387.
76. Benveniste, K., Salaun, J. P. and Durst, F., Phytochem. (1977) 16, 69.
77. Lamoureux, G. L. and Rusness, D. G., (1976), 172nd National ACS Meeting, Aug. 29–Sept. 3, San Francisco, Calif.
78. Frear, D. S., In: "Herbicides, Chemistry and Mode of Action," Vol. 2, (Edited by Kearney, P. C. and Kaufman, D. D.), Marcel Dekker Inc., New York, N.Y. (1976).
79. Eastin, E. F., Weed Sci. (1971) 19, 261.
80. Eastin, E. F., Weed Sci. (1972) 20, 255.
81. Biswas, P. K. and Hamilton, W., Weed Sci. (1969) 17, 206.
82. Kadunce, R. E., Stolzenberg, G. E. and Davis, D. G. (1974), 168th National ACS Meeting, Sept. 8–13, Atlantic City, N.J.
83. Beynon, K. J. and Wright, A. N., J. Sci. Food Agric. (1969) 20, 250.
84. Frehse, H., In: "Terminal Residues of Organophosphorus Insecticides in Plants," Pesticide Terminal Residues, Butterworths, London (1971).

85.  Shimabukuro, R. H., Lamoureux, G. L., Swanson, H. R.,
     Walsh, W. C., Stafford, L. E. and Frear, D. S.,
     Pest. Biochem. Physiol. (1973) 3, 483.
86.  Frear, D. S. and Swanson, H. R., Pest. Biochem. Physiol.
     (1973) 3, 473.
87.  Diesperger, H., Muller, C. R. and Sandermann, H., Jr.,
     FEBS Letters (1974) 43, 155.
88.  Kearney, P. C., J. Agric. Food Chem. (1965) 13, 561.
89.  Blake, J. and Kaufmann, D. D., Pest. Biochem. Physiol.
     (1975) 5, 305.
90.  Nimmo-Smith, R. H., Biochem. J. (1960) 75, 284.
91.  Williams, C. H. and Jacobson, K. H., Toxicol. Appl.
     Pharmacol. (1966) 9, 495.
92.  Mahavdevan, S. and Tappel, S. A., J. Biol. Chem. (1967)
     242, 2369.
93.  Still, C. C. and Kuzirian, O., Nature (1967) 217, 799.
94.  Frear, D. S. and Still, G. G., Phytochem. (1968) 7, 913.
95.  Matsunaka, S., Science (1968) 160, 1360.
96.  Hoagland, R. E., Graf, G. and Handel, E. D., Weed Res.
     (1974) 14, 371.
97.  Hoagland, R. E. and Graf, G., Weed Sci. (1972) 20, 303.
98.  Ray, T. B. and Still, C. C., Pest. Biochem. Physiol.
     (1975) 5, 171.
99.  Hoagland, R. E. and Graf, G., Phytochem. (1972) 11, 521.
100. Akatsuka, T., Noyaku Kaguka (1973) 1, 55.
101. McRae, D. H., Yih, R. Y. and Wilson, H. E., Weed Sci. Abs.
     (1964) 87.
102. Baldwin, B. C., In: "Xenobiotic Metabolism in Plants, Drug
     Metabolism from Microbe to Man," (Edited by Parke, D. V.
     and Smith, R. L.), Taylor Francis Ltd., London (1977).
103. Menzie, C. M., In: "Metabolism of Pesticides," Bureau of
     Sport Fisheries and Wildlife Special Scientific Report,
     Washington, D. C. (1969).
104. Smith, R. J. and Tugwell, N. P., Weed Sci. (1975) 23, 176.
105. Adachi, M., Tonegawa, K. and Ueshima, T., Pest. Tech. Tokyo
     (1966) 14, 19.
106. Ishizuka, K. and Mitsui, S., Abstr. Ann. Mts. Agr. Chem. Soc.
     Japan (1966).
107. Bowling, C. C. and Hudgins, H. R., Weeds (1966) 14, 94.
108. Hoagland, R. E., Plant and Cell Physiol. (1978) 19 (In
     press).
109. Hoagland, R. E., Phytochem. (1975) 14, 383.
110. Akatsuka, T. and Kasakura, N., Ibaraki Daigaku Nogakubu
     Gakujutsu Hokoku (1972) 20, 17.
111. Tavener, R. J. A. and Laidman, D. L., Phytochem. (1972) 11,
     989.
112. Mendoza, C. E., Grant, D. L. and McCully, K. A., J. Agric.
     Food Chem. (1969) 17, 623.
113. Seifert, J. and Davidek, J., Pest. Biochem. Physiol. (1978)
     8, 10.

114. Veerabhadrappa, P. S. and Montgomery, M. W., Phytochem.
     (1971) 10, 1171.
115. Clifford, D. R., Hislop, E. C. and Shellis, C., Pestic. Sci.
     (1977) 8, 13.
116. Galliard, T. and Dennis, S., Phytochem. (1974) 13, 2463.
117. Veerabhadrappa, P. S. and Montgomery, M. W., Phytochem.
     (1971) 10, 1175.
118. Thomas, H. and Bingham, M. J., Phytochem. (1977) 16, 1887.
119. Fedtke, C. and Schmidt, R. R., Weed Res. (1977) 17, 233.
120. Roberts, T. R., Pest. Biochem. Physiol. (1977) 7, 378.
121. Jeffcoat, B. and Harries, N., Pestic. Sci. (1973) 4, 891.
122. Leather, G. R. and Foy, C. L., Pest. Biochem. Physiol.
     (1977) 7, 437.
123. Casida, J. E. and Lykken, L., Ann. Rev. Plant Physiol.
     (1969) 20, 607.
124. Rowlands, D. G., Residue Rev. (1967) 17, 105.
125. Spencer, E. Y., Residue Rev. (1965) 9, 153.
126. Eto, M., In: "Organophosphorus Pesticides: Organic and
     Biological Chemistry," CRC Press Inc., Cleveland, Ohio
     (1974).
127. Rowlands, D. G., J. Sci. Food Agric. (1966) 17, 90.
128. Rowlands, D. G., J. Sci. Food Agric. (1965) 16, 325.
129. Menzie, C. M., In: "Metabolism of Pesticides, An Update,
     U. S. Dept. Int. Fish and Wildlife Serv., Special Scientific
     Report, Washington, D. C. (1974).
130. Frear, D. S., In: "Herbicides, Chemistry, Degradation and
     Mode of Action," Vol. 2 (Edited by Kearney, P. C. and
     Kaufmann, D. D.), Marcel Dekker, New York, N.Y. (1976).
131. Frear, D. S. and Swanson, H. R., (1977) 173rd National ACS
     Meeting, March 21-25, New Orleans, La.
132. Boyland, E. and Chasseaud, L. F., Advan. Enzymol. (1969)
     32, 173.
133. Chasseaud, L. F., Drug Metab. Rev. (1973) 2, 195.
134. Arias, J. M. and Jakoby, W. B., In: "Glutathione:
     Metabolism and Function," Kroc Foundation Series, Vol. 6,
     Raven Press, New York (1976).
135. Shimabukuro, R. H., Lamoureux, G. L. and Frear, D. S.,
     In: "Chemistry and Action of Herbicide Antidotes," (Edited
     by Pallos, F. M. and Casida, J. E.), Academic Press Inc.,
     New York, N.Y. (1978).
136. Hutson, D. H., In: "Glutathione Conjugates, Bound and
     Conjugated Pesticide Residues," ACS Symposium Series 29
     (Edited by Kaufmann, D. D., Still, G. G., Paulson, G. D.
     and Bandal, S. K.), ACS, Washington, D. C. (1976).
137. Lamoureux, G. L., Shimabukuro, R. H., Swanson, H. R. and
     Frear, D. S., J. Agric. Food Chem. (1970) 18, 81.
138. Lamoureux, G. L., Stafford, L. E. and Shimabukuro, R. H.,
     J. Agric. Food Chem. (1972) 20, 1004.
139. Still, G. G. and Rusness, D. G., Pest. Biochem. Physiol.
     (1977) 7, 210.

140. Rusness, D. G. and Still, G. G., Pest. Biochem. Physiol. (1977) 7, 220.
141. Shimabukuro, R. H., Lamoureux, G. L., Swanson, H. R., Walsh, W. C., Stafford, L. E. and Frear, D. S., Pest. Biochem. Physiol. (1973) 3, 483.
142. Frear, D. S. and Swanson, H. R., Pest. Biochem. Physiol. (1973) 3, 473.
143. Frear, D. S. and Swanson, H. R., Phytochem. (1970) 9, 2123.
144. Lay, M. M. and Casida, J. E., Pest. Biochem. Physiol. (1977) 6, 442.
145. Lamoureux, G. L. and Rusness, D. G. (1976) 172nd National ACS Meeting, Aug. 29-Sept. 3, San Francisco, Calif.
146. Burkholder, R. R. S., Plant Glutathione S-Transferase, M. S. Thesis, N. D. State University, Fargo, N. D. (1978).
147. Shimabukuro, R. H., Frear, D. S., Swanson, H. R. and Walsh, W. C., Plant Physiol. (1971) 47, 10.
148. Frear, D. S. Unpublished data.
149. Bedford, C. T., Crawford, M. J. and Hutson, D. H., Chemosphere (1975) 5, 311.
150. Lamoureux, G. L., Stafford, L. E., Shimabukuro, R. H. and Zaylskie, R. E., J. Agric. Food Chem. (1973) 21, 1021.
151. Tan, K. H. and Lovrien, R., J. Biol. Chem. (1972) 247, 3278.
152. Lay, M. M. and Casida, J. E., Science (1975) 189, 287.
153. Lay, M. M. and Casida, J. E., In: "Chemistry and Action of Herbicide Antidotes," (Edited by Pallos, F. M. and Casida, J. E.), Academic Press Inc., New York (1978).
154. Frear, D. S. and Swanson, H. R., Pest. Biochem. Physiol. (1976) 6, 52.
155. Rusness, D. G. and Still, G. G., Pest. Biochem. Physiol. (1977) 7, 232.
156. Miller, L. P., Contrib. Boyce Thompson Inst. (1941) 12, 25.
157. Miller, L. P., Contrib. Boyce Thompson Inst. (1941) 12, 15.
158. Pridham, J. B., Phytochem. (1964) 3, 493.
159. Glass, A. D. M. and Bohm, B. A., Phytochem. (1970) 9, 2197.
160. Frear, D. S., In: "Pesticide Conjugates-Glycosides, ACS Symposium Series 29 (Edited by Kaufmann, D. D., Still, G. G., Paulson, G. D. and Bandal, S. K.), American Chemical Society, Washington, D. C. (1976).
161. Yamaha, T. and Cardini, C. E., Arch. Biochem. Biophys. (1960) 86, 127.
162. Pridham, J. B. and Saltmarch, M. J., Biochem. J. (1963) 87, 218.
163. Wojciechowski, A. Z., Phytochem. (1974) 13, 2091.
164. Fang, T. Y. and Baisted, D. B., Phytochem. (1976) 15, 273.
165. Baisted, D. B., Phytochem. (1978) 17, 435.
166. Adler, G. and Kasprzyk, Z., Phytochem. (1975) 14, 627.
167. Storm, D. L. and Hassid, W. C., Plant Physiol. (1974) 54, 840.
168. Yamaha, T. and Cardini, C., Arch. Biochem. Biophys. (1960) 86, 133.

169. Hodgson, R. H., Dusbabek, K. E. and Hoffer, B. L.,
     Weed Sci. (1973) 21, 542.
170. Barber, G. A., Biochem. (1962) 1, 463.
171. Tabone, D., Compt. Rend. (1955) 241, 1521.
172. Jacobelli, G., Tabone, M. J. and Tabone, D., Bull. Soc.
     Chim. Biol. (1958) 40, 955.
173. Corner, J. J. and Swain, T., Nature (1965) 207, 634.
174. Shindy, W. W., Jordan, L. S. and Jolliffe, V. A., J. Agric.
     Food Chem. (1973) 21, 629.
175. Kopcewicz, J., Ehmann, A. and Bandurski, R. S., Plant
     Physiol. (1974) 54, 846.
176. Frear, D. S., Phytochem. (1968) 7, 381.
177. Frear, D. S., Swanson, C. R. and Kadunce, R. E., Weeds
     (1967) 15, 101.
178. Murakoshi, I., Ikegama, F., Kato, F. and Haginiwa, J.,
     Phytochem. (1975) 14, 1269.
179. Colby, S. R., Science (1965) 150, 619.
180. Minale, L., Piatelli, M., DeStefano, S. and Nicolaus, R. A.,
     Phytochem. (1966) 5, 1037.
181. Beck, A. B. and Knox, J. R., Aust. J. Chem. (1971) 24, 1509.
182. Kruezaler, F. and Hahlbrock, K., Phytochem. (1973) 12, 1149.
183. Shimabukuro, R. H., Walsh, W. C., Stolzenberg, G. E. and
     Olson, P. A. (1975) Weed Sci. Soc. Amer. Meetings,
     Washington, D. C.
184. Dutton, A. J., Roberts, T. R. and Wright, A. N., Chemosphere
     (1976) 3, 195.
185. Hahlbrock, K., FEBS Letters (1972) 28, 65.
186. Liu, T. Y. and Castelfranco, P., Plant Physiol. (1970) 45,
     424.
187. Frear, D. S., Swanson, H. R. and Stolzenberg, G. E. (1977)
     174th National ACS Meeting, Aug. 28-Sept. 4, Chicago, Ill.
188. Hideaki, S. and Noguchi, M., Phytochem. (1975) 14, 1255.
189. Machackova, I., Ganceva, K. and Zmrhal, Z., Phytochem.
     (1975) 14, 1251.
190. Wright, B. J., Dowsett, J. R., Rubery, P. H., Baillie, A. C.
     and Corbett, J. R., Pestic. Sci. (1973)
191. Still, G. G., Rusness, D. G., Mansager, E. R., In:
     "Mechanism of Pesticide Action," ACS Symposium Series 2,
     ACS, Washington, D. C., (1974), 117.
192. Lamoureux, G. L. and Rusness, D. G., Unpublished data.

RECEIVED December 20, 1978.

# Animals

# Techniques for Studying the Metabolism of Xenobiotics by Intact Animal Cells, Tissues, and Organs In Vitro

ROBERT E. MENZER

Department of Entomology, University of Maryland, College Park, MD 20742

Researchers studying the fate of xenobiotics in mammals have tended to concentrate their efforts either on the whole animal or on liver homogenate systems such as microsomes. Each, of course, has its advantages. The response of a whole animal most closely represents what is likely to occur upon exposure of man to a compound. Liver homogenates are useful in that the liver is the principal organ responsible for the degradation and elimination of xenobiotics from mammalian systems, and liver microsomes appear to be the principal site within the mammal where metabolic conversions take place. These systems allow a rapid, inexpensive evaluation of metabolic events which are likely to take place in the mammal for any xenobiotic. The combination of studies in whole animals and liver microsomal systems generally provides a good understanding of the fate of a xenobiotic in a mammalian system.

Occasionally, however, a compound will be investigated in which the events taking place in a liver microsomal system do not entirely mirror what occurs in the whole organism. Furthermore, the use of microsomal systems does not provide information on the pharmacodynamics involved in the absorption, distribution, and elimination of a xenobiotic from an organism. Other techniques are available which will provide additional information on the fate of a xenobiotic in a mammal that would be difficult to obtain either with liver microsomal systems or in whole organisms. In this paper we will examine the use of perfused organ systems, with particular emphasis on liver and lung perfusion; tissue slices, particularly from lung and liver; cell culture systems, both primary cell cultures and established cell lines; and finally, the promising new technique of isolated hepatocyte preparations. For each technique we will examine the methodology currently in use and evaluate the ease by which an investigator inexperienced in the use of the technique would be able to adopt it for studies on specific compounds. The application of each of these techniques to the study of xenobiotics, with particular emphasis on pesticides, will be illustrated.

0-8412-0486-1/79/47-097-131$05.00/0

Organ Perfusion

As is the case with most *in vitro* mammalian preparations,
organ perfusion was originally developed to study the physiology
and biochemistry of the organ itself and the functional position
of the organ in the metabolism of the normal animal. Organ perfusion studies are an intermediate step between studies in the
whole animal and experiments with isolated subcellular preparations. By observing the response of a viable organ isolated from
the system in which it resides, one is able to assess the part
which the organ plays in the metabolism of any given system. It
is frequently possible to observe specific steps in metabolic
processes in an isolated organ when in the whole animal only substrate and final product are observable. It is in the ability
of the researcher to isolate individual reactions that perfused
organs have their principal utility. Another advantage of perfused organ preparations is that blood flow, gas exchange, and
temperature are under direct control. This enables the researcher
to deliberately manipulate these parameters to assess the effect
of, for example, reduced blood flow, anoxia, hypothermia, changes
in blood pH, or osmolarity on the metabolic process being studied.
For background information and descriptions of the methodology
available for organ perfusion one may refer to a number of books
dealing with the subject. Two examples are Ritchie and Hardcastle (11) and Ross (12).
Perfusion may be defined as the passage of a fluid medium or
blood through the vascular bed of an organ. It is easy to see
how one can utilize a perfusing organ to study the metabolism of
a xenobiotic by the simple introduction of the chemical into the
perfusate and observation of the effect which the organ has on
the chemical. The possibilities for continuous sampling of the
perfusate, continuous addition or pulse addition of the chemical
to the perfusate, and studies of the interactions of more than
one chemical in organs are readily apparent.
For workers studying xenobiotics the two most important
organ perfusion systems are those for the liver and the lungs.
The liver is probably the most frequently perfused organ and is
used for a wide variety of studies. The techniques for liver
perfusion presently most frequently used are those developed by
Miller *et al*. (7) as illustrated in Figure 1. The apparatus
designed by Miller and co-workers is now commercially available.
Techniques for perfusion of the lung have been more recently
developed, the system of Niemeier and Bingham (8) being most frequently referred to by workers in this area (9). Niemeier and
Bingham developed a system for the perfusion of rabbit lungs which
allows the use of undiluted autologous whole blood as the perfusate. Lung perfusion is more complicated than liver since one is
able to provide both a circulating liquid perfusate as well as
being able to ventilate the isolated lung with a gas system. In

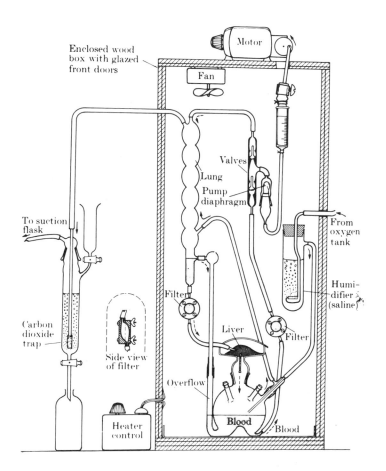

Journal of Experimental Medicine

*Figure 1. Liver perfusion apparatus. The apparatus is enclosed in a temperature-regulated cabinet and is composed of a system for pumping the perfusate (blood) at constant hydrostatic pressure and a system for oxygenating the blood (7, 12).*

a lung, therefore, one can introduce a xenobiotic to the system either through the perfusion system itself or through the gas ventilating system, thus approximating the introduction of the xenobiotic either through the circulatory system or the respiratory system in the whole animal. The use of lung perfusion is particularly advantageous because the estimation of substrate utilization by the lung is very difficult *in vivo*. Lung tissue slices or other *in vitro* preparations do not seem to approximate the physiological state of the whole organ as well as comparable preparations from the liver; the need for oxygen and the problem of diffusion are particular problems in the lung. Isolated perfused lung systems overcome these problems and will be particularly useful in the future for the study of the metabolism by the lung of xenobiotics introduced by inhalation.

Xenobiotic metabolism in perfused liver may be illustrated with parathion. Both parathion and paraoxon were studied to assess the metabolic relationships of these compounds in the liver (3). It was shown that 68% of the administered parathion was metabolized to water soluble compounds. These water soluble compounds were found to be conjugates of p-nitrophenol, the bulk of which was in the circulating perfusate, not associated with the liver tissue or excreted via the bile. An additional 2.5% was paraoxon and there were traces of unconjugated p-nitrophenol. Administered paraoxon was degraded almost entirely (98.5%) to water soluble compounds, which again were conjugates of p-nitrophenol.

Another type of experiment possible using perfused organ systems is illustrated by a study of mirex-induced suppression of biliary excretion of polychlorinated biphenyls (5). In this study it was shown that 50 mg/kg/day of mirex-pretreatment of the rats whose livers were perfused suppressed the biliary excretion of 4-chlorobiphenyl and its metabolites by 92%. Furthermore, the rate of metabolism of 4-chlorobiphenyl was decreased slightly by mirex pretreatment. The reason for this phenomenon was theorized to be that transport of otherwise readily excretable metabolites from the hepatocytes into the bile canaliculi was affected by mirex. The fact that mirex causes changes in the ability of the liver to excrete xenobiotics has implications for the possible effect of this compound on the toxicology of other compounds.

A number of recent studies of xenobiotics in perfused lung systems have been reported: aldrin and dieldrin (6), parathion, methadone, imipramine, chlorcyclizine, and pentobarbital (4), trichloroethylene (2), and carbaryl (1). These studies illustrate well the potential for important results which can be obtained from organ perfusion studies.

Perfused rabbit lungs were used to study the metabolism and binding properties of aldrin and dieldrin. The compounds were added to the system via the perfusion medium and samples were withdrawn at several intervals. It was noted that aldrin was epoxidized to dieldrin, but dieldrin was not further metabolized

in the system; no epoxide hydrase activity could be detected.
The uptake of aldrin and dieldrin was by diffusion. The rate of
uptake was biphasic, consisting of an initial rapid phase followed by a slower one, related to conversion of aldrin to dieldrin
in the case of aldrin. These studies show that the lungs are
not a significant storage site for either compound (6).

The metabolism of parathion, methadone, imipramine, chlorcyclizine, and pentobarbital was compared in a rabbit perfused
lung preparation with rabbit lung and liver microsomal preparations. In the perfused lung parathion, methadone, and pentobarbital were oxidatively metabolized. Parathion was extensively
metabolized to paraoxon and water soluble metabolites, which were
not further identified. No accumulation of parathion was observed in the system. With increasing perfusion time there was a
decrease in the appearance of parathion, methadone, and pentobarbital metabolites. This was more likely associated with
decreasing substrate or depletion of cofactor than to denaturation or destruction of the lung system. No significant differences were observed between the drug metabolizing activities of
the microsomes of lung or liver and the perfused lung system (4).

An interesting example of the use of the perfused lung
system to study the metabolism of a xenobiotic by the inhalation
route is given by Dalbey and Bingham (2). They studied the
metabolism of trichloroethylene in a rabbit perfused lung system.
Trichloroethylene was generated into the air supplied to the
isolated perfused lungs, and the compound and its metabolites
were measured periodically in the perfusate and in the lung
tissue following a three-hour perfusion period. Trichloroethylene
was extensively metabolized to trichloroethanol, trichloroethanol
glucuronide, and trichloroacetic acid. It was postulated that
chloral hydrate was an intermediate in the metabolism of trichloroethylene but it was not isolated in this system.

Carbaryl metabolism in the perfused rabbit lung was shown to
be rapid. The pharmacokinetics of carbaryl uptake demonstrated
simple diffusion. After 30 minutes of perfusion 1-naphthol was
seen in the perfusate extracts. Since its concentration in the
perfusate decreased during the course of the experiment, it was
concluded that the 1-naphthol which was taken up by the lungs was
formed by nonenzymatic hydrolysis of carbaryl in the perfusate.
4-Hydroxycarbaryl appeared in the perfusate at 30 minutes and increased in concentration until 60 minutes, after which it decreased. Other metabolites were isolated but no attempt was made
to identify them (1).

Comparative studies (10) have shown that perfused organs,
especially the liver, parallel changes which occur in the whole
organism. Thus, the technique can be a useful bridge between
other *in vitro* studies and *in vivo* studies.

## Tissue Slices

The techniques for tissue slice studies of metabolism were probably first introduced by Otto Warburg in 1923 (19). The method caught on rapidly and was used by many workers so extensively that Krebs and Henseleit, writing in 1932 (15), noted that between the two methods available for studying metabolism in animal tissues, they preferred tissue slices over perfusion. This judgment probably represented a reaction to the lack of reproducibility of perfusion techniques and the complicated systems then in use. By comparison, tissue slices coupled with manometry offered a simple, producible, flexible method for studying metabolism. While the judgment made by Krebs and Henseleit would probably not be valid today, the intervening years have seen a great deal of fine work using the isolated tissue slice technique.

Again, the liver is the principal organ which has been studied using tissue slices. However, many other organs have also been used in a variety of studies. Of particular note for xenobiotic metabolism studies in addition to the liver are kidneys, lungs, and intestines. The key to the preparation of viable tissue slices is to obtain reproducible, thin slices, generally less than 0.5 mm thick. This is most frequently done at present using a microtome or similar instrument. The viability of the tissue and standardization to determine reproducibility are frequently evaluated using Warburg respirometry (16).

Thin slice techniques have been used extensively for the study of pesticide metabolism, and examples of a variety of studies follow. One of the earliest establishments of the need for conversion of an organophosphorus insecticide to an active anticholinesterase metabolite used the liver slice technique in combination with Warburg respirometry (14). Liver slices were used to demonstrate the conversion of dimefox, a phosphoramidate, to an active inhibitor using rat brain cholinesterase as the substrate. Inhibition of cholinesterase was measured in the Warburg apparatus, and inhibition of cholinesterase was taken as indirect evidence for metabolism of dimefox by the liver slice. Liver slices 0.5 mm thick and 5 mm square, washed twice with 0.9% sodium chloride, were used in each Warburg flask. Substrate and enzyme sources were added from side arms, and cholinesterase inhibition was assayed by standard methodology.

The herbicides propham and chloropropham were studied in the rat *in vivo* and metabolism was compared in liver slices and kidney slices (13). These herbicides were metabolized *in vivo* to two major and three minor metabolites; both oxidative and hydrolytic mechanisms were evident. Liver and kidney slices, however, did not hydrolyze the chain moiety as observed *in vitro*. Only liver slices converted the herbicides to their oxidative metabolites.

Rat renal cortical slices and rat liver slices were used to assess the mechanism for excretion of dichlorodiphenylacetic acid (DDA) from animals (18). It was hypothesized that DDA is excreted

via the organic acid system.  It was shown that DDA was avidly
accumulated by liver and by kidney slices.  DDT or organic bases
did not inhibit the accumulation of DDA, indicating that the
organic acid excretion system is indeed responsible for the elimination of DDA from the mammalian system.  This ultimately, of
course, is the method for the elimination of DDT from the system
since DDT is first converted to DDA before it is excreted.

An interesting study of carbaryl metabolism has been reported
using an isolated intestinal tissue (17).  For this study the
small intestine between the bile duct and the cecum was removed
from male rats, rinsed in isotonic saline, and divided into three
approximately equal parts.  The sections were everted and maintained over ice in fresh saline plus glucose solution until the
serosal compartment was filled with serosal fluid.  The filled
sacs were then transferred to a flask containing mucosal fluid
and incubated with agitation for one or two hours.  Analysis of
the products of carbaryl incubation indicated the production of
1-naphthol, again apparently by nonenzymatic mechanisms.  At least
seven metabolites were identified.  The principal water soluble
metabolite (60%) was 1-naphthol glucuronide.

Although much useful information about xenobiotic metabolism
has been obtained with liver slice techniques, most workers today
prefer to use other methods, probably because of difficulties of
reproducibility using the technique.

## Cell Culture

Mammalian cells in culture have been used for over one-half
century to study various aspects of biology.  Since Harrison first
successfully propagated medullary tissue *in vitro* in 1907, cell
cultures have been utilized in the study of radiobiology, cell
division, and genetic cytology as well as other areas of cell biology.  Mammalian cell cultures have also been used to study the
correlation of cytotoxicity of drugs with other pharmacological
attributes.  The primary use of cell cultures has been to provide
a method for investigating the direct action of drugs and other
chemicals on cells in the absence of the complex interactions
which apply in the whole animal.  A high correlation, for example,
has been found between *in vitro* cytotoxicity and *in vivo* antitumor
activity of a number of chemotherapeutic agents screened for anti-
cancer activity.

A wide variety of cell types have been cultured and maintained *in vitro*.  Both normal cells from many different organs and
tissues of many different animal species and abnormal cells isolated from tumors or other abnormal tissues have been utilized.
Cells have been successfully explanted from animals in all stages
of development, from the embryo to the adult.

One of the problems which must be recognized in working with
cell cultures is the difference which is likely to exist between
these cell strains and the tissue from which they originated.

Cell strains or cell lines, so called, consist of cells which may have been growing *in vitro* for a considerable length of time and which have undergone many subcultures or dilutions of cell numbers. Generally they have a different pattern of metabolism, are capable of supporting the growth of a wide variety of viruses and microorganisms, and are frequently polyploid. Such divergences from normal tissue must be considered when evaluating experimental results.

Some of the difficulties in working with cell lines are eliminated by working in primary cell cultures. These are cells which have not undergone even a single passage or subculture since having been explanted from the donor animal. Such cultures have been shown to retain enzymatic activities similar to those of the *in vivo* donor tissue. The activity usually lasts through a few initial subcultures before receding to decreased levels.

Cells of both types, cell lines and primary cell cultures, are commercially available. The techniques for maintaining and using cells are simple, although rigorous sterile technique is absolutely necessary to avoid contamination of cell cultures by invading microorganisms of all types. The media used for cell cultures are ideal for the growth of microorganisms, which, if they contaminate the cultures, lead to artifacts in the experimental results. Rigorous attention to sterile technique is a prerequisite to accurate interpretation of the results of research using cell cultures.

Only a few papers appear in the literature reporting the results of studies of pesticide metabolism in cultured mammalian cells. The various studies have used human embryonic lung L-132 cells, HeLa S cells, mouse fibroblast L-929 cells, and mouse L-5178 lymphoma cells. All of these are established cell lines. In addition, studies have been conducted using primary human embryonic lung cells.

DDT metabolism has been studied in HeLa S cells [22], mouse L-5178 lymphoma cells [29], and primary human embryonic lung cells [28]. The variation in the susceptibility of a compound to metabolism by various cell types is illustrated in these studies. Mouse lymphoma cells grown for 72 hours in the presence of DDT failed to metabolize the compound. At the other end of the spectrum, HeLa S cells metabolized DDT to DDD, DDE, DBM, and DBP. DDE was the metabolite present in the highest quantity after 24 hours of incubation and was postulated to be the terminal metabolite in this system. It is noted in the paper, however, that the conversion of DDT to DDE could have been enhanced by the iron porphyrin complexes in the medium. Primary human embryonic lung cells metabolized DDT only to DDD (38%) and DDA (4%). No other metabolites were found in this cell culture system.

Carbaryl has been studied in both a human embryonic lung cell line, the L-132 strain [20, 21] and in primary human embryonic lung cells [23]. The HEL cell line was apparently active in conjugating carbaryl metabolites. The water soluble aglycones re-

sulting from beta-glucuronidase and aryl sulfatase treatment were
4-hydroxycarbaryl and 5,6-dihydro-5,6-dihydroxycarbaryl.  In
addition, hydroxylation at the C-4 position in conjunction with
hydrolysis of the carbamate group resulted in the formation of
naphthalene-1,4-diol.  The interesting metabolite, 1-naphthyl
methylcarbamate-$N$-glucuronide, was also reported in this study.
The results obtained in primary HEL cells agreed very closely
with those from the HEL cell line.  In the primary cell cultures
1-naphthol was the principal metabolite isolated.  Others included naphthalene-1,4-diol, naphthalene-1,5-diol, 4-hydroxycarbaryl,
5-hydroxycarbaryl, and 5,6-dihydro-5,6-dihydroxycarbaryl.  In
addition significant amounts of the administered carbaryl were
present in extracts as conjugates.  Acid hydrolysis freed 4-
hydroxycarbaryl, naphthalene-1,4-diol, and 5,6-dihydro-5,6-di-
hydroxycarbaryl.  On the other hand, beta-glucuronidase treatment
of the aqueous material did not free aglycones.  This result was
in agreement with the earlier work in which Baron and Locke postulated the formation of an $N$-glucuronide in the cell culture
system.  The use of both primary and established HEL cells is an
important link in understanding the metabolism of carbaryl in
mammalian systems.

The utility and value of cell culture studies is illustrated
well by a study of dimethoate metabolism in primary human embryonic lung cells (27).  In this study the cells were shown to
oxidize dimethoate with no interference from competing hydrolytic
reactions.  Thus, the progression of dimethoate metabolism from
the phosphorodithioate to the phosphorothioate, concomitant with
oxidative $N$-dimethylation of both the phosphorodithioate and
phosphorothioate, could be demonstrated (Figure 2).  The relationships existing between these three metabolites and their parent
compound could not be established so well in a system in which
hydrolytic reaction were competing with the oxidative ones.

Studies of the acaracide chlorphenamidine (24), and the
related phenylurea herbicides, chlorotoluron, fluometuron, and
metobromuron, (25) revealed striking differences in the susceptibility of these materials to metabolism by the cells.  On the
one hand, chlorphenamidine was very susceptible to oxidative
metabolism in HEL cells with the formation of nearly 82% of the
$N$-formyl metabolite and 2% of 4-chloro-$o$-toluidine as well as
small quantities of other metabolites.  While the herbicides were
very resistant to metabolism (less than 2% of the applied compound
was metabolized in 72 hours in each case), the small quantities
of metabolites that were formed were the result of oxidative
reactions in cells.  It was in this cell culture system that the
formation of $N$-formyl derivatives of chlorotoluron was first observed, a result later corroborated in liver microsomal preparations and in rats *in vivo* (26).  The chromatographic behavior
of the formyl derivatives made their detection difficult in
systems which more actively metabolized the compound because of
interfering materials on thin layer chromatographic plates.

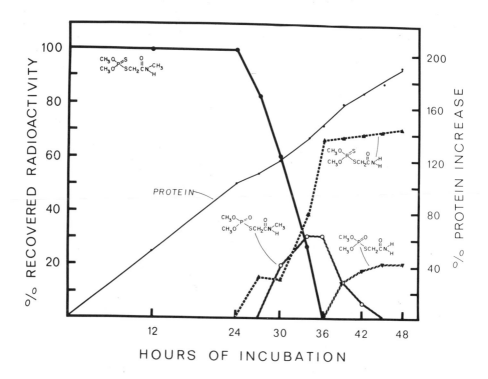

*Figure 2. Dimethoate disappearance, organoextractable metabolite formation, and percentage of protein increase in HEL cell cultures incubated with $^{14}$C-dimethoate. Disappearance of dimethoate corresponds with the appearance of the des-N-methyl metabolite and the oxygen analog, which in turn disappears corresponding with the increase of its des-N-methyl derivative (27).*

Cell culture techniques are useful in the study of xenobiotic metabolism.  They cannot be used to establish quantitative
relationships between xenobiotics and their metabolites, particularly when reference to the whole animal is desired, but they
can be invaluable in studying the mechanisms of metabolism and
in characterizing metabolites which may appear in only minor
quantities in other mammalian systems.

## Isolated Hepatocytes

The preparation and use of isolated hepatocytes is a recent
innovation in the study of xenobiotic metabolism and should prove
to be most useful.  The technique is basically a simple one.
Liver cells are dissociated from the protein matrix of the organ
and are isolated in viable condition for use much as if they were
isolated cells in culture as described earlier.  A variety of
methods have been developed for the isolation of hepatocytes,
although the techniques have not yet reached the routine stage so
that all researchers agree on the same basic methodology for
their preparation.  Earlier techniques involved either (1) the perfusion of liver with calcium chelators or alkaline hyperosmolar
salt solutions, (2) the digestion of liver pieces in tetraphenyl-
boron, a potassium chelator, (3) the use of enzymes as dissociat-
ing agents, notably trypsin for fetal or neonatal material, and
(4) collagenase/hyaluronidase digestion.  Various combinations of
these techniques have also been tried (40).  Currently there
appear to be basically two methods for the preparation of hepatocytes in general use.  One involves the perfusion of isolated
liver with Hank's buffer for approximately 15 minutes followed by
the addition of collagenase to the perfusate for an additional 10
to 15 minutes.  This treatment collapses the liver, after which
it is minced, centrifuged, washed, and resuspended in Hank's
buffer for immediate use (45, 46, 47).  The other technique eliminates the necessity for perfusion and uses enzymatic dissociation by treatment of liver with collagenase/hyaluronidase in
Hank's balanced salt solution followed by centrifugation, washing,
and resuspension (32, 40).  The latter technique has the advantage of simplicity and low cost since no special perfusion apparatus is needed.  Furthermore, it would be possible to prepare
hepatocytes from pieces of fresh liver which might, for example,
be available from biopsies without the need for the whole organ
as required in the perfusion technique.  Both techniques appear
to give good yields of viable cells which can be used for metabolism studies.  As for most *in vitro* methods, most of the early
developmental work on isolation of viable hepatocytes has been
done with rat livers.  However, there is no reason why the techniques developed cannot be applied to the livers of other species
as well, perhaps with very little modification.  In fact chicken
hepatocytes have been isolated using the rat liver techniques and
were shown to carry out normal biochemical functions (37, 38).

The criteria of viability of isolated liver cells are a
matter of considerable concern for metabolism studies since reproducibility demands a technique for standardization of preparations made at different times or by different methods. The
most universally used technique to assess viability of isolated
hepatocytes is the trypan blue exclusion test (31, 45). The test
depends on the fact that the intact plasma membrane excludes dyes
such as trypan blue, but damaged cells are stained, particularly
intensely in the nucleus. Unfortunately, this actually measures
structural integrity, not viability *per se*. Other tests have
been used in addition, including electron microscopy, the content
of adenine nucleotides, the activities of various enzymes, and
the ability to synthesize various compounds. It seems to this
reviewer that one must establish for his own type of experiments
whether the cells are viable using criteria particularly applicable to the type of research being conducted. For example, in
a metabolism study one might choose a particular substrate which
could be used as a positive control in all preparations, whose
metabolism could be conveniently measured and quantified for
comparison between various preparations.

It is somewhat surprising to report that no studies have yet
been published involving the metabolism of a pesticide in isolated hepatocytes. However, the technique has been widely applied in studies of drug metabolism and several reports on the
metabolism of air pollutants and industrial chemicals have now
appeared. Examples of drug metabolism studies are the reports of
Billings *et al.* (33) on α-1-acetylmethadol, propoxyphene, buta-
moxane, ethinimate, 8-methoxybutamoxane, and *p*-nitrophenol;
Erickson and Holtzman (39) on ethylmorphine; Hayes and Brendel
(42) on quinine sulfate, dansylamide, and antipyrine; and
Aarbakke *et al.* (30) on antipyrine. In general, the drugs studied were metabolized by the isolated hepatocytes by *N*- and *O*-
demethylation, aromatic and aliphatic hydroxylation, and sulfate
and glucuronic acid conjugation. These studies show that the
metabolism of drugs in isolated hepatocytes correlates with *in
vivo* drug metabolism better than does the liver homogenate 9000*g*
supernatant or microsomal fraction. The results obtained from
hepatocytes were more comparable to liver perfusions than to subcellular fractions in terms of the relative rates of individual
reactions, which were sometimes faster and sometimes slower in
hepatocytes than in microsomes.

Aromatic hydrocarbons are readily hydroxylated by isolated
hepatocytes (34, 35, 43). Bock and co-workers showed that naphthalene was converted to 1-naphthol and to 1,2-dihydro-1,2-di-
hydroxynaphthalene and its sulfate and glucuronic acid conjugates
(34). The isolated hepatocytes were more efficient in carrying
out these conversions than microsomes, the reason being that the
enzymes responsible, mixed function oxygenase, epoxide hydratase,
and glucuronyl transferase, are all located in the same membranes. Benzo(a)pyrene was converted into arene oxides, phenols,

quinones, and dihydrodiols as initial products and later sulfate, glucuronide, and glutathione conjugates were isolated (35). The monohydroxylated compounds and sulfate esters accumulated intracellularly, the 4,5- and 7,8-dihydrodiols were distributed evenly between the cells and the medium, and the 9,10-dihydrodiol accumulated in the medium. In these experiments significant amounts of radioactivity were bound irreversibly to cellular macromolecules (43).

The sequential formation of metabolites by isolated hepatocytes is illustrated by studies on the 4-hydroxylation of biphenyl and the subsequent conjugation of the metabolite (44). Figure 3 illustrates the fact that hydroxylation preceded glucuronide formation and that the removal of 4-hydroxybiphenyl by conjugation was necessary to stimulate a second phase of hydroxylation.

Fry *et al.* (41) have compared isolated cells from rat liver and kidney in terms of their ability to metabolize ethoxycoumarin, biphenyl, benzo(a)pyrene, 4-methylumbelliferone, and benzoic acid. The level of metabolism in the kidney cell suspension was extremely low compared with liver cells for initial oxidative reactions, but the pattern and extent of conjugations were very similar between the two types of cells. The difference in the ability of these cells to metabolize these compounds may relate to a different specificity of the renal cytochrome P-450, which is not adapted to xenobiotic metabolism.

The ability to retain active cytochrome P-450 in isolated hepatocytes is crucial to the use of this system to study xenobiotic metabolism. Cytochrome P-450 declines rapidly in isolated hepatocytes, but recently it was discovered that the addition of certain hormones to a primary hepatocyte culture retained the cytochrome P-450 activity at optimum levels for up to 24 hours (36). These workers used primary hepatocyte cultures derived from collagenase preparation with added hormones to study the metabolism of aflatoxin $B_1$.

Although isolated hepatocytes have not as yet been extensively used in metabolism studies, they clearly offer great promise in this area.

## Conclusion

When one compares the various *in vitro* techniques used to study the fate of xenobiotics in mammals, one must be impressed by the fact that no one of the methods available is adequate to a complete understanding of the metabolism of a compound. However, when all methods are taken together, a rather complete picture can be assembled. Using carbaryl, one of the most extensively studied pesticides, as an example, one can see that the total *in vitro* results rather completely mirror *in vivo* metabolism. In fact, certain metabolites found *in vitro* have not been isolated following *in vivo* studies, the *N*-glucuronide noted from cell

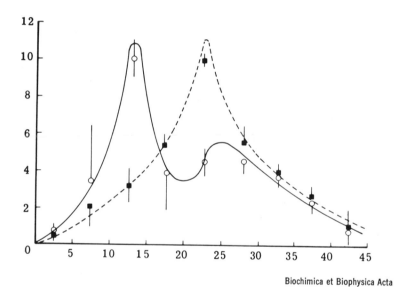

*Figure 3. Rate of formation of 4-hydroxybiphenyl and its glucuronide conjugate in viable isolated hepatocytes. The rates of formation of (○), 4-hydroxybiphenyl and (■), its glucuronide conjugate are average rates for the respective 5-min intervals. Each point represents the mean of three values obtained from different experiments (± S.D.) (44).*

cultures. The principal metabolite, 1-naphthol, is found in all systems studied. The 5,6-dihydro-5,6-diol, 5-hydroxy, 1,5-diol sequence is observed in cell cultures, while the 4-hydroxy metabolite is observed in perfused organs and cell cultures. The 1,4-diol was also isolated from cell cultures as were several glycoside conjugates.

One might compare the relative merits of the four techniques considered in this paper, adding microsomes to complete the picture, from four points of view: (1) ease of preparation, (2) flexibility of experimental use, (3) reproducibility of results, and (4) the extent to which the results obtained mirror *in vivo* results (Table I).

Table I. Relative merits of *in vitro* techniques for studying the metabolism of xenobiotics.

| | Microsomes | Organ Perfusion | Tissue Slices | Cell Culture | Isolated Hepatocytes |
|---|---|---|---|---|---|
| **Ease of Preparation** | | | | | |
| Requirement for Special Equipment | - | - | o | + | o |
| Requires special training of personnel | + | - | + | o | - |
| Time for preparation | - | o | + | + | - |
| Expense | + | + | + | - | + |
| **Flexability of Experimental Use** | - | o | - | + | + |
| **Reproducibility of Results** | + | + | o | + | + |
| **Mirrors *in vivo* results** | - | - | o | - | + |

+ Favorable, positive aspect of this technique
o Neutral
- Negative aspect of this technique

Although the assignment of values for each category is arbitrary and subjective, one must conclude from this exercise that each technique will be useful for some purposes in some researcher's hands. Ultimately our understanding of the fate of xenobiotics in mammals will be enhanced by accumulating data from all sources and applying each bit of data to obtain the complete picture.

Acknowledgement

Scientific Article No. A2519  Contribution No. 5551  of the Maryland Agricultural Experiment Station, Department of Entomology.

The author thanks Miss Figen Ünlü for her assistance in the preparation of this paper and Dr. Judd O. Nelson for his helpful advice in its development.

## Abstract

Techniques considered include isolated whole living cells; cell, organ, and tissue culture; organ slices; and isolated perfused organs. Whole cell techniques serve as an important link between studies using purified enzymes and subcellular fractions and studies using whole organisms. The use of cells, tissues, and organs in culture is growing since they allow the researcher to explore the nature of metabolites and to research an understanding of the mechanisms of metabolism taking place within the cells or organs without the complicating regulatory influences of the whole organism. Both primary cells in culture and established cell lines have been used to study xenobiotic degradation. Conversely, the effects of xenobiotics on the cell can also be conveniently studied. The combination of the two types of studies allows one to ascertain whether the cell's metabolism of a xenobiotic is accomplished by a healthy cell or as the result of or in combination with some cellular defect. The use of whole organs, such as perfused liver, provides the opportunity to extend a metabolism experiment over a longer period of time than is possible with either subcellular fractions or isolated cells. Whole organs or organ slices allow the introduction of a higher degree of cellular organization and differentiation than the single cell, but without the complications of external regulation. The use of isolated hepatocytes is a recent innovation in the study of xenobiotic metabolism and should be most useful.

## Literature Cited

### Perfused Organs

1. Blase, B. W., and Loomis, T. A.  Toxicol. Appl. Pharmacol.
   (1976) 37, 481.
2. Dalbey, W., and Bingham, E.  Toxicol. Appl. Pharmacol. (1978)
   43, 267.
3. Fuhremann, T. W., Lichtenstein, E. P., Zahlten, R. N.,
   Stratman, F. W., and Schnoes, H. K.  Pestic. Sci. (1974) 5,
   31.
4. Law, F. C. P., Eling, T. W., Bend, J. R., and Fouts, J. R.
   Drug Metab. Disp. (1974) 2, 433.
5. Mehendale, H. M.  Toxicol. Appl. Pharmacol. (1976) 36, 369.
6. Mehendale, H. M., and El-Bassiouni, E. A.  Drug Metab. Disp.
   (1975) 3, 543.
7. Miller, L. L., Bly, C. G., Watson, M. L., and Bale, W. F.  J.
   Exp. Med. (1951) 94, 431.

8.  Niemeier, R. W., and Bingham, E. Life Sci. (1972) 11, part
    II, 807.
9.  Orton, T. C., Anderson, M. W., Pickett, R. D., Eling, T. C.,
    and Fouts, J. R. J. Pharmacol. Exp. Therap. (1973) 186,
    482.
10. Popov, T. A., and Kagan, Y. S. Gig. Sanit. (1977) 40.
    [CA 87:904]
11. Ritchie, H. D., and Hardcastle, J. C. (eds.) "Isolated
    Organ Perfusion", University Park Press, Baltimore, 1973.
12. Ross, B. D., "Perfusion Techniques in Biochemistry",
    Clarendon Press, Oxford, 1972.

*Tissue Slices*

13. Fang, S. C., Fallin, E. and Freed, V. H. Toxicol. Appl.
    Pharmacol. (1973) 25, 493.
14. Fenwick, M. L., Barron, J. R. and Watson, W. A. Biochem. J.
    (1957) 65, 58.
15. Krebs, H. A., and Henseleit, K. Hoppe-Seyler's Z. Physiol.
    Chem. (1932) 210, 33.
16. O'Neil, J. J., Sanford, R. L., Wasserman, S., and Tierney,
    D. F. J. Appl. Physiol.: Respirat. Environ. Exercise
    Physiol. (1977) 43, 902.
17. Pekas, J. C. Am. J. Physiol. (1971) 220, 2008.
18. Pritchard, J. B. Toxicol. Appl. Pharmacol. (1976) 38, 621.
19. Warburg, O. Biochem. Z. (1923) 142, 317.

*Cell Culture*

20. Baron, R. L., and Locke, R. K. Bull. Environ. Contam.
    Toxicol. (1970) 5, 287.
21. Locke, R. K., Bastone, V. B., and Baron, R. L. J. Agr. Food
    Chem. (1971) 19, 1205.
22. Huang, E. A., Lu, J. Y., and Chung, R. A. Biochem. Pharmac.
    (1970) 19, 637.
23. Lin, T. H., North, H. H., and Menzer, R. E. J. Agr. Food
    Chem. (1975) 23, 253.
24. Lin, T. H., North, H. H., and Menzer, R. E. J. Agr. Food
    Chem. (1975) 23, 257.
25. Lin, T. H., Menzer, R. E., and North, H. H. J. Agr. Food
    Chem. (1976) 24, 756.
26. Muecke, W., Menzer, R. E., Alt, K. O., Richter, W., and
    Esser, H. O., Pestic. Biochem. Physiol. (1976) 6, 430.
27. North, H. H., and Menzer, R. E. Pestic. Biochem. Physiol.
    (1972) 2, 278.
28. North, H. H., and Menzer, R. E. J. Agr. Food Chem. (1973)
    21, 509.
29. Spalding, J. W., Ford, E., Lane, D., and Blois, M. Biochem.
    Pharmacol. (1971) 20, 3185.

## Isolated Hepatocytes

30. Aarbakke, J., Bessesen, A., and Morland, J.   Acta Pharmacol.
    Toxicol. (1977) 41, 225.
31. Baur, H., Kasperek, S., and Pfaff, E.   Hoppe-Seyler's Z.
    Physiol. Chem. (1975) 356, 827.
32. Bellemann, P., Gebhardt, R., and Mecke, D.   Anal. Biochem.
    (1977) 81, 408.
33. Billings, R. E., McMahon, R. E., Ashmore, J., and Wagle, S.
    R.   Drug Metab. Disposition (1977) 5, 518.
34. Bock, K. W., VanAckeren, G., Lorch, F., and Birke, F. W.
    Biochem. Pharmacol. (1976) 25, 2351.
35. Burke, M. D., Vodi, H., Jernström, B., and Orrenius, S.   J.
    Biol. Chem. (1977) 252, 6424.
36. Decad, G. M., Hsieh, D. P. H., and Byard, J. L.   Biochem.
    Biophys. Res. Commun. (1977) 78, 279.
37. Dickson, A. J., and Langslow, D. R.   Biochem. Soc. Trans.
    (1975) 3, 1034.
38. Dickson, A. J., and Langslow, D. R.   Biochem. Soc. Trans.
    (1977) 5, 983.
39. Erickson, R. R., and Holtzman, J. L.   Biochem. Pharmacol.
    (1976) 25, 1501.
40. Fry, J. R., Jones, C. A., Wiebkin, P., Bellemann, P., and
    Bridges, J. W.   Anal. Biochem. (1976) 71, 341.
41. Fry, J. R., Wiebkin, P., Kao, J., Jones, C. A., Gwynn, J.,
    and Bridges, J. W.   Xenobiotica (1978) 8, 113.
42. Hayes, J. S., and Brendel, K.   Biochem. Pharmacol. (1976) 25,
    1495.
43. Jones, C. A., Moore, B. P., Cohen, G. M., Fry, J. R., Biochem.
    Pharmacol. (1978) 27, 693.
44. Jones, R. S., Mendis, D., and Parke, D. V.   Biochim. Biophys.
    Acta (1977) 500, 124.
45. Seglen, P. O.   "Methods in Cell Biology", D. M. Prescott
    (ed.), Vol. 8, Academic Press, New York, 1976, pp. 29-83.
46. Wagle, S. R.   Life Sci. (1975) 17, 827.
47. Wagle, S. R., and Ingebretsen, Jr., W. R.   Methods in
    Enzymol. (1975) 35, 579.

RECEIVED December 20, 1978.

# The Use of Animal Subcellular Fractions to Study Type I Metabolism of Xenobiotics[1]

RONALD W. ESTABROOK, JURGEN WERRINGLOER, and JULIAN A. PETERSON

Department of Biochemistry, Southwestern Medical School, University of Texas Health Science Center, Dallas, TX 75235

The genius of man has resulted in the synthesis of a vast number of organic compounds during the last century. The quest to seek new drugs, synthetic polymers for industrial use, insecticides and pesticides -- to name but a few areas of chemical development -- has provided both beneficial as well as detrimental results which touch the lives of each of us. The last decade has seen a surge of activity directed toward the evaluation of a wide array of organic chemicals which have the potential of negatively modifying the homeostasis of cells and organs. Nearly every day the popular press identifies yet another agent which can be shown in experimental animals or bacterial test systems to cause mutagenesis and cellular dysfunction or neoplasia. It is now well established that many of these chemicals are merely precursors of metabolic products which are the true causative agents of cellular changes. Therefore considerable effort is now being expended to identify and characterize the requisite enzyme systems responsible for the metabolic transformation of such chemicals.

The purpose of this presentation is to review the methodology employed and the results obtained when studying one such enzyme system -- an enzyme complex which has a broad specificity for the oxidative alteration of a variety of both natural and synthetic organic chemicals. Central to this enzyme complex is a family of hemeproteins called cytochromes P-450. It is the properties and reactions of this type of hemeprotein and its associated electron transport carrier proteins which will serve as the primary emphasis of the present report.

[1] Supported in part by a research grant from the United States Public Health Service National Institutes of Health (GM-16488).

The Characterization of Cytochrome P-450

Cytochrome P-450 is widely distributed in nature spanning
the phylogenetic tree from bacteria to the human organism. It
has been observed in yeast, flowering plants, insects, reptiles, birds and animals (1,2). Indeed, it is interesting that
the first report of cytochrome P-450 occurred as a consequence
of studying the respiratory pigments of the mid-gut of the
silkworm (3). The ease of detecting cytochrome P-450, using
spectrophotometric methods to assess the characteristic absorbance band of the carbon monoxide adduct of the reduced hemeprotein, has greatly facilitated the quantitative evaluation of
this cellular pigment (4,5). In organisms other than some
specialized bacteria, cytochrome P-450 is a membrane bound
protein -- a property which until recently has rendered it
refractory to isolation and purification. Methodologies are
now available, however, which permit the solubilization and
stabilization of the hemeprotein permitting its characterization as a homogeneous protein species.

It is possible to generalize and identify two basic types
of cytochrome P-450 depending on the associated electron
transport carrier proteins responsible for transferring electrons (reducing equivalents) from reduced pyridine nucleotides
to the hemeprotein. As shown in Figure 1, we have designated
these as Class A or B. The Class A type of cytochrome P-450 is
found associated with the mitochrondria of many cell types
where it functions together with an iron-sulfur protein and a
flavoprotein (6). The reactions of cholesterol metabolism in
steroidogenic organs such as the adrenal, testis, and placenta
are catalyzed by this class of cytochromes P-450.

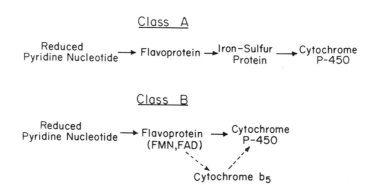

Figure 1.   Two general classes of cytochrome P-450 based on the type of electron
carriers functional in the transfer of reducing equivalents from reduced pyridine
nucleotides

Best characterized (7,8) are the reactions for the oxidative
degradation of camphor by the bacterium Pseudomonas putida
where this class of cytochrome P-450 plays a key role in the
initiation of the metabolism of this complex molecule.

The Class B type of cytochromes P-450 is generally associated with the endoplasmic reticulum (or its membrane equivalent) where it functions in concert with a flavoprotein which
contains both FMN and FAD as prosthetic groups (9-11).  This
class of cytochrome P-450 is generally found associated with a
second hemeprotein, cytochrome $b_5$.  Although the role of
cytochrome $b_5$ in the cyclic function of cytochrome P-450 (see
below) is controversial, the parallelism of cellular association lends credence to its possible action as an electron
transport carrier required for reduction of an intermediate
formed during the course of cytochrome P-450 reactions.

The description provided in a later section of this presentation will emphasize those reactions of cytochrome P-450
which occur during its interaction with the substrate to be
metabolized as well as molecular oxygen.  A common pattern has
emerged for the sequence of reaction steps involving cytochrome
P-450 whether it is the pigment of either Class A or B.  The
principal difference resides in the manner of donation of
electrons transported from reduced pyridine nucleotide rather
than the reaction intermediates formed during oxygen activation
and substrate transformation.

## Methodologies of Study

An evaluation of the reactions occurring during the mixed
function oxidation of many xenobiotics requires a suitable
source of the enzyme system as well as appropriate instrumental
apparatus.  The most frequently employed enzyme system which
has been studied in greatest detail is the one associated with
the microsomal fraction of liver.  This organ source is rich
in the electron transport carriers which function in the
activation of oxygen for xenobiotic metabolism, in part because
of the role of the liver in serving as the primary recipient
of chemicals absorbed from the intestinal tract.  Further the
requisite enzyme constituents, notably cytochrome P-450, are
rapidly synthesized in liver as a result of exposure of animals
to various inducing agents such as barbiturates or polycyclic
hydrocarbons.  Thus, the content and composition of cytochromes
and flavoproteins associated with liver microsomes can be
readily altered to permit biologically differing conditions
which assist in the delineation of the pattern of enzymatic
reactions occurring.  Studies with liver microsomes have
served as the pattern for comparable studies of xenobiotic
metabolism in other tissues such as the lung, kidney, intestine,
etc.

The Preparation of Liver Microsomes. Rather standard
techniques of differential centrifugation of liver homogenates
have been developed for routine use in the preparation of
microsomal fractions for study.

Most important is the need to recognize the multitude of
factors which can influence the subsequent experimental results
obtained when using this source of the enzyme system. The
investigator should be cognizant of the variations introduced
when using animals that are not controlled for alterations
resulting from diet, inadvertent exposure to inducers (such as
insecticides commonly used indiscriminately in animal quarters)
and stress to name but a few. Further, the choice of age,
sex, species, and genetic characteristics all introduce
variables which lead to differences in the enzymatic characteristics measured.

In general animals are decapitated and the livers perfused
in situ with cold isotonic saline to remove as much blood as
possible. After homogenization in the presence of a polyhydroxy compound, such as 0.25 M sucrose, the microsomal fraction
is isolated by differential centrifugation after first removing
unbroken cells, nuclei, and mitochondria. If precautions are
taken, the enzyme activity of microsomes isolated in this way
remains relatively stable for 48 to 72 hrs.

The Spectrophotometric Analysis of Microsomal Pigments.
The microsomal fraction is composed of membrane vesicles
originating from disruption of the endoplasmic reticulum.
Therefore special instrumentation should be employed to accurately evaluate the spectrophotometric properties of the
hemeproteins associated with these turbid membrane suspensions.
A number of different types of commercial spectrophotometers
are available for the measurement of difference spectra when
using samples that have high light scattering characteristics.
A schematic diagram for one such instrument is shown in Figure
2. Basically, the principal involved requires light from a
tungsten filament lamp to be appropriately attenuated and
dispersed by a split grating to generate two beams of mono-
chromatic light which can impinge on a pair of cuvettes containing the membrane fragments to be analyzed. These cuvettes
are positioned near the surface of the light detector to
include the greatest solid angle of scattered transmitted
light. Suitable electronic demodulation permits the accurate
evaluation of differences in light absorption between the
pigments in a sample cuvette minus those in the reference
cuvette. Coupled together with wavelength scanning capabilities, the difference absorbance spectrum can be readily
obtained. In addition to the capability of recording difference spectra, using the "split-beam" mode, such an instrument can be modified to measure the kinetics of absorbance
changes at a predetermined wavelength, relative to a

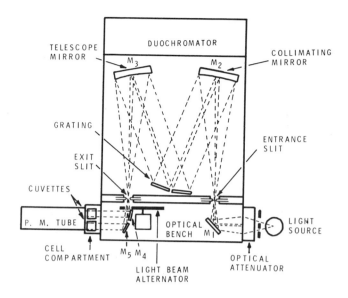

TELESCOPE MIRROR

DUOCHROMATOR

COLLIMATING MIRROR

$M_3$

$M_2$

GRATING

ENTRANCE SLIT

EXIT SLIT

CUVETTES

P. M. TUBE

OPTICAL BENCH $M_1$

LIGHT SOURCE

CELL COMPARTMENT

$M_5$ $M_4$

LIGHT BEAM ALTERNATOR

OPTICAL ATTENUATOR

American Instrument Company

*Figure 2. Representation of the duochromator optical configuration of the Aminco-DW2a spectrophotometer in the split-beam mode (12)*

reference wavelength (usually an isosbestic point), as a function of time. A number of articles have been written describing the application of this methodology and many of the pitfalls and limits which may influence the interpretation of such spectrophotometric techniques (13,14).

Determination of Reaction Products. Measurements of the overall rates of xenobiotic metabolic transformations have been limited in the past to the colorimetric evaluation of products that can be readily derivatized or made reactive in coupled enzymatic oxidation-reduction reactions. For example, formaldehyde is easily measured colorimetrically during the N- or O-demethylation of many drug substrates (15). Other compounds, such as polycyclic hydrocarbons, form fluorescent products during metabolism and these can be readily quantitatively measured (16,17,18). In other cases radioactive compounds can be employed and use of differential solubility, as a consequence of the more hydrophilic characteristics of the metabolic products, provides an additional means of evaluating reaction rates (19).

In recent years the introduction of high pressure liquid chromatography has opened a new and powerful method for product identification. This method is rapid, sensitive, and, with proper precautions, quantitative. One of the major new contributions to our knowledge of xenobiotic metabolism, which has resulted from the application of HPLC methods, is the recognition that multiple products are formed and that initial products formed may be rapidly further metabolized to secondary or tertiary products (20,21,22). The more general application of this methodology will undoubtedly have a profound influence on the current rather simplistic viewpoint which prevails regarding the oxidative transformation of many organic compounds.

## The Cyclic Function of Cytochrome P-450

The primary function of cytochrome P-450 is to interact with molecular oxygen in a manner that permits the cleavage of the oxygen molecule to form an atom of oxygen with electrophilic characteristics. This "activated oxygen" is then presumed to react with a molecule of the organic substrate, which is at or near the site of oxygen bound to the hemeprotein, so that the substrate molecule is transformed to a higher oxidation state. This may be evaluated, for example, by the formation of an epoxide with aromatic compounds, by the N- or O-dealkylation of secondary or tertiary amines as well as ethers, or by the incorporation of oxygen into alkanes. Many of the reaction steps for the mixed function oxidation of substrates have been delineated and the reactive intermediates characterized. The following description briefly summarizes our current state of knowledge of these reactions.

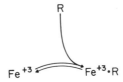

*Figure 3*

The Interaction of Substrate. The initial step in the function of cytochrome P-450 is the binding of the organic substrate to be metabolized to the oxidized form of the hemeprotein, as illustrated in Figure 3. Associated with this interaction is a change in the properties of the heme of cytochrome P-450. In the absence of a substrate molecule, the heme is in the low-spin, hexacoordinate form and it is characterized by an optical absorbance spectrum with a major absorbance band whose maximum is about 418 nm (Figure 4). The presence of a single unpaired electron in the ferric iron of low spin cyto-

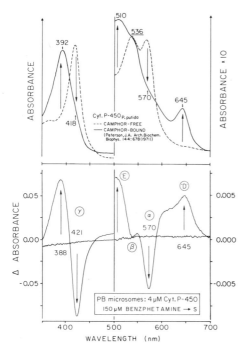

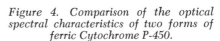

Acta Biologica et Medica Germanica

Figure 4. Comparison of the optical spectral characteristics of two forms of ferric Cytochrome P-450.

(Top) The absolute spectra of soluble Cytochrome P-450 isolated from Pseudomonas putida in the presence and absence of the substrate camphor (23). (Bottom) The difference spectra obtained when benzphetamine interacts with Cytochrome P-450 of liver microsomes (24).

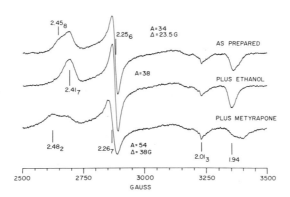

Annals of the New York Academy of Sciences

Figure 5. EPR spectra of Cytochrome P-450 of liver microsomes and the influence of ethanol and the dipyridyl derivative, metyrapone. Rat liver microsomes from phenobarbital treated animals were examined using an E-4 Varian EPR spectrometer (29).

chrome P-450 renders it paramagnetic.  This is reflected by an
electron paramagnetic resonance spectrum (shown in its first
derivative form) of the type illustrated in Figure 5.  Considerable interest and debate has centered on the interpretation
of this EPR spectrum and the possible presence of unique
ligands, such as sulfur, coordinated to the heme of cytochrome
P-450 (25,26,27,28).

The addition of an excess of substrate (R) to be metabolized, to cytochrome P-450 results in a marked change in the
absorbance spectrum of the ferric hemeprotein (Figure 4)
leading to a pigment with its major absorbance band located at
about 390 nm.  The basis for this hypsochromic effect of the
substrate on the spectral properties of oxidized cytochrome P-
450 is related to the spin state change of the heme iron.  This
is confirmed by the appearance of an absorbance with a g value
of about 8 when the substrate complexed form of ferric cytochrome P-450 is examined by low temperature EPR spectroscopy
methods (30,31).  One interpretation of these changes in the
physical properties of the heme protein is the binding of the
organic substrate molecule in the hydrophilic heme pocket of
the hemeprotein, thereby perturbing the electron density distribution of the heme to form the pentacoordinate, high-spin
complex (32,33).  Such an interpretation (supported by studies
using spin-labeled organic compounds (34)) would place the
substrate molecule in close proximity to the heme iron and thus
in a spatial configuration where it is appropriately located
for interaction with the "active oxygen" generated during the
cycle of cytochrome P-450 function.

The optical spectral changes associated with substrate
binding provide a rather simple technique to measure this first
step in cytochrome P-450 action.  Since many systems under
study involve the membrane bound form of cytochrome P-450, the
technique of difference absorbance spectrophotometry has been
applied (see discussion in Section II).  As illustrated in
Figure 6, the addition of increasing concentrations of a substrate (in this example, the steroid androstanedione has been
added to a cytochrome P-450 containing preparation of liver
microsomes) results in a progressive decrease in absorbance
at about 420 nm concomitant with an increase in absorbance
at about 385 nm.  This form of absorbance change has been
termed "Type I" (36) and many substrates metabolized by
cytochrome P-450 can be shown to cause this alteration in
the spectral properties of the hemeprotein.  In a number of
instances, the magnitude of spectral change observed can be
related to the concentration of substrate added to the reaction mixture and one can then estimate the affinity of
cytochrome P-450 for each type of substrate examined.
However, a satisfactory interpretation of substrate interaction with ferric cytochrome P-450 (based solely on optical
absorbance difference spectrophotometry of the membrane

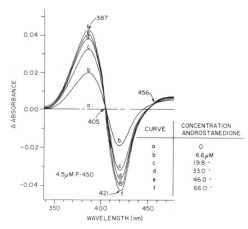

| CURVE | CONCENTRATION ANDROSTANEDIONE |
|-------|-------------------------------|
| a | 0 |
| b | 6.6 μM |
| c | 19.8 " |
| d | 33.0 " |
| e | 46.0 " |
| f | 66.0 " |

*Figure 6. Effect of increasing concentrations of substrate on the optical density changes observed during the spin state transition of ferric Cytochrome P-450.*

*Liver microsomes from phenobarbital treated rats were suspended to a protein concentration of 2 mg/mL. Various concentrations of androstanedione were added to the contents of the sample cuvette and the resultant difference spectra recorded.*

enzyme) is sometimes lacking. This is due in part to complications arising from the presence of "endogenous substrates" associated with the membrane fragments (24, 37–40), extraneous solvent effects which presumably alter the hydrophobic heme environment of the hemeprotein (41,42), as well as temperature dependent changes in the properties of the membrane (31).

The general concept that oxidized cytochrome P-450 reacts with the substrate to be metabolized as the first step in the function of the hemeprotein appears to be generally accepted. The detailed interpretation of the changes in the physical properties of the hemeprotein accompanying the binding of substrate remains largely speculative and serves as an area of research currently under active investigation.

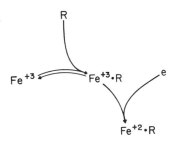

*Figure 7*

Reduction of cytochrome P-450. The complex of ferric
cytochrome P-450 with substrate undergoes a one electron reduction (Figure 7) to form the ferrous hemeprotein. In reactions
involving the Class A type of cytochrome P-450, this electron
is donated by a reduced iron-sulfur protein. The initial
source of this electron is from reduced pyridine nucleotides
(either NADPH or NADH depending on the system under study)
which interacts with a specific flavoprotein that serves also
as an iron-sulfur protein reductase ($\underline{6},\underline{43}$, $\underline{44}$). In the case of
the Class B type of cytochrome P-450, the flavoprotein, NADPH-
cytochrome P-450 reductase, mediates the transfer of the
electron from NADPH to the ferric hemeprotein ($\underline{45}$). This
flavoprotein has attracted a great deal of interest because of
its unusual property of containing two flavin prosthetic groups
(FMN and FAD) and the ability to generate stable free radical
forms of the enzyme during NADPH oxidation ($\underline{9},\underline{10},\underline{11}$). Recent
experiments have indicated that the sequence of electron trans-
port by this flavoprotein involves first the reduction of FAD
followed by the reduction of FMN ($\underline{46}$), i.e., a form of reduced
FMN is envisioned as the agent donating an electron to reduce
cytochrome P-450. However, the ability to form a number of
different states of reduction of this flavoprotein (Figure 8)
and the need to transfer only one electron for the reduction of
cytochrome P-450 ($\underline{47},\underline{48}$), leaves unresolved the possible role
of other free radical forms of the flavoprotein from partici-
pating in this or other reactions.

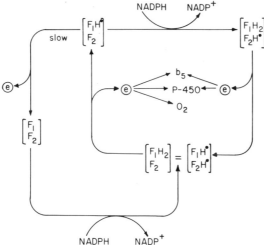

*Figure 8. Schematic proposal for the various states of reduction of the flavo-
protein, NADPH–Cytochrome P-450 reductase. $F_1$ is presumed to represent FAD
and $F_2$ to represent FMN. The existence of various free radical species is indicated.*

Table I

Concentration of Microsomal Electron Transfer Components

|  | P-450 | FMN | FAD | RATIO |
|---|---|---|---|---|
|  | nmoles/mg protein | | | P-450/FMN |
| RATS |  |  |  |  |
| control | 0.71 | 0.075 | 0.15 | 9.5 |
| phenobarbital |  |  |  |  |
| pretreatment | 2.1 | 0.08 | 0.13 | 26.3 |
| MICE |  |  |  |  |
| C57BL/6J | 0.51 | 0.021 | 0.094 | 24.3 |
| DBA/2J | 0.53 | 0.013 | 0.090 | 40.8 |

Recently interest has developed in the area of membrane structure and the spatial relationship of this flavoprotein to cytochrome P-450 (49). A consideration of the stoichiometry (Table I) of the flavoprotein to cytochrome P-450 reveals a surfeit of hemeprotein molecules relative to its electron donating partner. The problem becomes even more complex when considering the amphipathic properties of the flavoprotein and its physical location on the surface of the membrane (50-54). The potential role of membrane fluidity facilitating the "pinball" like motility of the flavoprotein as it services the dispersed pool of hemeprotein molecules is a hypothesis (55, 56) which stands in contrast to the proposal (49,57-59) of clusters or patches of multienzyme complexes based on hydrophobic interactions in the membrane. Clearly, a more detailed understanding of membrane structure is a prerequisite to the delineation of the process of reduction of the high spin form of oxidized cytochrome P-450 bound by substrate.

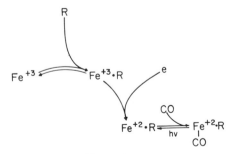

*Figure 9*

Reaction with Carbon Monoxide. Reduced cytochrome P-450 reacts rapidly with carbon monoxide (Figure 9) to form a complex which serves as the hallmark for this class of cellular pigment (60-62). A characteristic absorbance band (Figure 10) at about 450 nm (hence the name P-450) is associated with this complex. The chemical basis for the unique absorbance band at 450 nm for the carbon monoxide adduct of the reduced hemeprotein is unknown although numerous studies have been carried out, in particular using model compound complexes of heme, which suggest that a form of sulfur participates as one of the ligands of the heme of cytochrome P-450 (25-28) and that this "soft ligand" may in part be responsible for this unusual property of this class of hemeproteins. The bathochromic shift in absorbance of reduced cytochrome P-450, when it reacts with carbon monoxide, stands in sharp contrast to other known hemeproteins where a hypsochromic spectral shift is observed (6). The ability of reduced cytochrome P-450 to form complexes with absorbance bands in the vicinity of 450 nm is not restricted to its reaction with carbon monoxide. Interaction of reduced cytochrome P-450 with the dipyridyl derivative, metyrapone, results in the formation of an absorbance at about 445 nm (63). Recently, it was shown that a number of other organic compounds (such as safrole, the class of amphetamines, SKF-525A, etc.) react with reduced cytochrome P-450 to form derivatives, called product adducts or metabolite complexes, with absorbance bands in the spectral region from 450 to 460 nm (64). The details of the chemistry of these types of reactions remains to be further studied. Suffice it to say that all of these studies strongly suggest the existance of an environment in the heme pocket of cytochrome P-450 which is atypical of other known hemeproteins (59).

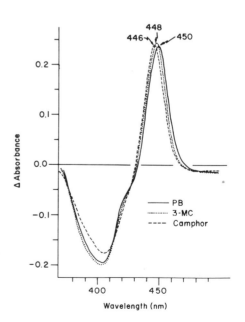

*Figure 10. Optical absorbance properties of the carbon monoxide complex of reduced Cytochrome P-450.*

*Cytochrome P-450 associated with liver microsomes prepared from animals pretreated with phenobarbital (PB) or 3-methylcholanthrene (3-MC) as well as Cytochrome P-450 isolated and purified from Pseudomonas putida (camphor) were reduced by sodium dithionite and examined by difference spectrophotometry. After gassing the contents of the sample cuvette with carbon monoxide, the various spectra were recorded. Differences in the location of the absorbance band maxima are indicated.*

Although the most commonly observed property for the
reduced cytochrome P-450 complex with carbon monoxide is an
absorbance band with a maximum at 450 nm, the exact locus of
this absorbance maximum can be subtly shifted depending on the
source of the hemeprotein. As shown in Figure 10, the absorbance band maximum is located at about 446 nm for the cytochrome
P-450 isolated and purified from the camphor grown bacterium,
Pseudomonas putida (43,65). The hemeprotein formed in liver
microsomes as a result of exposure of animals to polycyclic
hydrocarbons such as 3-methylcholanthrene has an absorbance
band at 448 nm (66). These differences undoubtedly result from
changes in the environment of the heme for each of these hemeproteins as a consequence of synthesis of proteins with modified
amino acid composition and primary structure (67). The result
has been a plethera of names, such as P-448, $P_1$-450, etc.,
which frequently confuse individuals not familiar with the
vagaries of a developing nomenclature which still seeks a
common base.

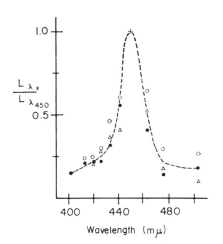

Science

*Figure 11.  Photochemical action spec-
trum for the light reversibility of carbon
monoxide inhibition of Cytochrome P-
450 catalyzed reactions.*

Rat liver microsomes were incubated with
(●), codeine; (○), aminopyrine; or (△),
acetanilide with various mixtures of carbon
monoxide and oxygen and NADPH and
irradiated with light of selected wavelengths
(69).

The property of reduced cytochrome P-450 reacting with
carbon monoxide served as the primary characteristic for
delineating the function of this hemeprotein in the oxidative
metabolism of many different substrates (68,69). Like other
hemeproteins, the reaction of carbon monoxide with the reduced
pigment is an equilibrium reaction which is photosensitive
(70). The first definition of a biological function for cytochrome P-450 was achieved by applying the photochemical action
spectrum methodology of Warburg during a study of the 21
hydroxylation of progesterone as catalyzed by the microsomal
fraction isolated from the adrenal cortex (68). Extension
of these studies to an examination of many mixed function
oxidation reactions catalyzed by liver microsomes (Figure 11)

confirmed the general role of this hemeprotein in the oxygen
activation required for the oxidative conversion of a broad
spectrum of organic compounds.

The fact that the carbon monoxide complex of reduced
cytochrome P-450 has an absorbance band in the Soret region
of the spectrum, which is significantly displaced from the
absorbance bands of comparable complexes of other reduced
hemeproteins, serves as a useful property in evaluating
spectrophotometrically changes in the cellular content of this
pigment following exposure of animals to a variety of chemicals.
As shown in Figure 12, treatment of animals with a barbiturate,
phenobarbital, results in a marked increase in the content of
cytochrome P-450 in the liver of these animals. This property
of "enzyme induction" can be accurately and rapidly monitored
spectrophotometrically. It is worth noting that data of the
type presented in Figure 12 illustrates the high content of

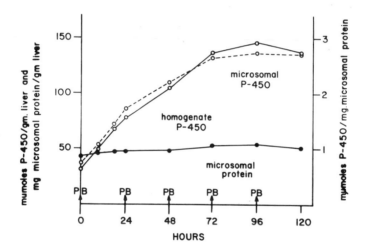

*Figure 12. Induction of liver microsomal Cytochrome P-450 following treatment
of rats with phenobarbital. Male rats (150–200 gm) were injected intraperitoneally
daily with 80 mg of phenobarbital/kg body weight. Animals were sacrificed at
the times indicated and the content of Cytochrome P-450 in (○ – – – ○), isolated
liver microsomes as well as (○—○), liver homogenates (13).*

cytochrome P-450 in an organ such as the liver. Subsequent to treatment of the animals for five days with phenobarbital, approximately 15 percent of the protein of the endoplasmic reticulum of liver is composed of this one class of protein (71). Likewise, as much as 5 percent of the protein of the liver can be cytochrome P-450. Truly, cytochrome P-450 is not a minor constituent in this and other organs - it is the domi-nant species of hemeprotein which is present at a concentration equivalent to that of myoglobin in some muscle tissue.

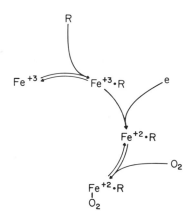

*Figure 13*

Reaction with Oxygen. In the presence of molecular oxygen reduced cytochrome P-450 reacts rapidly to form an intermediate (Figure 13) termed oxycytochrome P-450. The existence of an oxygenated form of reduced cytochrome P-450 was predicted from the early experiments designed to determine those factors which influence the extent of carbon monoxide inhibition of cytochrome P-450 catalyzed reactions (68). These studies had clearly shown that carbon monoxide was an inhibitor which was competi-tive with oxygen, i.e., the magnitude of inhibition observed is dictated by the ratio of carbon monoxide to oxygen rather than simply the concentration of carbon monoxide in the reaction system.

Studies by Ishimura et al. (72,73) as well as Gunsalus et al. (74,75), using the soluble and purified cytochrome P-450 isolated from Pseudomonas putida, clearly demonstrated the presence of a reasonably stable derivative of the reduced hemeprotein when exposed to oxygen. This complex was identi-fiable spectrophotometrically, as shown in Figure 14, and

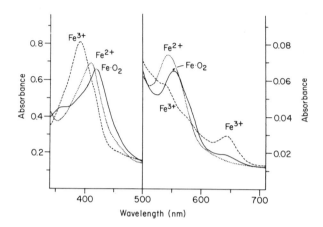

*Figure 14. Absorption spectra of oxidized, reduced, and Oxycytochrome P-450. Samples of purified Cytochrome P-450 isolated from* Pseudomonas putida *were examined spectrophotometrically in the presence of the substrate camphor (73).*

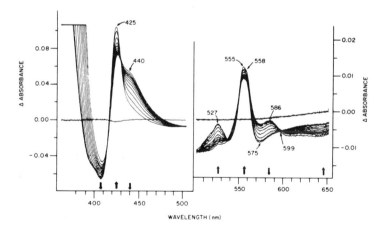

*Figure 15. Repetitive scan difference spectral measurements of liver microsomal Cytochrome P-450 during the NADPH supported steady state metabolism of hexobarbital. Liver microsomes from phenobarbital treated male rats were diluted to 1 mg of protein/mL in a buffer mixture containing 50mM TRIS chloride (pH 7.5), 150mM KCl, 10 mM MgCl₂, and 2mM hexobarbital. NADPH (0.5mM final concentration) was added to initiate the reaction and the difference spectra recorded every 30 sec. The absorbance band at about 440 nm is attributed to Oxycytochrome P-450.*

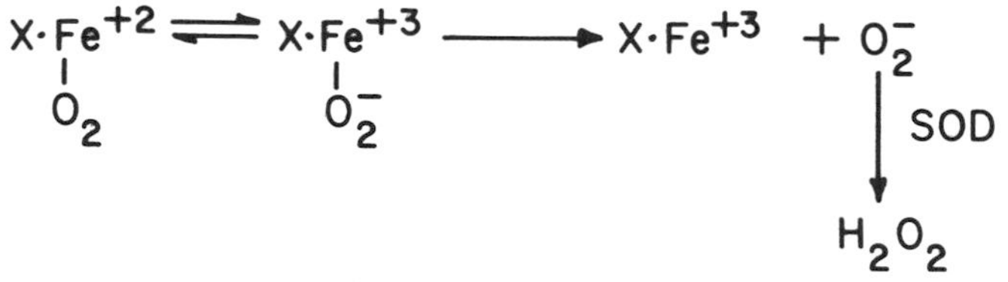

$$X \cdot Fe^{+2} \rightleftharpoons X \cdot Fe^{+3} \longrightarrow X \cdot Fe^{+3} + O_2^-$$

with $O_2$ and $O_2^-$ groups below, and:

$$\downarrow SOD$$

$$H_2O_2$$

*Figure 16.    Possible valence states of Oxycytochrome P-450 and its dissociation to form superoxide*

was recognized to resemble the oxygenated form of other heme-proteins (76-79).   The ability to demonstrate the presence of oxycytochrome P-450 during the functioning of the integrated and membrane bound electron transport system of microsomes (the Class B type of cytochrome P-450) is more complex and subject to many variables.   Repetitive scan spectrophotometric measure-ments during the NADPH supported aerobic steady state oxidation of a variety of substrates by liver microsomes reveals (Figure 15) the presence of an absorbance band with a rather broad maximum at about 440 nm in the difference spectrum (80,81). This absorbance band is similar to the spectral intermediate seen with the purified cytochrome P-450 from Pseudomonas putida.   The magnitude of this absorbance band of oxycytochrome P-450, when studied using liver microsomes, is markedly in-fluenced by the type of substrate studied, the associated activity of NADPH-cytochrome P-450 reductase, i.e., the balance of addition of the first electron versus the second electron (see below) for the function of cytochrome P-450, and the presence of excess NADPH and oxygen.   As shown in Figure 15, the concentration of oxycytochrome P-450 progressively de-creases as the oxygen concentration in the reaction medium decreases.

Oxycytochrome P-450 can be considered to be an equilibrium between two ternary complexes.   In one case (Figure 16), the ferrous hemeprotein can be envisioned as complexed with a molecule of superoxide.   The latter can be visualized as de-caying giving rise to the high spin ferric hemeprotein sub-strate complex and the superoxide anion (or its protonated form, the perhydroxyl radical).   The presence of adventitious superoxide dismutase associated with the microsomal fraction

would then catalyze the formation of hydrogen peroxide. It is
now well established that hydrogen peroxide is formed during
NADPH oxidation by liver microsomes (82,83). Although the
source of this hydrogen peroxide remains speculative, the
decomposition of oxycytochrome P-450 seems a very likely possibility and recent studies (83-85) have supported the hypothesis
that superoxide is generated during the function of cytochrome
P-450. Thus, one can consider an "oxidase type" cycle for
cytochrome P-450 (Figure 17) whereby electrons originating from
NADPH are diverted to the reduction of oxygen for the formation
of hydrogen peroxide rather than for the mixed function oxidative metabolism of xenobiotics. In vitro studies using isolated liver microsomes have revealed the ability of many
compounds to stimulate the rate of formation of hydrogen
peroxide formation concomitant with their oxidation via cytochrome P-450 (86,87). In the few cases studied using halogenated hydrocarbons (88,89) it is apparent that a significant
diversion of electrons occurs resulting in an uncoupling of

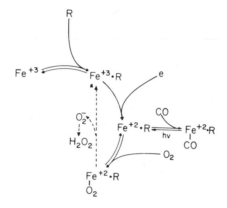

*Figure 17. Dissociation of superoxide from Oxycytochrome P-450 for the forma-
tion of hydrogen peroxide*

oxygenation reactions. This may be of particular interest to
those concerned with pesticides because of the frequent use of
compounds, such as Lindane.

The Second Electron. Oxycytochrome P-450, to which a
molecule of substrate is bound, undergoes further reduction
to an intermediate termed peroxycytochrome P-450 (Figure 18).
Like oxycytochrome P-450, the proposed intermediate peroxycytochrome P-450 can be written in a variety of equivalent
electron valence forms. The inability to isolate and characterize this proposed intermediate has impeded further
understanding of its chemistry and physical properties

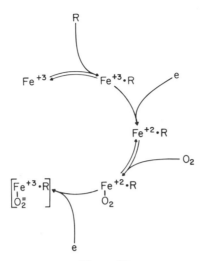

*Figure 18*

although its existence as a transient intermediate in the
function of cytochrome P-450 has been generally assumed. The
stoichiometry of mixed function oxidation reactions requires
the participation of two electrons; the reduction of the ferric
cytochrome P-450 complex has been established (47,48) to be a
one electron transfer reaction. Studies with the purified
bacterial cytochrome P-450 have shown (7) the transformation of
oxycytochrome P-450 by the addition of the reduced iron sulfur
protein, putidaredoxin. Further, the ability to observe
spectrophotometrically intermediates formed during the reaction
of ferric cytochrome P-450 with organic hydroperoxides, such as
cumene hydroperoxide, which differ from oxycytochrome P-450
substantiates the existence of additional oxygen containing
complexes of cytochrome P-450 (90).

Protonation of peroxycytochrome P-450 and the direct
release of hydrogen peroxide concomitant with the formation of
the ferric cytochrome P-450 complex with substrate (Figure 19)
is an alternative means of explaining the formation of hydrogen
peroxide during NADPH oxidation by liver microsomes. Considerable work has centered on distinguishing the two alternatives
for the formation of hydrogen peroxide, i.e., the decomposition
of oxycytochrome P-450 with the release of superoxide which
then undergoes dismutation or the protonation of peroxycytochrome P-450 and the direct formation of hydrogen peroxide. An
examination of the reaction scheme shown in Figure 19 reveals a
major difference between these two options which should delin-
eate the dominant pathway for hydrogen peroxide formation. As
discussed above, two electron transfer steps are required to
form peroxycytochrome P-450 while only one electron transfer

step is needed to generate oxycytochrome P-450. Previous
studies of drug metabolism by the cytochrome P-450 containing
liver microsomes revealed a "synergistic effect" of NADH

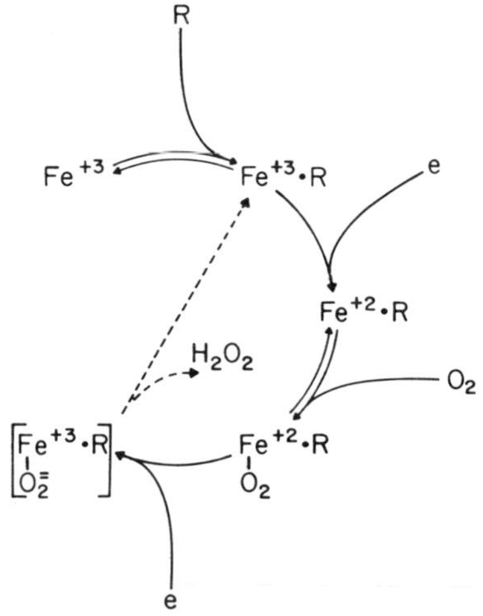

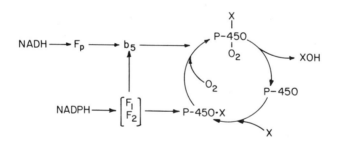

Figure 19.  *Proposed formation of hydrogen peroxide from Peroxycytochrome
P-450*

Figure 20.  *Scheme showing the proposed role of reduced Cytochrome $b_5$ as the
donor of the electron required for the reduction of Oxycytochrome P-450 and the
formation of Peroxycytochrome P-450*

when supplementing the NADPH dependent mixed function oxidation of various substrates.  This "synergistic effect"
elicited by NADH (91-94) was attributed to a role for reduced
cytochrome $b_5$ as the donor of the second electron required for
the cyclic function of cytochrome P-450.  This is illustrated
in Figure 20.  The presence of NADH would spare reducing
equivalents originating from NADPH needed for the reduction of

cytochrome $b_5$ and it would also increase the extent of steady state reduction of this hemeprotein. Comparable studies were carried out to determine whether a "synergistic effect" by NADH on the NADPH dependent formation of hydrogen peroxide also occurred. These results were negative (83,85). This suggests that the principal pathway for the formation of

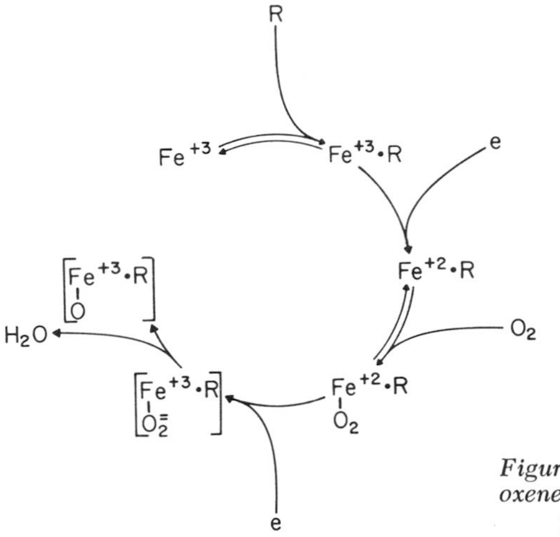

*Figure 21. Proposed formation of an oxene-type intermediate during the cyclic function of Cytochrome P-450.*

hydrogen peroxide was the decay of oxycytochrome P-450 rather than the protonation of peroxycytochrome P-450. Obviously, more definitive experiments will have to be carried out but the present limitation in methodologies precludes the design of such unequivacol studies.

    Other Possible Intermediates. The sequence of reactions involved in the "activation of oxygen" from peroxycytochrome P-450 are unknown. Much has been written and many speculative hypotheses have been proposed but no experimental verification exists to better define possible intermediates. One such hypothesis, which is very attractive, proposes the formation of an oxene complex of cytochrome P-450 resulting from the protonation of peroxycytochrome P-450 and the release of a molecule of water (95,96). This is illustrated in Figure 21. The existence of an oxenoid species of oxygen would fulfill the requirement of a highly electrophilic atom which could participate in hydroxylation reactions. Recently, the presence of free-radical species has also been deduced from deuterium isotope experiments (97). However, the failure to detect any measureable concentration of free radicals during the microsomal catalyzed oxidative metabolism of any substrate yet examined indicates the absence of a steady state concentration of such proposed free radicals. Additional intermediates such as the carbanion form of some substrates, the

existence of a carbene form of the substrate, and the generation of epoxides should all be considered as possibilities
until our level of knowledge is sufficiently expanded to
permit choices based on experimental rather than theoretical
considerations.

## The Role of the Membrane

Cytochrome P-450 present in mammalian tissues is recognized to be intimately associated with membranes.  Studies of
membrane bound enzymes have the disadvantage that special
methodologies, such as the use of difference spectrophotometry
as described earlier, as well as the presence of high concentrations of lipid can introduce variables that are difficult
to fully evaluate.  The latter, i.e., the presence of lipid,
can perturb the pattern of metabolism because of a non-specific
sequestering of the highly lipophilic substrates that are
oxidatively transformed during the function of cytochrome P-
450 (31,98).  Recently considerable interest has centered on
the spatial and structural organization of cytochrome P-450
and its associated electron transfer proteins within the
mileau of the microsomal membrane.  The unique stoichiometry
of flavoproteins and cytochromes (cf. Table I) have provided
the opportunity to evaluate the role of the membrane in regulating and modifying the types of reactions catalyzed and the
influence of restricted mobility of protein within the lipid
mosaic of the membrane.  It has been proposed (49,58,59)
that cytochrome P-450 exists as clusters (Figure 22) which

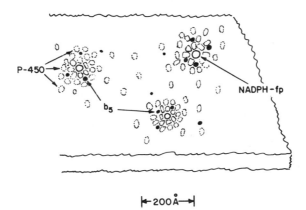

P-450

$b_5$

NADPH-fp

|←200Å→|

*Figure 22.  Schematic of the microsomal membrane showing clusters of mole-
cules of Cytochrome P-450 surrounding the flavoprotein reductase*

can form patches of electron transport complexes within or
withon the membrane.  Much controversy surrounds this inter-

pretation (55,56) and the extent of membrane fluidity, as it
influences the cytochrome P-450 dependent metabolism of substrates, remains as an area requiring further study.  The
solution of this intriguing problem will undoubtedly influence
our further understanding of the reactions involved and the
relationship of studies carried out in vivo to those that have
been experimentally ascertained by in vitro studies.  The
importance of the membrane to studies of the metabolism of
xenobiotics cannot be underestimated.  Most of the compounds
which are oxidatively transformed are highly lipophilic.
Further, the lipid composition of the microsomal membrane can
be readily modified by the type of diet employed as well as
the age and sex of the experimental animal system under study.

## Multiple Types of Cytochrome P-450

Any consideration of the factors which influence the role
of cytochrome P-450 in the metabolism of xenobiotics must
account for the ever increasing body of evidence which shows
the multiple types of cytochrome P-450 that exist in a single
cell type, such as the hepatocyte.  It has been known for many
years that various inducing agents can cause a preferential
stimulation in the metabolism of drug substrates.  The basis
for this difference was clearly delineated by the observation
(66) that treatment of animals with the inducing agent, 3-
methylcholanthrene, resulted in the synthesis of a hemeprotein
associated with liver microsomes which had optical absorbance
properties distinct from a similar pigment induced upon treatment of animals with phenobarbital (cf. Figure 10).  The
last decade has seen major advances in the isolation and
purification of different types of cytochromes P-450.  Differences in response to specific antibodies, protein structure,
and molecular weights are all subjects of current research
(99-104).  A direct demonstration of the change in the pattern
of types of cytochrome P-450 associated with liver microsomes
isolated from animals subjected to different inducing agents
is shown by the polyacrylamide gel electrophoresis results
presented in Figure 23.  Dramatic alterations in the magnitude
as well as mobility of proteins in the molecular weight range
between 45,000 and 50,000 can be seen after exposure of animals
to the inducing agents, phenobarbital or pregnenolong-16-
alpha-carbonitrile.  Thus one must consider, when discussing
the in vivo enzymatic activity of cytochrome P-450, not only
the influence of the membrane and the availability of cofactors such as reduced pyridine nucleotides and oxygen but
also the presence of unique types of cytochrome P-450.

A logical extension of these studies is to postulate the
presence of unique types of cytochrome P-450 which possess a
specificity for various classes of substrates.  As of this
writing, the demonstration of substrate specificity has not

been proven although substrate preference can be shown, i.e.,
the cytochrome P-450 isolated from liver microsomes of animals

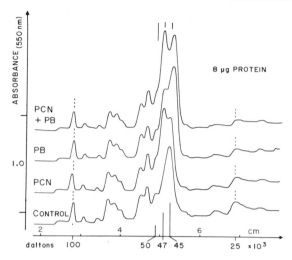

Figure 23.   PAGE patterns of proteins present in liver microsomes from untreated
animals (control), pregnenolone-16 α-carbonitrile (PCN)-, or phenobarbital (PB)-
treated male rats. Microsomes were isolated and treated with SDS prior to electrophoresis and staining with Coomassie blue.

pretreated with a polycyclic hydrocarbon has a high activity
in the metabolism of benzo(a)pyrene but also catalyzes the
oxidative metabolism of drugs such as benzphetamine.  This
puzzle becomes even more intriguing when evaluating the
recognized competitive effects of various types of substrates
when rates of metabolism are measured using the membrane bound
form of the enzyme.  Clearly, the integration of knowledge
gained from studies with various types of purified cytochrome
P-450 as well as the electron transport complexes existent in
the membrane will be required before a meaningful assessment
of the in vivo transformation of xenobiotics can be accomplished.

Concluding Remarks

     The delineation of the sequence of events which occurs as
the hemeprotein, cytochrome P-450, reacts sequentially with a
molecule of substrate to be metabolized, an electron derived
from NADPH and transferred via the flavoprotein, NADPH-cytochrome P-450 reductase, a molecule of oxygen, and then a second
electron has been briefly discussed in the foregoing sections.

The resulting overall scheme shown in Figure 24 attempts to synthesize our present understanding of this cyclic process. One must recognize, however, that much remains to be revealed if we are to gain sufficient knowledge which may permit the development of agents that can predictably perturb this

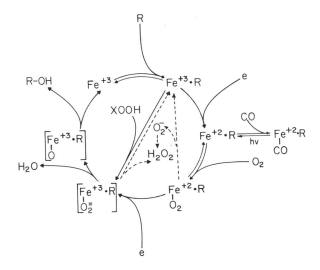

*Figure 24. Scheme of intermediates formed during the cyclic reaction of Cytochrome P-450 associated with the metabolism of many xenobiotics. The possible sites of formation of hydrogen peroxide as well as the pathway of metabolism initiated by organic hydroperoxides are illustrated.*

reaction system. Indeed, achievement of this knowledge is a necessary prerequisite to attainment of the goal of predicting the oxidative transformation of xenobiotics to highly toxic agents (many with the known potential of serving as carcinogens) or to products that are not detrimental to cellular function. The inventory of questions which remain unanswered is long and includes such items as follows:

a) What is "active oxygen" and how does it perform the necessary chemistry to interact with such a broad spectrum of chemicals as those known to be metabolized by cytochrome P-450?

b) What is the unique chemistry of cytochrome P-450 that permits it to react with oxygen and the substrate molecules in a manner that permits the catalysis of xenobiotic transformation?

c) Do the multiple forms of cytochrome P-450, which are selectively induced by various chemicals, reflect more than a single mechanism for the activation of oxygen?

d) What constraints are imposed by the hydrophobic environs of the membrane and associated problems of protein polarity, fluidity, or existence as clusters?

e) What factors dictate the pattern of electron transport from reduced pyridine nucleotides and how are these reflected in the case of substrate metabolism?

f) Is the concomitant formation of hydrogen peroxide, known to occur during the cytochrome P-450 metabolism of substrates, of any significance to cellular activity?

These and many more questions are under intensive investigation in many laboratories. Undoubtedly, new results will reveal the fragile foundation on which our current hypotheses are developed. The importance of knowning how this enzyme system functions is at the forefront of scientific concern during the present time when a great deal of attention has been focused on the wide spread dissemination in our environment of xeno-biotics. The future holds great promise to bring forth new ideas and new concepts. It will be interesting to reflect back on the meager beginning where we stand now.

## Abstract

The oxidative conversion of many lipophilic chemicals which are xenobiotics occurs by means of an enzyme system where the hemeprotein, cytochrome P-450, functions as an oxygenase. The importance of these types of reactions is now recognized as the primary step in the metabolic formation of many toxic agents including carcinogens. The details of our current understanding of cytochrome P-450 interaction with the organic substrate molecule, oxygen, and electrons derived from reduced pyridine nucleotides is described in the present paper. Particular attention is directed toward the sequence of reactions occurring and the attendent problems of defining the parameters which regulate the functionality of the mem-brane bound enzyme complex. The methodologies employed for studies to define the role of cytochrome P-450 in the metab-olism of drugs, steroids, and chemicals which can be converted to carcinogens, have been described and typical results illustrated. The extension of these studies to better define the specificity of the reaction system as well as the prop-erties of reactive intermediates poses the direction for future experimentation.

## Literature Cited

1. Omura, T., in Cytochrome P-450, edited by Sato, R. and Omura, T., p. 7, Academic Press, New York (1978).
2. Pan, H. P. and Fouts, J. R., Drug Metab. Rev. (1978) 7, 1.
3. Estabrook, R. W., in Handbook of Experimental Pharmacology Vol. 28/2, edited by Brodie, B. B. and Gillette, J. R., p. 264, Springer-Verlag, Berlin-Heidelberg-New York (1971).
4. Omura, T. and Sato, R., J.Biol. Chem. (1964) 239, 2370.
5. Omura, T. and Sato, R., J. Biol.Chem. (1964) 239, 2379.
6. Omura, T., Sato, R., Cooper, D. Y., Rosenthal, O., and Estabrook, R. W., Fed. Proc. (1965) 24, 1181.
7. Peterson, J. A. and Mock, D. M., in Cytochromes P-450 and b_5, edited by Cooper, D. Y., Rosenthal, O., Snyder, R., and Witmer, C., p. 311, Plenum Press, New York and London (1975).
8. Gunsalus, I. C., in The Structural Basis of Membrane Function, edited by Hatefi, Y. and Djavadi-Ohaniance, L., p. 377, Academic Press, New York (1976).
9. Iyanagi, T. and Mason, H. S., Biochemistry (1973) 12, 2297.
10. Iyanagi, T., Makino, N., and Mason, H. S., Biochemistry (1974) 13, 1701.
11. Masters, B. S. S., Prough, R. A., and Kamin, H., Biochemistry (1975) 14, 607.
12. Operators Manual, DW-2a UV-VIS Spectrophotometer, Instruction 1710, American Instrument Company, Silver Spring, Maryland.
13. Estabrook, R. W., Peterson, J. A., Baron, J., and Hildebrandt, A. G., in Methods in Pharmacology, Vol. 2, edited by Chignell, C. F., p. 303, Appleton-Century-Crofts, New York (1972).
14. Estabrook, R. W. and Werringloer, J., in Methods in Enzymology Vol. 52C, edited by Fleischer, S. and Packer, L., p. 212, Academic Press, New York (1978).
15. Werringloer, J., in Methods in Enzymology Vol. 52C, edited by Fleischer, S. and Packer, L., p. 297, Academic Press, New York (1978).
16. Wattenberg, L. W., Leong, J. L., and Strand, P. J., Cancer Res. (1962) 22, 1120.
17. Ullrich, V. and Weber, P., Hoppe-Seyler's Z. Physiol. Chem. (1972) 353, 1171.
18. Prough, R. A., Burke, M. D., and Mayer, R. T., in Methods in Enzymology Vol. 52C, edited by Fleischer, S. and Packer, L., p. 372, Academic Press, New York (1978).
19. DePierre, J. W., Johannesen, K. A. M., Moron, M. S., and Seidegard, J., in Methods in Enzymology Vol. 52C, edited by Fleischer, S. and Packer, L., p. 412, Academic Press, New York (1978).
20. Thacker, D. R., Yagi, H., and Jerina, D. M., in Methods in Enzymology Vol. 52C, edited by Fleischer, S. and Packer, L., p. 279, Academic Press (1978).

21. Prough, R. A., Patrizi, V. W., and Estabrook, R. W., Cancer Res. (1976) 36, 4439.
22. Capdevila, J., Estabrook, R. W., and Prough, R. A., Biochem. Biophys. Res. Commun. (1978) 82, 518.
23. Peterson, J. A. Arch. Biochem. Biophys. (1971) 144 678.
24. Werringloer, J., Kawano, S., and Estabrook, R. W., Acta. Biol. Med. German., in press (1978).
25. Blumberg, W. E. and Peisach, J., in Advances in Chemistry, Vol. 100, edited by Gould, R. F., p. 271, American Chemical Society Publications, New York (1971).
26. Chevion, M., Peisach, J., and Blumberg, W. E., J. Biol. Chem. (1977) 252, 3637.
27. Collman, J. P., Sorrell, T. N., Hodgson, K. O., Kulschrestha, A. K., and Strouse, C. E., J. Am. Chem. Soc. (1977) 99, 5180.
28. Collman, J. P. and Sorrell, T. N., in Drug Metabolism Conceptes, edited by Jerina, D. M., ACS Symposium Series No. 44, p. 27, American Chemical Society, Washington (1977).
29. Estabrook, R. W., Mason, J. I., Baron, J., Lambeth, D., and Waterman, M., Ann. N. Y. Acad. Sci. (1973) 212, 27.
30. Waterman, M. R., Ullrich, V., and Estabrook, R. W., Arch. Biochem. Biophys. (1973) 155, 355.
31. Ebel, R. E., O'Keeffe, D. H., and Peterson, J. A., J.Biol. Chem. (1978) 253, 3888.
32. Estabrook, R. W., Martinez-Zedillo, G., Young, S. Peterson, J. A., and McCarthy, J., J. Steroid Biochem.. (1975) 6, 419.
33. Estabrook, R. W., Werringloer, J., Capdevila, J., and Prough, R. A., in Polycyclic Hydrocarbons and Cancer, Vol. 1, edited by Gelboin, H. and T'so, P. O. P., p. 281, Academic Press, New York (1978).
34. Griffin, B. W., Smith, S. M., and Peterson, J. A., Arch. Biochem. Biophys. (1974) 160, 323.
35. Griffin, B. W., Peterson, J. A., Werringloer, J., and Estabrook, R. W., Ann. N. Y. Acad. Sci. (1075) 244, 197.
36. Schenkman, J. B., Remmer, H., and Estabrook, R. W., Mol. Pharmacol. (1971) 68, 1042.
37. Diehl, H., Schadelin, J., and Ullrich, V., Hoppe-Seyler's Z. Physiol. Chem. (1970) 351, 1359.
38. Vore, M., Lu, A. Y. H., Kuntzman, R., and Conney, A. H., Mol. Pharmacol. (1974) 10, 963.
39. Holtzman, J. L., Rumack, B. H., and Erickson, R. R., Arch. Biochem. Biophys. (1976) 173, 710.
40. Powis, G., Jansson, I., and Schenkman, J. B., Arch. Biochem. Biophys. (1977) 179, 34.
41. Leibman, K. C. and Estabrook, R. W., Mol. Pharmacol. (1971) 7, 26.
42. Nebert, D. W., Kumaki, K., Sato, M., and Kon, H., in Microsomes and Drug Oxidations, edited by Ullrich, V., Roots, I., Hildebrandt, A. G., Estabrook, R. W., and

Conney, A. H., p. 224, Pergamon Press, Oxford (1977).

43. Katagiri, M., Ganguli, B. N., and Gunsalus, I. C., J. Biol. Chem. (1968) 243, 3543.

44. Baron, J. in Cytochromes P-450 and b$_5$, edited by Cooper, D. Y., Rosenthal, O., Snyder, R., and Witmer, C., p. 55, Plenum Press (1975).

45. Masters, B. S. S., Baron, J., Taylor, W. E., Isaccson, E. L., and LoSpalluto, J., J. Biol. Chem. (1971) 246, 4143.

46. Vermilion, J. L. and Coon, M. J., in Flavins and Flavoprotein, edited by Singer, T. P., p. 674, Elsevier, Amsterdam (1976).

47. Peterson, J. A., White, R. E., Yasukochi, Y., Coomes, M. L., O'Keeffe, D. H., Ebel, R. E., Masters, B. S. S., Ballou, D. P., and Coon, M. J., J. Biol. Chem., (1977) 252, 4431.

48. Cooper, D. Y., Cannon, M. D., Schleyer, H., and Rosenthal, O., J. Biol. Chem. (1977) 252, 4755.

49. Estabrook, R. W., Werringloer, J., Masters, B. S. S., Jonen, H., Matsubara, T.,Ebel, R., O'Keeffe, D., and Peterson, J. A., in The Structural Basis of Membrane Function, edited by Hatefi, Y. and Djavadi-Ohaniance, L., p. 429, Academic Press, New York (1976)

50. Ito, A. and Sato, R., J. Cell. Biol. (1969) 40, 179.

51. Nilsson, O. and Dallner, G., FEBS Lett. (1975) 58, 190.

52. Welton, A. F., Pederson, T. C., Buege, J. A., and Aust, S. D. Biochem. Biophys. Res. Commun. (1973) 54, 161.

53. Vermilion, J. L. and Coon, M. J., Biochem. Biophys. Res. Commun. (1974) 60, 1315.

54. Yasukochi, Y. and Masters, B. S. S., J. Biol. Chem. (1976) 251, 5337.

55. Yang, C. S., Strickhart, F. S., and Kicha, L. P., Biochim. Biophys. Acta (1977) 465, 362.

56. Yang, C. S., Life Sci. (1977) 21, 1047.

57. Franklin, M. R. and Estabrook, R. W., Arch. Biochem. Biophys. (1971) 143, 318.

58. Peterson, J. A., Ebel, R. E., O'Keeffe, D. H., Matsubara, T., and Estabrook, R. W., J. Biol. Chem. (1976) 251, 4010.

59. Peterson, J. A., O'Keeffe, D. H., Werringloer, J., Ebel, R. E., and Estabrook, R. W., in Microenvironments and Metabolic Compartmentation, edited by Srere, P. A. and Estabrook, R. W., p. 433, Academic Press, New York (1978).

60. Klingenberg, M., Arch. Biochem. Biophys. (1958) 75, 376.

61. Garfinkel, D., Arch. Biochem. Biophys. (1958) 77, 493.

62. Omura, T. and Sato, R., J. Biol. Chem. (1962) 237, 1375.

63. Hildebrandt, A. G., in Biological Hydroxylation Mechanism, edited by Boyd, G. S. and Smellie, R. M. S., p. 79, Academic Press, London (1972).

64. Werringloer, J. and Estabrook, R. W., in The Induction of Drug Metabolism, edited by Estabrook, R. W. and Lindenlaub, E., F. K. Schattauer Verlag, Stuttgart and New York, in press (1978).

65. Peterson, J. A., Arch. Biochem. Biophys (1971) 144, 678.
66. Alvares, A. P., Schilling, G., Levin, W., and Kuntzman, R., Biochem. Biophys. Res. Commun. (1967) 29, 521.
67. Guengerich, F. P., Biochem. Biophys. Res. Commun. (1978) 82, 820.
68. Estabrook, R. W., Cooper, D. Y., and Rosenthal, O., Biochem. Z. (1963) 338, 741.
69. Cooper, D. Y., Levin, S., Narashimhulu,, S., Rosenthal, O., and Estabrook, R. W., Science (1965) 147, 400.
70. Warburg, O., Heavy Metal Prosthetic Groups and Enzyme Action, Clarendon Press, Oxford (1949).
71. Estabrook, R. W., Franklin, M. R., Cohen, B., Shigamatzu, A., and Hildebrandt, A. G., Metabolism (1971) 20, 187.
72. Ishimura, Y., Ullrich, V., and Peterson, J. A., Biochem. Biophys. Res. Commun. (1971) 42, 140.
73. Peterson, J. A., Ishimura, Y., and Griffin, B. W. Arch. Biochem. Biophys. (1972) 149, 197.
74. Gunsalus, I. C., Tyson, C. A., and Lipscomb, J. D., in Oxidases and Related Systems Vol. 2, edited by King, T. E., Mason, H. S., and Morrison, M., p. 583, University Park Press, Baltimore (1973).
75. Yu, C. A., Gunsalus, I. C., Katagiri, M., Suhara, K., and Takemori, S., J. Biol. Chem. (1974) 249, 94.
76. Sidwell, A. E., Jr., Munch, R. H., Barron, E. S. G., and Hogness, T. R., J. Biol. Chem. (1938) 123, 335.
77. Yamazaki, I., Yokota, K., and Shikama, K., J. Biol. Chem. (1961) 239, 4151.
78. Ishimura, Y., Nozaki, M., Hayaishi, O., Nakamura, T., Tamura, M., and Yamazaki, I., J. Biol. Chem. (1970) 245, 3593.
79. Fujisawa, H., Hiromi, K., Yueda, M., Nozaki, M., and Hayaishi, O., J. Biol. Chem. (1971) 246, 2320.
80. Estabrook, R. W., Hildebrandt, A. G., Baron, J., Netter, K. J., and Leibman, K., Biochem. Biophys. Res. Commun. (1971) 42, 132.
81. Estabrook, R. W., Matsubara, T., Mason, J. I., Werringloer, J., and Baron, J., Drug Metab. Disp. (1973) 1, 98.
82. Hildebrandt, A. G. and Roots, I., Arch. Biochem. Biophys. (1975) 171, 385.
83. Werringloer, J., in Microsomes and Drug Oxidations, edited by Ullrich, V., Roots, I., Hildebrandt, A. G., Estabrook, R. W., and Conney, A. H., p. 261, Pergamon Press, Oxford (1977).
84. Kuthan, H., Tsuji, H., Graf, H., Ullrich, V., Werringloer, J., and Estabrook, R. W., FEBS Lett. (1978) 91, 343.
85. Estabrook, R. W., Kawano, S., Werringloer, J., Kuthan, H., Tsuji, H., Graf, H., and Ullrich, V., Acta Biol. Med. German. in press (1978).
86. Hildebrandt, A. G., Speck, M., and Roots, I., Biochem. Biophys. Res. Commun. (1973) 54, 968.
87. Estabrook, R. W. and Werringloer, J., in Microsomes and

Drug Oxidations, edited by Ullrich, V., Roots, I., Hildebrandt, A. G., Estabrook, R. W., and Conney, A. H., p. 748, Pergamon Press, Oxford (1977).

88. Ullrich, V. and Diehl, H., Eur. J. Biochem. (1971) 20, 509.
89. Staudt, H., Lichtenberger, F., and Ullrich, V., Eur. J. Biochem. (1974) 46, 99.
90. Rahimtula, A., O'Brien, P. J., Hrycay, E. G., Peterson, J. A., and Estabrook, R. W., Biochem. Biophys. Res. Commun. (1974) 60, 695.
91. Cohen, B. S. and Estabrook, R. W., Arch. Biochem. Biophys. (1971) 143, 46.
92. Hildebrandt, A. G. and Estabrook, R. W., Arch. Biochem. Biophys. (1971) 143, 66.
93. Mannering, G. J., Kuwahara, S., and Omura, T., Biochem. Biophys. Res. Commun. (1974) 57, 476.
94. Werringloer, J. and Estabrook, R. W., Biochem. Biophys. Res. Commun. (1976) 71, 834.
95. Ullrich, V. and Staudinger, Hj., in Biochemie des Sauerstoffs, edited by Hess,B. and Staudinger, Hj., p. 229, Springer-Verlag, Berlin (1968).
96. Ullrich, V., in Biological Reactive Intermediates, edited by Jollow, D. J., Kocsis, J. J., Snyder, R., and Vainio, H., p. 65, Plenum Press, New York (1977).
97. Groves, J. T., McClusky, G. A., White, R. A. and Coon, M. J., Biochem. Biophys. Res. Commun. (1978) 81, 154.
98. Parry, G., Palmer, D. N., and Williams, D. J., FEBS Lett. (1976) 67, 123.
99. Welton, A. F. and Aust, S. D., Biochim. Biophys. Acta (1974) 373, 197.
100. Haugen, D. A., Coon, M. J., and Nebert, D. W., J. Biol. Chem. (1976) 251, 1817.
101. Haugen, D. A., van der Hoeven, T. A., and Coon, M. J., J. Biol. Chem. (1975) 250, 3567.
102. Thomas, P. E., Lu, A. Y. H., Rayan, D., West, S. B., Kawalek, J. and Levin, W., J. Biol. Chem. (1976) 251, 1385.
103. Johnson, E. F. and Muller-Eberhard, U., in Drug Metabolism Concepts, edited by Jerina, D., p. 72, American Chemical Soc., Washington, D. C. (1977).
104. Ryan, D.. E., Thomas, P. E., and Levin, W., Mol. Pharmacol. (1977) 13, 521.

RECEIVED December 20, 1978.

# The Use of Animal Subcellular Fractions to Study Type II Metabolism of Xenobiotics

MAUREEN J. CRAWFORD and DAVID H. HUTSON

Shell Research Ltd., Shell Toxicology Laboratory (Tunstall), Sittingbourne Research Centre, Sittingbourne, Kent, ME9 8AG, U.K.

Type II biotransformations or conjugation reactions are enzyme-catalysed energy-requiring biosyntheses. The ultimate reaction requires a high-energy donor substrate, an acceptor substrate and an appropriate transferase. The high-energy substrate may contain the endogenous conjugating agent (conjugand) (e.g. glucuronic acid, as in UDPGA) or it may contain the xenobiotic (e.g. 4-chlorobenzoic acid, as in 4-chlorobenzoyl-CoA). If the xenobiotic is to be activated to become a donor substrate, other enzymes and high energy substrates (e.g. ATP) are called into action. If we assume for the moment that the low molecular weight substrates for these reactions have equal access to every component in the cell, then the subcellular location of the transferring enzyme will be the controlling factor in the sub-cellular distribution of the conjugation reaction.

## History of the Technique

The metabolism of foreign compounds has been studied in various subcellular fractions from about 1950. Brodie and coworkers (1) presented the first overview of the enzyme-catalysed metabolism of these compounds in 1958. In the inter-vening years, the properties of microsomes and other subcellular fractions in relation to the metabolism and toxicity of drugs, pesticides and, more recently, 'environmental' chemicals have received an enormous amount of study. However, it is interesting to note that the best of the earlier reviews of the enzymology of foreign compound metabolism by J. R. Gillette in 1963 (2) contains the essential details of each of the conjugation reactions referred to below. Progress has not been even: it has proved difficult to keep our treatment of glucuronyltransferase within reasonable limits, yet amino acid conjugation, despite some very interesting species differences, has received very little attention at the enzyme level.

For our practical purposes, the animal cell can be regarded as composed of nucleus, endoplasmic reticulum, mitochondria

0-8412-0486-1/79/47-097-181$12.25/0

and lysosomes suspended together in water containing dissolved
proteins and small molecules. One of the values of studying
type II reactions at the subcellular level lies in the information gained about the role of these components and the mechanism
of the reactions. When the cell is fragmented and the various
organelles are separated, the conjugation reaction under investigation may not be observed in any of the fractions because
enzymes have been separated from mandatory cofactors. For
example, glucuronidation reactions are not observed in the isolated endoplasmic reticulum (which contains the transferase)
because the high-energy donor substrate, uridine diphospho-
glucuronic acid (UDPGA), is located in the soluble fraction.
Thus the effort required to reconstitute the conjugation reactions
at the subcellular level has been vital to the full understanding of their mechanisms.

   None of this could have happened without the efforts of
biochemists who have developed an understanding of intermediary
metabolism and subcellular fractionation procedures. Differential centrifugation is still the main method used and therefore
the steady development of preparative-scale centrifuges has also
been very important.

## The Preparation of Subcellular Fractions

   Subcellular fractionation is usually carried out by differential centrifugation. However, other methods such as precipitation and chromatography have been investigated for the
isolation of specific fractions.

### 2.1 Differential Centrifugation

   Differential centrifugation is by far the most widely used
technique. It is effective, clean and gentle and although it
could have been displaced at one time by a faster technique, the
availability of preparative ultra-centrifuges capable of up to
500,000 g has cut down preparation times to a very competitive
level. The machines now also operate at acceptable noise levels.
Fresh tissue is homogenised in buffered salt solution and the
resultant homogenate is centrifuged at about 600 g to remove
unbroken cells and cell debris. The supernatant is then centrifuged at 8000-10,000 g for about 20 min to sediment the mitochondria. Some lysosomes are sedimented at this stage. The
supernatant is then centrifuged at about 200,000 g for 20 min
to sediment the fragmented endoplasmic reticulum (microsomal
fraction) together with some lysosomes. The resulting supernatant is the soluble fraction (cytosol). Each of the particulate fractions may be further purified by washing and
recentrifugation. They may be individually further purified by
density gradient centrifugation. The isolation of microsomes has
received a lot of attention from drug metabolism researchers
because of the importance of the microsomal mono-oxygenase
system in xenobiotic metabolism (see preceding Chapter). When

the routine procedure outlined above is carried out there is
inevitably some contamination of one fraction by another. This
is best seen by considering a fractionation of rat liver carried
out in our laboratory by Wright and coworkers (3) during studies
on the effect of the ingestion of dieldrin on hepatocytes. The
fractionation procedure was monitored by measuring the activities
of several enzymes in each fraction, including succinic dehydrogenase (mitochondrial), and glucose-6-phosphatase and chlorfenvinphos dealkylase (microsomal). Some of these results are
illustrated in Figure 1.

Often we require samples of only the microsomal and
cytosolic fractions, in which case we routinely prepare 20%
homogenates in 0.1 M potassium phosphate buffer pH 7.4, centri-
fuge at 10,000 g for 20 min and use this supernatant to prepare
microsomes (190,000 g/30 min/pellet) and cytosol (supernatant)
(4). Protein concentrations are required in order that enzyme
specific activities can be calculated. These are measured using
either the sensitive procedure describes by Lowry et al (5)
or the simple modification of the biuret reaction described
by Robinson and Hodgen (6).

Precipitation
Rapid methods for the preparation of microsomal fractions
have been looked for in recent years. Isoelectric precipitation
of liver microsomes from post-mitochondrial supernatant at pH
5.4 is a useful such method (7). Mono-oxygenase characteristics
in the product compare very well with those of conventional
microsomes but the status of the glucuronyl transferase was
not reported. These preparations contain about 45% more protein
than do conventional preparations and their possible contamination by cytosol enzymes, such as the glutathione transferases,
requires further investigation. A calcium ion sedimentation
method was accidently discovered during a preparation of plasma
membranes which became contaminated with aggregated microsomes.
The method was then developed specifically for microsomes (8).
Mono-oxygenase characteristics were similar to those in
conventionally-prepared microsomes but again glucuronyl transferase was not tested (9)(10). The method has been applied to
rat and rabbit kidney and lung tissue. Microsomal yields from
the latter differ from those obtained by centrifugation in that
there is a higher yield of protein with lower specific activity
(11).

Gel Filtration Chromatography
Microsomes and cytosol of rat liver 13,000 g supernatant
have been separated by gel filtration through Sepharose 2B;
the microsomes were collected in the exclusion volume (Vo) and
the cytosol, between Vo and Vt (12). The method has been applied
to rat lung with remarkable success giving microsomes with very
high specific activities (for oxidative reactions) (13). An
example of one of our own separations using this technique is
shown in Figure 2 (10 ml of 10,000 g supernatant from 40% rat

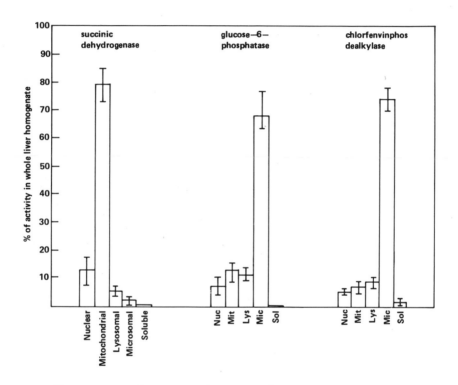

*Figure 1.   Distribution of marker enzymes between subcellular fractions*

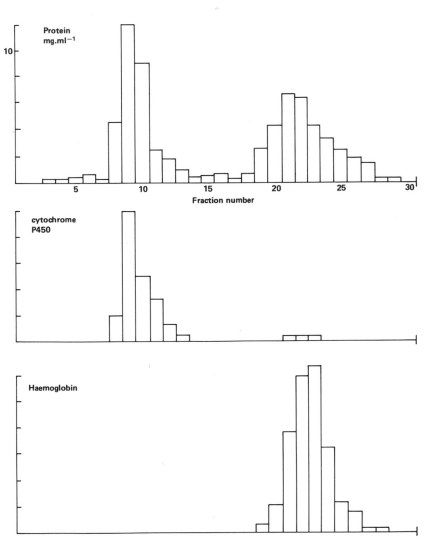

*Figure 2.    Gel filtration of rat liver 10,000 g supernatant on Sepharose 2B*

liver homogenate applied to a 2.5 cm x 25 cm column run at 4-5$^\circ$, upward flow, 1 ml/min; 5 ml fractions collected).

## Advantages of the Subcellular Fractions

Individual subcellular fractions, supplemented with the appropriate cofactors, usually afford information on discrete steps in metabolic pathways in a way that is not possible using animals, organs or cells. The study of cofactor requirements provides information on the mechanism of each reaction, as do studies with isolated purified enzymes. The conditions for the reaction to be studied can be optimised and further metabolism can, if necessary, be blocked so that an intermediate of interest can be isolated.

In a converse sense, now that we know something about the mechanisms of the more common conjugation reactions, a study of the subcellular location and cofactor requirements of the biotransformation of a xenobiotic offers useful information on the metabolism of that compound. It is important to know each discrete step in the biotransformation of a xenobiotic because we then have a chance of identifying intermediates that may prove hazardous under certain circumstances. It is important also to know the effect of toxicants on the function of a particular cell organelle. This requires the study of subcellular fractions.

Another important advantage of subcellular techniques is that the fractions are relatively easy to prepare and they are reasonably robust provided that correct conditions are used. Conditions are described in some detail in the individual sections below.

## Disadvantages of the Technique

The difficulties that may be experienced in working with subcellular fractions are detailed below in the sections on the individual conjugation reactions. However, some useful general-isations may be made. The extrapolation back to the situation in vivo from subcellular systems is a long one. We tend to base our comparisons on enzyme activity measured under conditions favouring good kinetics (e.g. zero order for cofactors, rate linear with time and protein concentrations). However, in vivo, cofactors and/or substrate concentration may be rate-limiting; penetration of substrate to enzyme may be restricted or facili-tated; natural modifiers may be present; interaction between metabolic processes may occur and affect reaction rates. The values $K_m$ (a measure of enzyme-substrate affinity) and $V_{max}$ (the capability of the enzyme when saturated with substrate) are valuable, particularly in a comparative sense. Their true relevance to a particular situation in vivo however is difficult to assess.

Another trap, but of our own making, must be considered.
A rapid assay system is very important in enzyme purification
and is very convenient in tissue and species-comparisons. It also
helps, but is less easy to arrange, in structure-activity studies.
There has been a tendency in xenobiotic enzymology for convenience
to dominate in the selection of substates. The newcomer to the
science of xenobiotic metabolism must surely be puzzled at the
central role occupied by p-nitrophenol. Unsuitable or restricted
substrate selection has led to the perpetration of some quite
unwarranted generalisations. In addition certain convenient substrates have proved unsuitable in a physico-chemical sense and
their use has led to some very complex kinetics dominated by the
properties of the substrate rather than those of the enzyme.
    Another difficulty, or rather a potential failure, of
approaches using separated subcellular fractions is that one may
miss an interaction between two processes. The most common
example of this is the production of a metabolite by oxidation
(i.e. a type I process) followed by its conjugation (type II
process). The two reactions may be more than simply consecutive.
Specific examples will be discussed below.

## Use in Xenobiotic Metabolism Studies

    Subcellular fractions have been used extensively to study
the discrete steps in xenobiotic metabolism. They are also very
useful in a comparative sense. Conjugation reactions, like other
biotransformations, may be affected by a number of factors.
These include species, tissue, sex, strain, stress, age, time,
chemicals (induction, inhibition, activation) and pregnancy. The
effects of these on a particular biotransformation are conveniently studied at the subcellular level. For example, if
species comparisons in vitro are shown to be valid in terms of
in vivo results across a range of experimental animals, they can
be usefully extended to human biopsy samples, thus furnishing
some metabolic data for man. The relationship between chemical
structure and metabolism is also very conveniently investigated
in vitro.
    These various aspects are exemplified below for the indivi-
dual conjugation reactions. The reactions requiring activated
conjugand (glucuronide formation, sulphation, phosphorylation,
acetylation and methylation) are discussed first followed by
those involving activation of the xenobiotic (amino acid conjugation). Glutathione conjugation, which depends upon the mutual
intrinsic reactivity of both substrates, is discussed last.

### Conjugation with Glucuronic Acid
Mechanism and location. Glucuronic acid conjugation is
probably the most quantitatively important of the Type II processes, both in terms of proportion of a particular xenobiotic
being so conjugated, and in the variety of compounds taking part

in the reaction. Phenols, alcohols, carboxylic acids and N-hydroxy
compounds all form O-glucuronides and a number of S- and N-
glucuronides have been detected. The process has recently been
reviewed in some detail by Dutton and co-workers (14)(15).

This process is an example of one in which the endogenous
conjugand (glucuronic acid) is activated to a high energy donor
(uridine-5'-diphospho-α-D-glucuronic acid, UDPGA). The transfer
of the α-D-glucopyranuronyl group from UDPGA to the acceptor,
forming β-D-glucopyranuronosides, is catalysed by UDPGA-
glucuronyl transferase (EC 2.4.1.17). The enzyme is located in
the endoplasmic reticulum of mammalian cells and therefore
appears, on subcellular fractionation, in the microsomes.

Isolation, properties and use. The components required for
an in vitro study: microsomes, UDPGA, xenobiotic and buffer, are
readily available. UDPGA is also available radiolabelled. This
simple system is perfectly adequate for many studies of pesticide
metabolism. It is inappropriate to review assay methods in great
detail in this chapter because, in xenobiotic metabolism, we are
so often interested in a specific compound or series of compounds
and the assay procedure will be based on the conversion of that
compound. There are, however, some recent methods that may be
generally useful. A method involving UDP[$^{14}$C]GA utilises an
Amberlite XAD-2 column to separate unchanged UDPGA, conjugate
and unchanged substrate (16). A continuous assay based on the
enzymatic assay of the UDP released during the transfer has also
been reported (17).

The isolation of the enzyme is achieved by the preparation
of microsomes as described above. The enzyme is relatively stable
in frozen 10,000 g supernatant and in frozen microsomal pellet.
If stored at -196°C (liquid nitrogen), rat and rabbit enzymes
can be kept for many days (18). Because the enzyme is closely
associated with the lipoprotein microsomal membranes, further
purification must be preceded by solubilisation. A recent method
(19) involves treatment of the microsomes with 1% Lubrol 12A9
(a condensate of dodecyl alcohol with approx. 9.5 mol of ethylene
oxide per mol) for 20 min at 4°C. The enzyme remained in the
supernatant after further centrifugation i.e. solubilisation
apparently occurred. It was then precipitated with ammonium
sulphate and further purified in the presence of 0.05% Lubrol
by DEAE cellulose chromatography. The product contained only 3
polypeptides; enzyme activities towards 2-aminophenol and 4-nitro-
phenol were increased 43- and 46-fold respectively. The purified
enzyme had much improved stability in comparison with the
microsomally-bound enzyme. Although there is much kinetic
evidence for the existence of several glucuronyl transferases
(15), very few pairs of aglycone specificites have been separated
physically. One such separation is that of the activities
towards 4-nitrophenol and morphine by Dell Villar et al (20).
It is in this area where purification of the enzymes is important.
Purification, however desirable in theory and however necessary

to the study of the enzyme, is rarely carried out in studies of pesticide conjugation. Our main concern is the fate of the pesticide in the whole animal and the role that the conjugation may play in the disposition of the pesticide. Nevertheless we have to be aware of some practical complications consequent on the particulate nature of this enzyme.

UDPGA-glucuronyl transferase is 'latent' in freshly prepared microsomes. Membrane-perturbing processes such as aging, freezing and thawing, and treatment with detergents, chaotropes, organic solvents, alkali, trypsin or phospholipases may activate the enzyme by a factor of 40 or more (15). This property, together with evidence derived from kinetic studies, some involving competitive substrates, indicates that the enzyme is deeply buried, possibly on the inner surface of the microsomal vesicle. For this reason it is advisable to pretreat microsomes with Triton X-100 (overall 0.05% solution) before adding the xenobiotic substrate. This treatment should fully activate the enzyme and remove errors due to unknown amounts of activation caused by age, storage, mechanical effects or even an effect of the xenobiotic substrate itself. The treatment should also allow access of both UDPGA and the xenobiotic to the enzyme. This may be restricted, particularly if an ionic substrate (e.g. a carboxylic acid) is being investigated. There are two further problems associated with its use however. The amount of activation is species-dependent. For example, the glucuronidation of 7-hydroxychlorpromazine (21) is activated twice as much in rat liver microsomes as it is in guinea-pig liver microsomes. Activation is also dependent on the concentration of Triton X-100 (see Figure 3).

Another problem is the destruction of UDPGA by pyrophosphorylase. This is partly inhibited by EDTA but a better solution is apparently the use of citrate buffer which virtually abolishes the pyrophosphorylase action (15).

The enzyme has a pH optimum of about 7.4 though this may vary somewhat with ionisable substrates. Reaction rates are linear for at least an hour at 37°C.

Examples of use. One of the most frequent uses of the glucuronidation system in our laboratory is in the biosynthesis of glucuronides of faecal metabolites. These are then chromatographically compared with suspected glucuronides found in the urine or in the bile of treated animals. Figure 4 illustrates the formation of the glucuronide of anti-12-hydroxy-[14C]endrin under the following conditions: volume, 5 ml; hydroxyendrin, 0.004 mM; UDPGA, 0.75 mM; washed rabbit liver microsomes (4.2 mg/ml) in 0.1 M TRIS-HCl buffer (pH 7.4 at 37°C); incubation temperature, 37°C. Portions (1 ml) were withdrawn at intervals and partitioned between benzene and water which were then radioassayed to afford the proportions of unchanged substrate and conjugate respectively (22). Triton X-100 had no effect on this reaction, possibly because the very lipophilic anti-12-

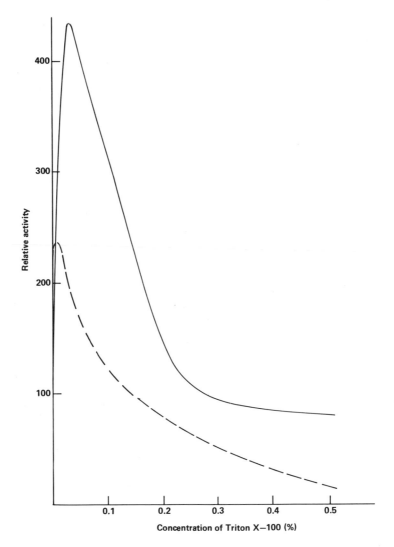

*Figure 3.*    *Effect of Triton X-100 on glucuronidation: (———), rat liver microsomes;*
*(— — —), guinea pig liver microsomes.*

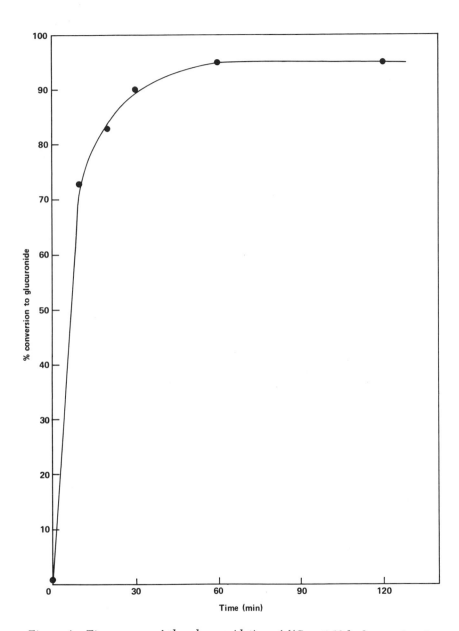

*Figure 4.   Time course of the glucuronidation of* [14]*C anti-12-hydroxyendrin by rabbit liver microsomes*

hydroxyendrin was readily accessible to the enzyme.

The common experimental animals, e.g. guinea-pig, rat, mouse, hamster and dog, all possess reasonable amounts of hepatic microsomal glucuronyl transferase. Litterst et al (23) have compared the hepatic enzyme in rhesus monkey (currently in short supply) with species which may be used as alternative test animals. Activities towards 4-nitrophenol (nmol per min per mg protein) were: rhesus monkey, 7; squirrel monkey, 8-11 (sex difference); common tree shrew (9-12); miniature pig (6-9); Sprague-Dawley rat (2-3). These measurements were made without the addition of detergent. Conditions were: substrate, 0.2 mM; UDPGA, 3.3 mM; protein, 1 mg/ml; Tris buffer pH 7.4, 1 mM. The cat and other Felidae excrete little or no glucuronide conjugates of xenobiotics (24). The high $K_m$ value for 4-nitrophenol with cat liver glucuronyl transferase compared to that with rat liver transferase (25) is in accord with this observation. Hens similarly do not excrete many glucuronide conjugates and have very low enzyme activities in liver. These are examples of the in vitro subcellular results comparing well with the situation in vivo. The occurrence of glucuronyl transferase in birds generally has not been studied. Fish excrete glucuronides (26) and have been shown to possess hepatic glucuronyl transferase activity towards 2-aminophenol (27) 3-trifluoromethyl-4-nitrophenol (26), and 4-nitrophenol (28). Glucuronide formation is important in man but the hepatic enzyme has not been examined in detail.

Another important use of in vitro techniques is for the comparison of biotransformation in different tissue types. However, after a survey using a sensitive methylumbelliferone assay, Aitio (29) concluded that liver is the most important organ of glucuronide synthesis. It was estimated that the whole gastrointestinal tract possessed only 15-20% of the enzyme activity found in liver. Some results are summarised in Table I.

Low enzyme activity has also been found in the placenta of several species, including man (30). The relative activities found for various tissues are partly a function of the choice of substrate. For example, brain, heart, fat and diaphragm possess very low activities towards methylumbelliferone (30) but quite high activites towards the carbaryl metabolite, 1-naphthol (31). This demonstrates that model substrates serve only as a guide; for relevant information on a specific chemical, only studies on that chemical will really suffice.

Toxicological significance. The value of glucuronidation lies in the dramatic change in polarity that the process confers. The glucuronides are also very readily secreted in bile or via the kidneys and thus removed from the body. Glucuronidation can also prevent certain types of metabolite from being further bioactivated to reactive species such as the quinones which may be formed from aromatic dihydrodiols (32). The process is almost always a detoxification, however in some important

cases the reverse is observed. The glucuronidation of N-hydroxy-
arylacetamides (e.g. N-hydroxyphenacetin, Figure 5) affords
chemically reactive molecules capable of interacting with tissue
macromolecules (33). The demonstration of this type of bioactivation is a valuable use of in vitro test systems.

Table I. Glucuronidation of methylumbelliferone
in rat tissues

| | Enzyme activity | |
|---|---|---|
| Tissue | nmol product per g wet wt. liver | nmol product per whole organ |
| Liver | 460 | 3200 |
| Duodenal mucosa | 260 | 96 |
| Adrenal glands | 170 | 63 |
| Kidneys | 150 | 120 |
| Spleen | 30 | 35 |
| Lungs | 28 | 34 |
| Thymus | 19 | 9 |
| Heart | 1.4 | 1.1 |
| Brain | 0.8 | 1.3 |

The use of separated subcellular fractions may fail to
reveal possible interactive effects or functional relationships
between the fractions. For example, the addition of UDPGA to
rat liver microsomes increases their rate of 12-hydroxylation of
dieldrin (34). The rationale for adding UDPGA to an oxidative
system was that syn-12-hydroxydieldrin (Figure 6), although more
hydrophilic than dieldrin, is still a very lipophilic molecule,
particularly in view of the hydrogen bonding of the hydroxyl
group to the epoxide oxygen. Thus, when formed as a metabolite
via the action of microsomal mono-oxygenase, it would remain near
its site of formation, possibly inhibiting further hydroxylation
of dieldrin. This effect was first noted by von Bahr and
Bertilsson (35) with demethylimipramine.

The functional relationship between microsomal mono-
oxygenase, epoxide hydratase and glucuronyl transferase has
recently been investigated in liver microsomes and in isolated
hepatocytes (32). The results provide a good illustration of one
of the limitations of the subcellular approach. In the hepatocyte and in microsomes fortified with NADPH and UDPGA, naphthalene is oxygenated to its 1,2-oxide which is cleaved to a
dihydrodiol (by epoxide hydratase) which, in turn, is conjugated
with glucuronic acid (Figure 7). However, microsomes afford the
dihydrodiol as the major metabolite; hepatocytes afford the
glucuronide. Only by using either more microsomal protein or the

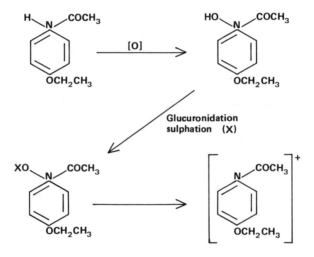

*Figure 5.   Conjugation in the formation of reactive metabolites from phenacetin*

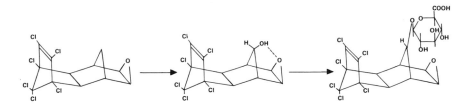

*Figure 6.    Hydroxylation and glucuronidation of dieldrin*

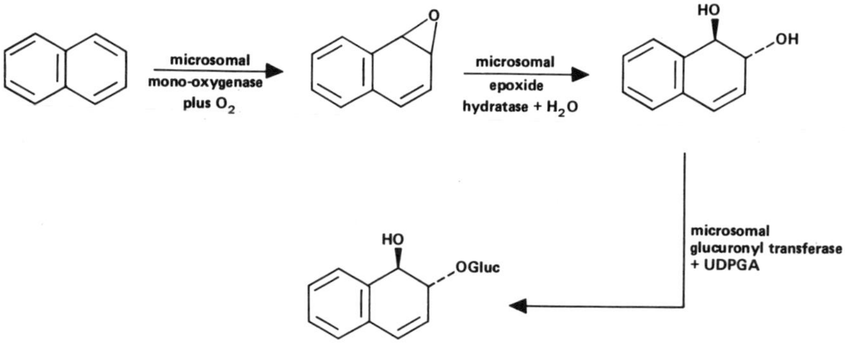

Figure 7.   Relationship between the enzymes affecting the metabolism of naphthalene

allosteric effector of glucuronyl transferase, UDP-N-acetyl-
glucosamine, could microsomes be forced to yield reasonable
quantities of glucuronide. This effector may also competitively
inhibit the destructive effect of the pyrophosphorylase on UDPGA
in vitro.

### Conjugation with Sulphate
Mechanism and location. Conjugation with sulphate is
mediated by the sulphotransferase enzymes (historically sulpho-
kinases). The donor substrate, which contains the activated
sulphate group, is 3'-phosphoadenosine-5'-phosphosulphate (PAPS).
Acceptor groups are principally phenolic but an alcoholic or
primary amine function can also be sulphated via the same
mechanism. Irrespective of the chemical nature of the final
sulphated product, sulphoconjugation follows the same general
pathway: activation of inorganic sulphate to yield first adeno-
sine 5'-phosphosulphate (APS) and then 3'-phosphoadenosine 5'-
phosphosulphate (PAPS), followed by transfer of the sulphate
group from PAPS to suitable acceptors:

$$ATP + SO_4^{2-} \longrightarrow APS + PP_i \qquad (1)$$

$$APS + ATP \longrightarrow PAPS + ADP \qquad (2)$$

$$PAPS + Acceptor \longrightarrow PAP + sulphated\ acceptor \qquad (3)$$

The enzymes catalysing these reactions are (1) ATP-sulphate
adenylyl transferase (ATP-sulphurylase); (2) ATP-adenylyl sulphate
3'-phosphotransferase (APS-kinase) and (3) an appropriate
sulphotransferase (EC 2.8.2). In mammalian cells the enzymes
responsible for the production of PAPS from sulphate are localised in the cytosol. Sulphotransferases are located in both the
microsomal and the cytosolic fractions of a wide variety of
tissues; their general tissue distribution resembles that of the
UDP-glucuronyltransferases, except that they are also abundant in
placenta. Boundaries of their specificities are more clear than
those of the glucuronyl transferases, and distinctive phenol,
steroid and arylamine sulphotransferase activities have been
detected. Other transferases deal apparently solely with endogenous compounds, e.g. cerebroside and polysaccharide sulphotransferases. Simple endogenous sulphates includes those of
steroids, adrenaline, tri-iodothyronine and serotonin. The
picture emerges (cf. the glucuronyl transferases) of the sulphotransferases responsible for the sulphation of small molecules
being freely soluble in the cytosol, whereas those that are
involved in the assembly of larger molecules are arranged,
together with other requisite biosynthetic enzymes, in assembly-
line fashion on the membranes of the endoplasmic reticulum and
the Golgi apparatus. It is extremely doubtful whether any of
these bound enzymes play any role in the metabolism of xenobiotics (36).

Isolation, properties and use. The uncertainty in the total
number, precise roles and specificities of the sulphotransferases
reflects the fact that they are exceedingly difficult to purify
and to separate from one another. Moreover, some of them aggregate and/or change conformation under certain conditions;
multiple peaks of similar activity, which may or may not be due
to the same enzyme, appear on chromatography columns and are a
constant hindrance to the experimentalist.

A sulphotransferase has been partially purified from bovine
kidney (acetone powder) using 4-nitrophenol as the assay substrate (37). The activity of the enzyme was measured using
[$^{35}$S]PAPS in the assay mixture. Substrate specificity was investigated and it was found to be relatively specific for simple aryl
sulphate formation as shown in Table II.

Table II. Relative substrate specificities for
bovine kidney sulphotransferase

| Substrate | Relative specificity |
|---|---|
| 4-Nitrophenol | 100 |
| 4-Hydroxybenzaldehyde | 75.9 |
| 4-Chlorophenol | 79.7 |
| 1-Naphthol | 32.5 |
| Phenol | 6.5 |
| o-Cresol | 21.7 |
| m-Cresol | 8.3 |
| 3-Nitrophenol | 49.8 |
| 3-Hydroxybenzaldehyde | 21.0 |

No activity could be demonstrated towards ethanol, propan-1-
ol, butan-1-ol, or towards a range of steroids.

The isolation of N-hydroxy-2-acetylaminofluorene (N-OH-2-
AAF) sulphotransferase has recently been achieved from the cytosol
fractions of male and female rat livers (the latter possess very
low activity) (38). A 2000-fold purification with a yield of over
12% was achieved using the following procedure: ammonium sulphate
fractionation, DEAE-cellulose column chromatography, hydroxyapatite column chromatography, sephadex G-200 gel filtration,
isoelectric focussing and, finally, more sephadex G-200 gel
filtration. The final preparation was homogenous on analytical
disc gel electrophoresis. The purified enzyme had activity
towards 4-nitrophenol with an approximately 1600-fold increase in
specific activity over the crude homogenate, but it had very low
activity towards endogenous steroids and serotonin. PAPS was used
as the sulphate donor in these assay mixtures and was synthesised
enzymatically (39). The pure enzyme was very unstable, especially
in dilute solutions. Thiol compounds were found to have a stabil-
ising effect and thiol blocking reagents were potent inhibitors.

The involved nature of these purifications suggests that the study of phase II sulphoconjugations using purified sulphotransferase from various animal species and animal tissues is impractical at present. An in vitro assay system for studying these reactions using crude subcellular fractions has been developed by Mulder et al (33). It comprises cytosol (600 μg protein/ml), xenobiotic (0.5 mM), Tris-HCl buffer (100 mM, pH 8.0) and a PAPS-generating system (PAPS-GS): 3'5'-adenosine diphosphate (PAP, 10 μM) and 4-nitrophenyl sulphate (10 mM). In this assay mixture 4-nitrophenyl sulphate is used to convert PAP into PAPS, a reaction presumably catalysed by a phenolsulphotransferase in the cytosol. The rate of formation of 4-nitrophenol is spectrophotometrically determined and is calculated by subtracting the amount of 4-nitrophenol released in a control incubation mixture (xenobiotic absent) from that released in the presence of the xenobiotic. The rate of sulphation may thus be indirectly calculated from the amount of 4-nitrophenol released using a molar extinction coefficient of 17,500 $M^{-1}$ $cm^{-1}$ (at pH 8.0). This assay procedure makes an important contribution to the field of xenobiotic metabolism in that it provides a cheap and simple method for studying the mechanisms and rates of phase II sulphate conjugation reactions using a PAPS-GS and cytosol. Hitherto PAPS has been commercially available in the labelled form only and its enzymic synthesis is a tedious process (39)(40). A more traditional assay procedure is that described by Wu and Straub (38) where PAPS is used at a concentration of approximately 0.3 mM when substrate concentration is 0.2 mM.

Examples of use. Harmol (Figure 8) is a good substrate for phenol sulphotransferase in rat liver 600 g fraction (41) but harmalol (Figure 8) is a very poor substrate. The reason for the difference in rate of sulphation of these two substrates is unknown, but the findings agree with the different rates and modes of conjugation (sulphation and glucuronidation) of the two compounds found in vivo.

The metabolism of harmol illustrates a problem that often arises when discussing the phase II conjugation of xenobiotics with sulphate. Sulphation of a xenobiotic or its metabolite is practically always accompanied by  conjugation with glucuronic acid. Glucuronic acid conjugation often predominates and this has been assumed to be due to a limited supply of sulphate in vivo. Mulder and coworkers have developed a method for the simultaneous measurement of UDP-glucuronyltransferase and phenolsulphotransferase from rat liver in vitro, using harmol as substrate and 600 g supernatant as the enzyme source (42). Triton X-100 was used to activate glucuronyl transferase (Section 5.1) and was shown to have no effect on the activity of phenolsulphotransferase. The amount of the conjugates formed was measured fluorometrically and the activities of the enzymes were expressed as arbitrary units of fluorescence recovered from a tlc analysis of the incubates. At low substrate concentrations

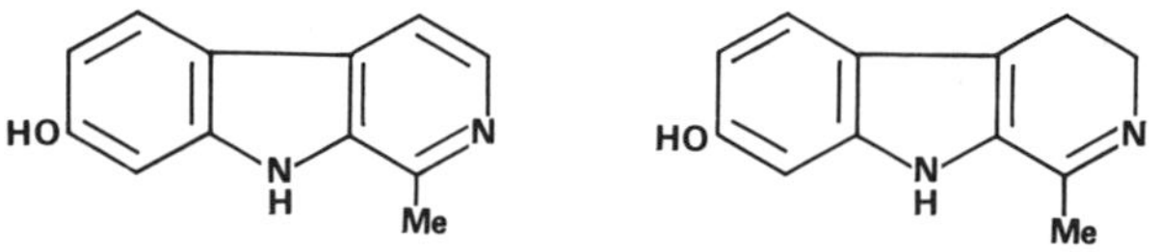

Figure 8.   Harmol and harmolol

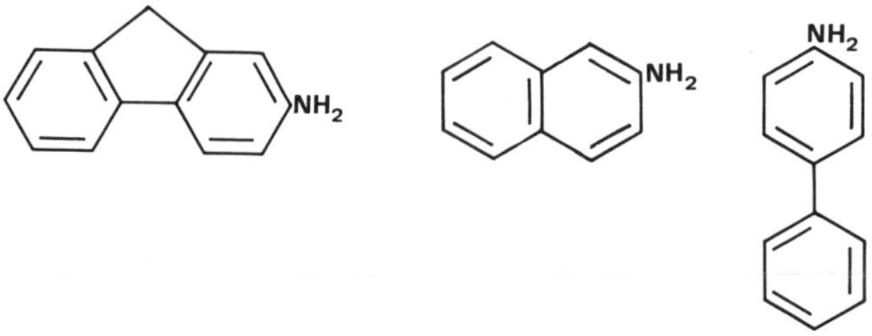

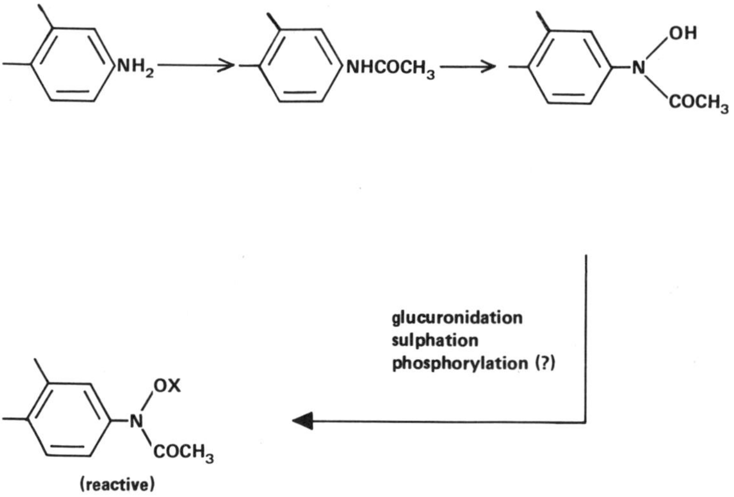

Figure 9.   Acetylation and conjugation in the activation of aromatic amines

(<40 μM) harmol was preferentially sulphated but with increasing substrate concentration, glucuronidation became more important. These results agree with earlier in vitro results (41) when the $K_m$ value for harmol of UDP-glucuronyl transferase was found to be 150 μM and of phenolsulphotransferase was <15 uM. Therefore, in some circumstances, the affinities of the enzymes for the substrate may control the relative amounts of conjugation. 2,6-Dichloro-4-nitrophenol may be used as a selective inhibitor of sulphation if glucuronic acid conjugation needs to be studied in the 10,000 g fraction of liver (43). Thus, using in vitro subcellular fractions containing even crude enzyme preparations, a greater understanding of in vivo findings is possible.

A second important facet of in vitro studies is the assessment of the relative importance of various animal organs in xenobiotic metabolism. Using rabbit lung soluble fraction, significant sulphation of 4-nitrophenol and 4-methylumbelliferone has been demonstrated (44). The former was sulphated by lung cytosol at about one third the rate found for liver cytosol (per mg protein). In these experiments PAPS was included in the incubation mixtures. This may account for the apparent disparity between these results and those of Gram et al (45) who could not detect any sulphotransferase activity towards 4-nitrophenol in rabbit lung supernatant. These authors utilised a PAPS-generating system in their experiments.

Sulphation of steroids has been studied in the cytosol of brain and liver from guinea-pigs and rats (46). [$^{35}$S]PAPS was used as the sulphate donor. 17-β-Oestradiol (E) and diethylstilbestrol (DES) were used as substrates. The following activities (pmol conjugate/mg tissue/20 min) were measured with brain preparations: rat: E, 0.6; DES, 2.0; guinea-pig: E, 0.1; DES, 4.1. Activities with guinea-pig liver were: E, 98; DES 333. Thus, with these substrates, the activity of the transferase in brain is only a small fraction of that of liver.

Toxicological significance. Conjugation of a xenobiotic with a completely ionised and highly hydrophilic moiety such as sulphate markedly alters its physico-chemical properties and this usually leads, like glucuronidation, to a complete loss of pharmacological or pesticidal activity. This and a rapid rate of excretion are the beneficial consequences of sulphoconjugation.

Several xenobiotics exert their toxic effects in mammals though the formation of reactive metabolites that combine with cellular macromolecules. The O-sulphation of N-OH-2-AAF has been postulated as an activation reaction (Figure 9) leading to the carcinogenic action of this compound (47). There is no direct evidence for the formation of these NO-sulphates in vivo; their instability precludes their isolation and characterisation. However, their transient existence has been demonstrated in vitro by the use of indirect methods, such as trapping the conjugates in situ by reaction with nucleophilic compounds (48). There is also indirect evidence that the sulphate conjugate of N-OH-2-AAF

is formed in rat liver in vivo (49). Mulder et al (33) have
recently used the PAPS generating system described earlier in this
section, to indirectly measure the rate of sulphation of N-OH-2-
AAF. The reaction rate was linear with cytosolic protein
concentration up to 1.2 mg/ml and was about 2.7 nmoles 4-nitro-
phenol formed per ml per mg soluble protein (at 31°C). These
results suggest that the NO-sulphate of N-OH-2-AAF had been
formed, but again isolation of the metabolite was not possible
because of its instability. Evidence that an NO-sulphate conjugate was formed in the incubation mixtures was obtained by
showing that the covalent binding of N-OH-2-AAF to macromolecules
increased dramatically during incubation with 4-nitrophenyl
sulphate and PAP. N-Hydroxyphenacetin, N-hydroxyacetanilide,
N-hydroxy-4-chloroacetanilide and N-hydroxy-2-acetylaminonaph-
thalene also formed sulphate derivatives at rates comparable to
that of N-OH-2-AAF. N-Hydroxyphenacetin and N-hydroxy-2-acetyl-
aminonaphthalene also became rapidly covalently bound after
sulphation of their N-hydroxy groups, but the O-sulphates of
N-hydroxy-4-chloroacetanilide and N-hydroxyacetanilide did not
react (Table III). DeBaun et al (48) have also extensively
studied this effect of sulphation on covalent binding of N-OH-2-
AAF, and the work is a good example of the use of subcellular
fractions in the investigations of mechanisms of carcinogenesis.

Table III. Conjugation rates and effect of conjugation
on covalent binding of some N-hydroxy-N-arylacetamides

| Substrate | Sulphation rate (nmoles/min/mg soluble protein) | Amount covalently bound (nmoles/ml) | |
|---|---|---|---|
| | | with 4-nitrophenylsulphate | without |
| N-hydroxyphenacetin | 2.6 | 25.0 | 0.2 |
| N-hydroxyacetanilide | 1.6 | 0.2 | 0.2 |
| N-hydroxy-4-chloro-acetanilide | 2.4 | 0.4 | 0.2 |
| N-hydroxy-2-AAF | 2.7 | 21.8 | 0.6 |
| N-hydroxy-2-acetylamino naphthalene | 2.0 | 1.9 | 0.2 |

This study shows clearly that the NO-sulphate of N-hydroxyphenacetin binds covalently to protein as soon as it is synthesised. Since phenacetin is N-hydroxylated by microsomal enzymes
(50)(51), it seems likely that the sulphation and glucuronidation pathways provide a reactive intermediate for covalent
binding. At the present time it is not clear whether either
reaction plays a role in causing the short-term toxic effects of

high doses of phenacetin in vivo (liver necrosis); however, this
work demonstrates the value of subcellular studies in the characterisation of enzymatic determinants of toxicity.

Phosphorylation

The excretion of di(2-amino-1-naphthyl)hydrogen phosphate
by dogs dosed with 2-naphthylamine (52) suggests that phosphorylation occurs in xenobiotic metabolism. However, only very few
examples have been found in the intervening 17 years. The process
has been postulated as a bioactivation step in carcinogenesis by
2-acetylaminofluorene (53). Monophenyl phosphate is excreted in
the urine of cats dosed with phenol (54). Rat liver mitochondria
contain an enzyme that catalyses the ATP-dependent phosphorylation
of 1-aminopropan-2-ol (55). These facts summarise most of our
knowledge on the phosphorylation of xenobiotics; they are stated
here to emphasise the apparently very minor role of this conjugation. The central role of phosphorylation in energy metabolism is presumably, of necessity, controlled by very substrate-
specific processes in which xenobiotics cannot readily
participate.

Acetylation

Mechanism and location. Acetylation is of relatively minor
importance in pesticide metabolism in comparison with glucuronidation, sulphation and glutathione conjugation. However, the
reaction must be expected whenever an aromatic amine is under
investigation per se or liberated during metabolism. The transfer
of acetate occurs from acetyl-coenzyme A and is catalysed by
arylamine N-acetyltransferase (EC 2.3.1.5). The enzyme is located
in the cytosol of mammalian cells. The reaction is general for
aromatic amines, sulphonamides, hydrazino compounds and some non-
aromatic amines (56). The enzyme operates via a simple ping-pong
mechanism of two consecutive steps: acetylation of the enzyme
by acetyl-CoA followed by transfer of acetate from acetyl-N-
acetyl-transferase to the acceptor substrate. This has been confirmed by the isolation of a [$^{14}$C]acetyl-N-acetyltransferase
protein capable of donating its acetyl group to isoniazid (57).
The reaction is important in the metabolism of endogenous amines,
including serotonin, tryptamine, histamine and phenylethylamine.
Man and rabbit exhibit a genetic polymorphism in N-acetylation
(58) (for example, of 4-aminobenzoic acid and isoniazid) and
individuals can be classified as 'rapid' or 'slow' acetylators.
The location of the N-acetyltransferases is not always cytosolic.
Those involved in the last stages of mercapturic acid formation
are located in the liver microsomal fraction (59).

In principle, O-acetylation and S-acetylation of foreign
compounds may occur (as they do in the formation of the endogenous substrates O-acetylcholine and S-acetyl-CoA); however,
they have not yet been demonstrated.

Isolation, properties and use. N-Acetyl transferase (to
aromatic amines etc.) is best used and measured in cytosol prepared by ultra-centrifugation. This may be dialysed before use.

Rabbit cytosol enzyme is stable for at least a month when frozen, and for 48 hours if stored at $4^o$ or $25^o$. It also withstands repeated freezing and thawing. Its pH optimum varies with substrate but lies between 6 and 8.5. A purification procedure from rabbit liver cytosol has been described by Weber and Cohen (60). This involved centrifugation to afford a 100,000 g supernatant, ammonium sulphate precipitation, Sephadex G-100 and DEAE-cellulose chromatography. Typical conditions for use are as follows: substrate (0.1 μmole), acetyl-CoA (0.5 μmole), 0.3 mM phosphate buffer pH 6.8 (perhaps higher), cytosol (0.5-5 mg protein) in a volume of 1 ml.

As usual, the assay system will depend on the substrate under investigation. However, a useful general method involves [$^{14}$C-1-acetyl]-acetyl-CoA, the products from which can be extracted into organic solvent and radioassayed either before or after chromatographic separation (61).

Examples of use. In vitro measurements (4-aminobenzoic acid) have been used to show a wide species distribution of N-acetyl-transferase (23). For example, the activity of the hepatic enzymes lies in the order: rhesus monkey = pig > squirrel monkey = tree shrew > rat. The industrial intermediate 2,4-toluenediamine is N-acetylated preferentially at the 4-amino group. The enzyme activity (in cytosol) is found in liver > kidney > intestinal mucosa > lung. The activity of the liver enzyme varies with species: hamster > guinea-pig > rabbit > mouse > rat > human (trace) > dog (zero) (62). The genetic polymorphism noted above was discovered at the in vivo level in man and rabbits. It is of the same type in both species (controlled as a simple autosomal Mendelian character with rapid acetylation dominant to slow (56)). It has been understood via subcellular studies. It is probably due to varying amounts of the same enzyme rather than to different enzymes (56). At least two N-acetyltransferases exist in the rabbit. They differ in their tissue distributions, substrate specificities and pH-activity profiles. The one responsible for the genetic polymorphism has a wide substrate specificity and is found mainly in the liver and gut (63).

Toxicological significance. N-Acetylation is very important in the inactivation of the pharmacological and biocidal properties of many amine drugs; however, this property is of minor importance in the pesticide field. Of greater interest and potential importance is the role that N-acetylation plays in the bioactivation of carcinogenic aromatic amines. 2-Aminofluorene, 4-aminobiphenyl and 2-aminonaphthalene (Figure 9), for example, are all thought to be N-acetylated in the first step on their metabolic routes to ultimate carcinogens. The enzyme activity is of course readily available in the liver cytosol of various species. It is of considerable interest that dog liver cytosol contains no detectable activity (Figure 10) (nor towards toluenediamine above) and that dog liver is not susceptible to the carcinogenic action of these compounds (64). When a variety of arylamines are

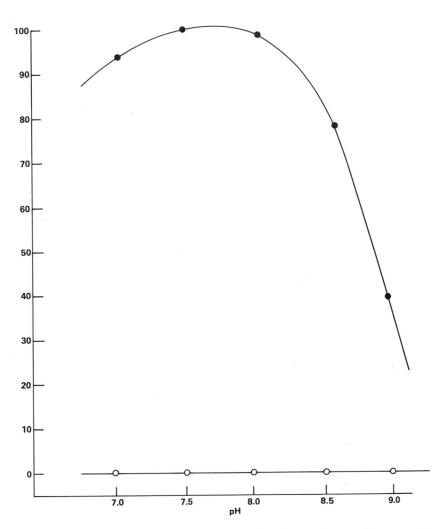

*Figure 10.* N-acetylation of 2-aminofluorene by dog and mouse liver cytosol: (●), mouse; (○), dog (64).

administered to dogs, only urinary bladder tumours are noted.
However, the administration of carcinogenic arylacetamides causes
both bladder and liver tumours. Clearly hepatic N-acetyl transferase is a determinant of liver carcinogenesis by arylamines.

The N-acetylation of isoniazid may also be a toxicating
reaction. An increased incidence of 'isoniazid hepatitis' has
been noted in rapidly acetylating humans (65).

Methylation

Mechanism and location. The methylation of phenols, thiols
and amines involves a methyl donor (S-adenosylmethionine) and
methyltransferases. Thus the mechanism is typical of type II
reactions although the result, in terms of increase in polarity,
is much less or even the reverse of the other type II processes.

O-Methylation. Catechol O-methyl transferase (66) (EC
2.1.1.6) is the most common O-methylating enzyme in xenobio-
chemistry. It is highly specific for the catechol (i.e. 1,2-
dihydroxybenzene) configuration, but given that, it is undemand-
ing in its other requirements (67). It is probably encountered
most commonly in xenobiotic metabolism at the and of the sequence:
arene → arene oxide → dihydrodiol → catechol → monomethylcatechol.
Most of the enzyme activity is present in the cytosol of various
tissues. Phenol O-methyltransferase, a microsomal enzyme, has
been detected in vitro (68) but its significance in vivo is
unknown because the O-methylation of monohydric phenols apparently
does not occur in vivo. A potentially useful general assay method
involving the use of the tritiated cosubstrate S-adenosyl-L-
[methyl-$^3$H]methionine has been described (69). The radioactive
methylated product is extracted into organic solvent for radio-
assay.

S-Methylation. S-Methylation is a general pathway of metabolism of the thiopyrimidone antithyroid drugs such as 6-propyl-
2-thiouracil. Tetrahydrofurfuryl mercaptan is also S-methylated
in an S-adenosylmethionine-dependent enzymatic reaction. The
enzyme was found in the microsomal fraction of liver, kidney and
small intestine (70). Thiophenol liberated during the metabolism
of dyfonate (Figure 11) is methylated (71). This reaction has not
been studied in vitro.

N-Methylation. Pyridine derivatives are N-methylated but the
reactions are quantitatively of minor importance. The most widely
studied N-methylation reactions are those involving the biogenic
amines. For example, phenylethanolamine N-methyltransferase (EC
2.1.1) (involved in the biosynthesis of epinephrine) has been
studied recently and found to methylate non-aromatic substrates
as well as aromatic ones (e.g. Figure 12, R = propyl, cyclohexyl,
cyclohex-3-enyl,cyclo-octyl). The enzyme has an absolute requirement for a hydroxyl group at the β-position on an ethyl side
chain (72).

Methylation reactions have not featured widely in pesticide
metabolism; however, there is enough information derived from
endogenous biochemistry and drug metabolism to be useful should

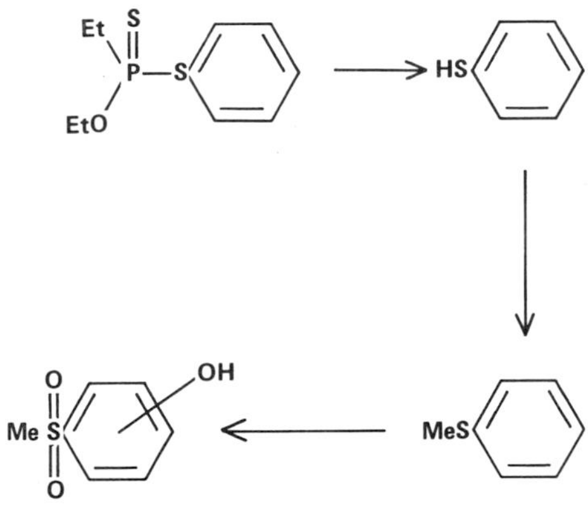

*Figure 11.   Methylation of thiophenol in the metabolism of dyfonate*

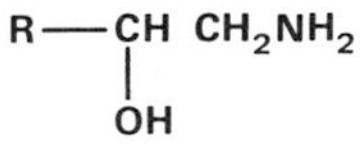

$$R \text{---} \underset{\underset{OH}{|}}{CH}\ CH_2NH_2$$

*Figure 12.   Substrate for phenylethanolamine N-methyltransferase*

it be necessary to study these reactions with particular
pesticides.

## Conjugation with Amino Acids

— Mechanism and location. Amino acid conjugation in pesticide
metabolism has recently been reviewed (73). Substrates for amino
acid conjugation are usually either aromatic carboxylic acids or
arylacetic acids. The most important conjugating amino acid is
glycine and, together with glutamine, accounts for the majority
of α-amino acid conjugates formed in mammals.

α-Amino acid conjugation occurs with the formation of an
amide bond. Thus, both the substrate and the metabolite possess
an ionisable carboxyl group. The first step of the reaction
occurs with the interactions of the xenobiotic with coenzyme A
(I). Conjugation of the activated xenobiotic with glycine occurs
in the second step and is catalysed by glycine N-acylase (EC
2.3.1.13) (II) (Figure 13). Thus, the formation of glycine conjugates may be contrasted with the mechanism of the other conjugation reactions discussed so far. It is the xenobiotic rather
than the endogenous conjugating moiety that is activated prior
to the transferase action.

Activation of benzoate into benzoyl-CoA is thought to be
catalysed by butyryl-CoA synthetase (EC 6.2.1.2) (74), which is
found in the mitochondrial matrix (75). Glycine N-acylase has
been prepared from mitochondria (76)(77) and has recently also
been found by Gatley et al (78) to be located in the mitochondrial
matrix. These authors have also shown that hydrolysis of benzoyl-
CoA occurs in situ and they postulate that the function of the
simultaneous activity of benzoyl-CoA synthetase and benzoyl-CoA
hydrolase is to prevent the accumulation of too much benzoyl-CoA.
This would occur if the supply of glycine, or its rate of conjugation, were limiting for hippurate synthesis and could thus
impair other CoA-requiring reactions (79). It is thought that
undissociated benzoic acid and hippuric acid cross the inner
membrane because of their lipid solubility. Further, Halling
et al (80) conclude that glycine crosses the inner membrane as a
zwitterion. Therefore the location of the enzyme does not
apparently impair the access of these substrates.

In addition to the conjugation of xenobiotics with amino
acids, endogenous compounds, notably the bile acids, conjugate
with glycine and taurine. Recently, arginine conjugates of bile
acids have also been identified (81).

Choloyl-CoA synthetase (EC 6.2.1.7), the enzyme responsible
for the formation of the activated bile acid intermediate, has
been located in the microsomal fraction of guinea-pig liver (82).
The intracellular location of the amino acid N-acyltransferase
enzymes responsible for the conjugation of the activated substrate with taurine or glycine has been in dispute for some time.
Siperstein and Murray (83) localised the enzyme(s) in the soluble
fraction of liver cells. Bremer (84) and Elliott (85) concluded
that they were located in the microsomal fraction and Schersten

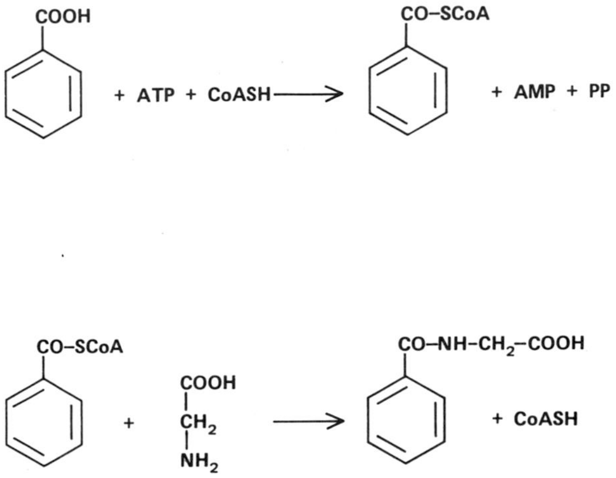


(I)

(II)

*Figure 13. Amino acid conjugation*

(86), in the lysosomal fraction. Vessey et al (87) have recently
found enzyme activity in the soluble fraction of bovine liver
cells and they have presented evidence for two distinct enzymes:
glycine N-acyltransferase and taurine N-acyltransferase.
Killenberg and Jordan (88) on the other hand have isolated a
single acyltransferase from rat liver which is capable of conjugating chemically synthesised bile acid - CoA derivatives with
glycine or taurine.
    Isolation, properties and use. There have been no recent
publications on the isolation of mitochondrial acyl-CoA syn-
thetases responsible for the activation of xenobiotics or their
metabolites. We have to turn to 'pure' biochemistry for information. Choloyl-CoA synthetase, as studied by Vessey and Zakim
(82), was stable for at least one month when the microsomal
fraction of guinea-pig liver was stored at $-50^{\circ}C$. The standard
assay procedure contained 16 $\mu M$ [$^{14}C$]cholate, 100 $\mu M$ CoA, 5 mM
$Mg^{2+}$, 5 mM ATP, 0.8 mg of microsomal protein/ml and 100 mM Tris/
HCl buffer, pH 7.3 in an assay volume of 0.1 ml. The identification of [$^{14}C$]choloyl-CoA was based on its comparison with
chemically synthesised choloyl-CoA on paper and thin-layer
chromatography. The pH optimum for its reaction was pH 7.2-7.3
and the reaction had an absolute requirement for bivalent cations,
$Mg^{2+}$ and $Mn^{2+}$ being the most effective. High concentrations of
ATP appeared to cause substrate inhibition. The enzyme could be
solubilised from the microsomal membrane in an active form by
treatment with Triton N-101. Inhibition studies were consistent
with the hypothesis that one enzyme is responsible for the
synthesis of the CoA-derivatives of all the major bile acids,
but that this enzyme is different from that metabolising fatty
acids to their CoA derivatives. These conclusions are supported
by the findings of Siperstein and Murray (83) that a preparation
of palmitoyl-CoA synthetase does not catalyse the synthesis of
choloyl-CoA.
    The enzyme responsible for the second step in the formation
of amino acid conjugates, is amino acid N-acyltransferase. It is
in this reaction that amino acid specificity would be expected
to influence the spectrum of conjugates seen in vivo. Glycine
N-acylase has been isolated from an acetone powder of beef liver
mitochondria (76). When tested with benzoyl-CoA as the acyl donor,
the enzyme was specific for glycine. After purification, a 53-
fold increase in the specific activity of the enzyme was realised
with an 11% recovery of the original activity. No loss of
activity was found when the enzyme was stored at $-25^{\circ}C$ for 5
months. Dilute solutions of the enzyme were stable at $0^{\circ}C$ for
several hours. Enzyme activity was measured spectrophotometrically,
based on the decrease in absorbance at 208 nm due to the
utilisation of benzoyl-CoA during the reaction (89).
    James and Bend (90) have shown from subcellular fractionation
studies that glycine N-acyltransferase activity was mainly
located in the mitochondrial fractions of rat and rabbit tissues.

Cytosol also contained significant levels of the enzyme but this fraction may have contained protein from the matrix of the mitochondrion. The enzyme is believed to be located in the mitochondrial matrix, but is probably not membrane bound.

As previously mentioned, Vessey et al (87) have concluded from their data that separate enzymes are responsible for the formation of taurocholic and glycocholic acids. Assays contained 50 mM phosphate buffer (pH 8.0) 0.8 mg of soluble fraction protein, $^{14}C$-labelled amino acid and 25 μM choloyl-CoA in a total volume of 0.1 ml. At this concentration of choloyl-CoA, the reaction with $[^{14}C]$taurine had a $K_m$ for taurine of 0.75 mM and a $V_{max}$ of 5.9 mol of conjugate synthesised/min/mg of cytosol protein. The reaction with $[^{14}C]$glycine had a $K_m$ for glycine of 0.4 mM and $V_{max}$ of 2.0 nmol/min/mg protein. Thus, in the bovine liver the maximum potential for taurine conjugation is greater than that for glycine, although glycine has greater affinity for the enzyme. Using the technique of alternative-substrate inhibition, the authors concluded that there were separate enzymes for the conjugation of cholic acid with glycine and taurine.

In a different approach to the problem, Killenberg and Jordan (88) have purified an enzyme from rat liver 20,000 g supernatant exhibiting amino acid N-acyltransferase activity. A 200-fold purification of the enzyme was achieved with a 6.5% recovery of the original activity. Polyacrylamide gel electrophoresis localised the glycine and taurine activities of the enzyme to a single band. Both activities were optimal at pH 7.8. Killenberg and Dukes (91) have purified chemically synthesised coenzyme A thioesters of cholic, chenodeoxycholic, deoxycholic and lithocholic acids. The biological activity of these thioesters was greater than 94%. In the presence of these substrates and at physiological concentration of taurine and glycine, taurine was shown to be the favoured substrate. This is consistent with the almost exclusive production of taurine conjugates seen in the rat in vivo.

A specific radiochemical method for the in vitro assay of the glycine conjugation of carboxylic acids has been developed using phenylacetyl-CoA-[carboxy-$^{14}C$] as the activated carboxylic acid acceptor (90). This compound is a commercially available radiochemical. The paper is noteworthy in that it describes the first attempt to really study glycine N-acyltransferase free from the complications of other (cofactor-synthesising) enzymes, e.g. an acyl-CoA synthetase.

Examples of use. In rabbit the specific activity of glycine N-acyltransferase (90) was found to be ten times higher in kidney mitochondria than in liver mitochondria. The relative quantitative roles of the two tissues in vivo is uncertain. In kidney mitochondria less than 1% of the adult activity was detected in the foetus at 20 days gestation and about 10% of the adult activity at 28 and 30 days gestation. After birth, activity rose very slowly to adult levels (10-14 weeks) (92). Using a similar

sensitive radiochemical procedure, enzyme activity was found to
be undetectable in rabbit lung (44).

Caldwell et al (93) have reported a rapid and sensitive
in vitro semi-micro method for the determination of hippuric acid
formation by human and rat cadaver tissue samples. Typical incubation mixtures (1 ml) contained [$^{14}$C]benzoic acid (200 nmol;
0.5 μCi), CoA (100 nmol), ATP (for kidney 2.5 μmol; for other
organs, 5 μmol), glutathione (20 μmol), MgCl$_2$ (3 μmol) and
glycine (60 μmol) with tissue homogenate (equivalent to 20 mg
tissue) in 0.2 M Tris buffer, pH 8.0. Human cadaver liver and
kidney samples formed hippuric acid conjugates, whereas brain,
intestine, heart and lung did not. Tissues from human and rat
corpses stored for 72 h at 4$^{o}$C were still capable of forming
hippuric acid. Hippuric acid formation in liver and kidney
samples of a 31 week old premature foetus was one half to one
third of that seen in comparable adult tissue, a finding similar
to that reported for liver by Irjala (94).

The most striking features of amino acid conjugation are the
variety of amino acids used and how these vary with species and
with structure of the xenobiotic. Hirom et al (95) have recently
reviewed amino acid conjugations in mammals; these and other
authors have noted the involvement of glycine, glutamine,
glutamic acid, serine, alanine and taurine in mammals, of
ornithine in birds and of several others in plants. Two examples
will serve to illustrate the effects of substrate and species.
1- and 2-Naphthylacetic acids are conjugated with glycine to
equal extents in the rat, but in the ferret a greater proportion of the 2-isomer is conjugated with glycine. The 1-isomer
is 63% conjugated with taurine by the ferret whereas the rat
excretes only a trace of this metabolite. The 2-isomer is conjugated with taurine equally in the two species (96) (Figure 14).
3-Phenoxybenzoic acid, liberated during the metabolism of the
pyrethroid insecticides permethrin and cypermethrin, is excreted
in different forms by four species so far studied (97)(98)(99).
Its major metabolite in cows is the glutamic acid conjugate, in
mice, the taurine conjugate and in dogs, the glycine conjugate;
in rats it is p-hydroxylated and sulphated prior to excretion
(Figure 15). These interspecies variations may be a consequence
of amino acid availability or of N-acylase specificity.

The situation in vivo is complicated by the fact that
carboxylic acids are also conjugated with glucuronic acid.
Dixon et al (100) have used a similar in vitro assay system to
that previously described (93) to study the physico-chemical,
structural and biological factors influencing the pattern of
conjugation reactions of arylacetic acids. Using phenylacetic
acid, 1-naphthylacetic acid, diphenylacetic acid and hydratropic
acid (methylphenylacetic acid) as substrates, they concluded
that the main factor influencing conjugation with glycine is the
chemical structure of the substrate. For example, α-substitution
of the methylene group of phenylacetic acids results in a

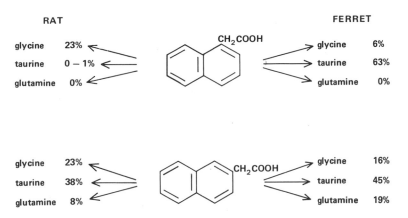

Figure 14.   *Amino acid conjugation of naphthylacetic acids*

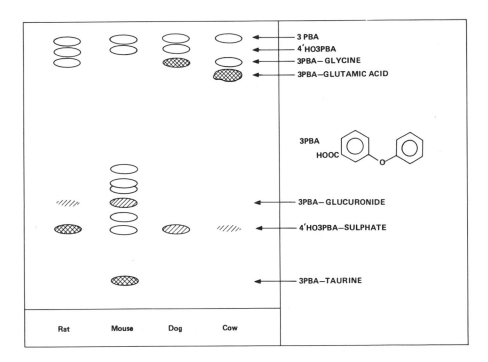

Figure 15.   *Species differences in the conjugation of 3-phenoxybenzoic acid*

blocking of amino acid conjugation in vitro. By contrast, glucuronic acid conjugation of arylacetic acid seems to be favoured by extensive non-specific entrapment by the endoplasmic reticulum, a process related more to lipid solubility than to chemical structure. These findings support in vivo metabolic profiles obtained when these acids are orally dosed to rats (101-106).

The explanation of these various differences will be found via the use of subcellular fractions, yet to date virtually no work directed to this end has been reported.

Toxicological significance. The change in physical properties effected by the amino acid conjugation of a carboxylic acid is not dramatic (although there is an obvious difference in the extreme case of, for example, 3-phenoxybenzoic acid to 3-phenoxybenzoyltaurine). However, one may expect a somewhat more efficient excretion of a conjugate compared with that of its parent acid. In the case of a bioactive acid (comparatively rare with respect to mammals in pesticide chemistry) conjugation is also likely to alter the molecular structure to diminish the activity. The species differences noted above are unlikely to have great consequences because amino acid conjugation is a relatively minor molecular change and it occurs usually near the end of a metabolic pathway.

Conjugation with Glutathione

Mechanism and location. Glutathione conjugation is the initiating step in mercapturic acid biosynthesis in mammals. The first step is the most important in detoxification because it confers hydrophilic character on the (usually) lipophilic xenobiotic and, in addition, the glutathione conjugates are readily secreted in bile and are thus readily eliminated from the animal. The second stage (γ-glutamyltransferase action) and third stage (peptidase action) are neglected areas of study in mercapturic acid biosynthesis, though some recent work has been published (107). They seem to occur in both liver and kidney. Both enzymes, for example, have been found in kidney microsomal fraction (108). The fourth stage is described in the Acetylation section above.

Glutathione conjugation is unique among the Type II processes in that a discrete high-energy substrate is not required. The chemical energy for the reaction is derived from the mutual reactivity of the nucleophilic sulphur of glutathione for an electrophilic centre in the xenobiotic substrate. The electrophilic centre may be present in the molecule per se or it may be generated by type I metabolism (see preceeding chapter). The conjugation step is catalysed by one or more of a number of glutathione transferases (EC 2.5.1.18) which are located in the cytosol of mammalian cells.

Isolation, properties and use. A very simple method of preparation from liver therefore consists of: homogenisation, centrifugation at 200,000 g for 30 min and dialysis against pH 7.4 buffer. These enzymes can be stored at -25°C for months. The demethylation of phosphoric acid triesters (with which we have

most experience) is retained after freeze-drying and storage at
4°C for months. However, the purified enzyme is, as usual, much
less stable. Whether fresh samples are dialysed or not, they must
be fortified with glutathione (to about 5 mM) for full activity.
The endogenous glutathione is lost during liver processing in
three ways: catabolism, oxidation and dilution. The acidity of
glutathione is sometimes overlooked by newcomers in this field.
It is essential to adjust the pH back up to 7.4 when preparing
the stock solution, even in 0.1 M phosphate buffer.

The history of the glutathione transferases is a classic
example of the dominant effect of substrate selection on research,
nomenclature and thinking. The electrophilic centres that are
subject to attack by glutathione include those in alkyl halides,
aralkyl halides, aryl halides, epoxides, alkenes, chlorotriazines,
nitrocompounds and compounds containing electrophilic nitrogen or
sulphur atoms. The situation in the early 1970s, reviewed by
Chasseaud (109)(110) and Hutson (111), was one in which the number
of enzymes was increasing with the increasing number of substrates
investigated. These enzymes (Figure 16) were not shown to be
discrete proteins but efforts were being made to separate the
various activities. Jakoby and coworkers then entered the field
and used the approach of separating rat liver cytosol proteins by
column chromatography and subsequently defining the activities of
the separated proteins. Their classification system (112)(113) is
based on the reverse order of elution from a carboxymethyl-
cellulose column which was the major step in the separation of
the transferases from one another. Seven proteins were isolated:
transferases AA, A, B, C, D, E, and M. Enzymes A, B. C and E have
molecular weights of 45,000 and are dissociable into two approximately equal sub-units. There is not much information available
on transferases AA (114), D or M. Whilst clarifying the situation
with respect to the protein, this work has not allowed a neat
correlation between protein and substrate type. There is considerable overlap in substrate specificity (112)(115) which is
illustrated in general terms in Figure 16. An earlier purification,
aimed specifically at 'dimethyl phosphoric acid triester –
glutathione methyl transferase' from rabbit liver, used a combination of ammonium sulphate precipitation, zinc salt formation,
calcium phosphate gel treatment and gel filtration on Sephadex
G150. A 45-fold purification was achieved (116) but the final
product, which also retained its activity towards methyl iodide,
was probably a mixture of all of the transferases (which form
about 10% of the liver cytosol). Four organophosphorus insecticide
-degrading enzymes have recently been separated from rat liver
cytosol by chromatography on hydroxyapatite (117). Transferase I
catalysed the demethylation of methylparathion; transferases III
and IV catalysed the demethylation and the de-arylation of methylparathion and the depyrimidinylation of diazinon. When different
groups of workers use different purification methods and assay
substrates it is difficult to correlate the results of the various

| 'Enzymes' classified by substrate | Jakoby's protein classification (AA,A,B,C,D,E,M) |
|---|---|
| Glutathione — | |
| S—alkyl transferase | $E \gg AA > B$ |
| S—aralkyl transferase | $A = C > E > M > B = AA$ |
| S—aryl transferase | $A > AA > B = C \gg E$ |
| S—epoxide (alkyl) transferase | $E \gg A$ |
| S—epoxide(aryl) transferase | $A = C = E > B > AA$ |
| S—alkene transferase | $C \gg A \gg B$ |
| S—triazinyl transferase | ? |
| nitro transferase | $C > AA > B > A$ |
| mercaptoalkyl transferase | $C > A = AA > B$ |

*Figure 16.   Glutathione transferases*

studies. Recently a study of the activity of transferases A, B,
C and E (115) in the demethylation of dimethyl 1-naphthylphosphate
revealed that this was an activity of transferase E (118). Therefore it is possible that transferase I (117) and transferase E
(115) are identical. Some encouraging results have been gained
recently by affinity chromatography on agarose to which glutathione
was attached by 1,6-diaminohexane spacer molecules. Transferases
AA, A and C were retained while transferase B appeared in the void
volume. The bound transferases could be recovered by affinity
elution with KCl/glutathione gradients (119). Bromosulphophthalein
-sepharose has also been used successfully for the pig cytosol
enzyme (120).

The selection of assay method depends, as usual, on whether
the priority for study is the enzyme activity or the reaction it
catalyses. Jakoby et al (112) have mostly used spectrophotometric
methods. Clarke et al (121) have worked out such a method for the
methylparathion methyl transferase. A reasonably convenient method
applicable to radioactive substrates (4) involves partition of the
reaction mixture between water and toluene and radioanalysis for
product and substrate respectively. A potentially useful partition
procedure employing [$^{35}$S]glutathione has been described by
Hayakawa et al (122). It is rather cumbersome but it is very sensitive and, of course, applicable to non-radioactive xenobiotic
substrates, thereby allowing much wider substrate selection for
structure-activity studies.

It is likely that high-pressure liquid chromatography will
be used increasingly in assays of glutathione conjugation. When
operated in the reverse-phase mode it is very suitable for the
analysis of polar conjugates, as has recently been demonstrated
(123). This method could operate with ultra-violet, fluorescence
or radioactivity detection, depending on circumstances.

A technical problem, particularly prevelant in glutathione
conjugation, is the tendency of the xenobiotic to react spontaneously with glutathione. This feature may give very high blank
rates which sometimes alter dramatically as the pH is increased
above 8. Therefore great care is needed in making allowances for
this in quantitative work.

Examples of use. A combination of methods, usually in vivo
studies supported by studies with subcellular fractions, has been
used to demonstrate the involvement of glutathione conjugation in
the metabolism of several classes of pesticide. These were
reviewed in some detail recently in this series (111) and only
more recent key references are given in the list of such reactions
shown in Table IV. Most of these are important detoxification
modes because they effect the alteration of the bioactive molecule.
An exception is the metabolism of the alkyl thiocyanates; in the
reaction between glutathione and the electrophilic sulphur atom,
cyanide ion is liberated and is probably responsible for the bioactivity of this class of compound. It should be noted that this
reaction is an example of glutathione reacting with an

electrophilic atom other than carbon. Glutathione conjugation also occurs frequently in the further metabolism of the primary bio-transformation products of various pesticides. Some examples are given below.

Table IV. Glutathione conjugation in pesticide metabolism

| Pesticide class | Reaction | Reference |
|---|---|---|
| Organophosphorus triesters | de-alkylation | (117) |
| | | (116) |
| | | (126) |
| | de-arylation | (117) |
| | de-pyrimidinylation | (127) |
| DDT | ? | |
| Hexachlorocyclohexanes | dehydrochlorination | (128) |
| Diphenyl ethers | de-arylation | (129) |
| Alkylthiocyanates | de-thiocyanylation | (130) (131) |
| Propachlor | de-chlorination | (129) |
| Haloacetamides | de-chlorination | (129) |
| Chloro-s-triazines | de-chlorination | (132) |
| Alkylmercapto-s-triazines | de-alkylsulphoxylation | (124) |
| Thiocarbamates | de-alkylsulphoxylation | (125) |

Two of the compound classes shown in Table IV, the alkyl-mercapto-s-triazines herbicides and the thiocarbamate herbicides, are good examples where the metabolism was studied at the sub-cellular level in order to explain the biotransformation pathways observed in vivo. Moreover, two reaction classes, in different subcellular fractions, used in a specific sequence, were needed to reconstruct and explain the overall reactions. A herbicidal methylmercapto-s-triazine was eliminated in rat urine as the s-triazinyl mercapturic acid and in rat bile as the s-triazinyl-glutathione conjugate. As the methylmercapto-s-triazine itself was not a substrate for cytosolic glutathione transferase, clearly an extra step was occurring in vivo. Incubation of the herbicide with rat liver microsomes (+ NADPH) afforded a new product, the herbicide S-oxide. When incubated with glutathione, the S-oxide reacted spontaneously to afford the same s-triazine conjugate as that observed in the bile (124). A similar sequence was discovered for the herbicides EPTC and butylate (N,N-dialkyl-S-alkyl thiocarbamates). The thiocarbamates were oxidised by microsomes to thiocarbamate sulphoxides. These compounds (which are reasonably stable) were substrates for a glutathione transferase-catalysed formation of S-(N,N-dialkylcarbamoyl) glutathiones (125). These sequences, illustrated in Figure 17, could not have been demonstrated easily be the use of a higher level of organisation such as whole cells.
    Glutathione has been shown to participate in

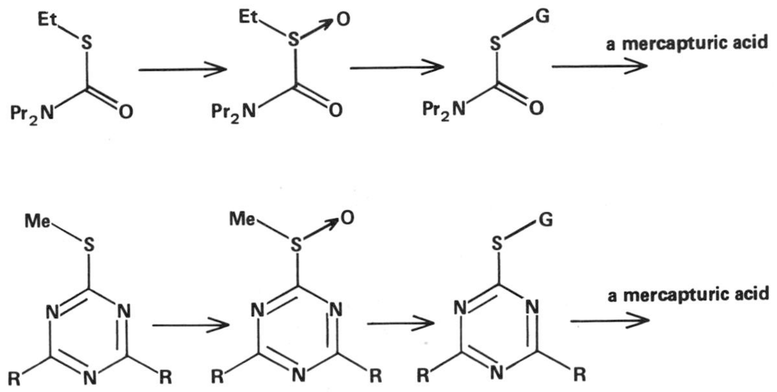

Figure 17. *Glutathione in the metabolism of thiocarbamate and thiotriazine herbicides*

biotransformation without being obvious in the final products. Even with the well-known glutathione-dependent demethylation of dimethylphosphate triester insecticides, most of the S-methylglutathione formed is metabolised to $CO_2$ and very little methylmercapturic acid is excreted. Clearly the use of subcellular fractions is indicated in discoveries of this type. The fate of the vinyl phosphate insecticide, dimethylvinphos, may be used to illustrate this point further. The main radioactive metabolites derived from $^{14}C$-phenyl labelling in vivo were de-methyldimethylvinphos and a metabolite derived from the phenylvinyloxy group, 1-(2,4-dichlorophenyl)ethanol (as glucuronide) (4). The demethylation, predictably, was effected by (dialysed) cytosol and glutathione.

2,4-Dichlorophenylethanol was assumed to be derived from 2,4-dichloroacetophenone which in turn was thought to be formed by the reductive dechlorination of the hydrolysis product of dimethylvinphos (2,4-dichlorophenacyl chloride). The mechanism of the reductive dechlorination was unknown until we studied the metabolism of the phenacyl chloride in rat liver fractions. The following sequence of reactions was discovered using cytosol: (i) spontaneous reaction of phenacyl halide with glutathione to afford 2,4-dichlorophenacyl-glutathione, (ii) enzyme-catalysed reaction of the latter with another molecule of glutathione to form oxidised glutathione and the phenacyl anion which rearranged to 2,4-dichloroacetophenone (133). Microsomes and NADPH simply reduced the keto group of 2,4-dichlorophenacyl chloride to give the chlorohydrin (not observed in the in vivo metabolism). Thus glutathione enters the metabolic pathways of dimethylvinphos at three points (Figure 18) but it is scarcely observed in the excreted metabolites. In this series of experiments we also used the in vitro technique to demonstrate that the administration of phenobarbital to rats (which protected them 10-fold against the acute oral toxicity of dimethylvinphos) induced the activity of the cytosol demethylating enzyme 2-fold. Dimethylvinphos exhibits a large  difference in acute toxicity to rat and dog (rat > dog); dog liver cytosol was shown to demethylate dimethylvinphos at about twice the rate of rat liver cytosol (4). Thus, the enzyme could have some role in the selective toxicity of dimethylvinphos.

This example illustrates several important features:
(i)   direct glutathione conjugation of parent molecule (effecting detoxification)
(ii)  glutathione conjugation after bioactivation by primary metabolism (hydrolysis in this case)
(iii) glutathione conjugation by attack on an electrophilic atom other than carbon (sulphur in this case)
(iv)  only traces of the glutathione-conjugated products (mercapturic acids) appearing in the excreted metabolites
(v)   use of subcellular fractions to investigate a species difference (rat versus dog)

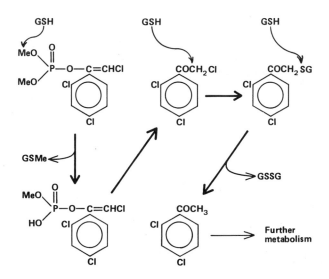

*Figure 18.   Glutathione in the metabolism of dimethylvinphos*

(vi) use of subcellular fractions to investigate the alteration
of drug-metabolising enzymes of an animal.

Studies of the liver enzyme have shown that glutathione
transferases occur in many other animals including rabbit (118),
pig (118), (23), monkey (23)(134)(135), tree shrew (23), sheep
(136), guinea-pig (122), horse (122), cow (122), mouse (122),
chicken (126), and man (137). Where detailed studies have been
carried out (135)(136) (137) the enzymes, including those of
man, have been shown to be very similar in physical properties.

Liver is the richest source of the enzymes. For example, a
recent study of Japanese monkey (Macaca fuscata) (134) was
typical in showing the following aryltransferase (1,2-dichloro-
4-nitrobenzene) activities (μmol/min/mg protein): liver, 18;
spleen, 2.6; kidney, 2.1; lung, 1.9; brain, 1.9; muscle, 1.8;
placenta, 0.3; pancreas, 0; erythrocytes, 0; blood, 0. Activity
has recently been reported in small intestines (138)(139) and in
leucocytes (140).

Enzyme measurements have also been used to assess glutathione
conjugation during development of the neonate. Alkyl transferase
activity in the rat neonate is very low for about 6 days and then
rises steadily for about 40 days to the adult level (141). Transferase B (measured as aryltransferase) is present at birth at
about one fifth of the adult level and rises steadily for about
40 days (142).

However, in all general statements about the presence of
glutathione transferase in various species, tissues or altered
states, the substrate used for assay must be noted before the
relevance to one's own work is assessed. The importance of
glutathione conjugation in limiting the cytotoxic, mutagenic and
carcinogenic action of electrophilic compounds (143) is generating much research into the species and tissue distribution of
the enzyme(s). However, too much reliance on results derived
from tests using substrates (e.g. polycyclic aromatic hydrocarbon
epoxides) unrelated to one's own problem may well prove to be
only of limited value.

Toxicological significance. Glutathione conjugation results
in a dramatic change in the physical properties of a molecule,
usually leading to a loss of bioactivity. The conjugate is
ideally structured for biliary secretion and therefore it is
efficiently removed from the liver. Other enzymes efficiently
convert the conjugate into a mercapturic acid that is readily
excreted via the urine. However, perhaps the most important
function of this conjugation process is the protection it affords
against electrophilic compounds, be they ingested as such or
generated within the organism via metabolism. Without this
protection mammals would be much more susceptible than they are
to low doses of teratogens, mutagens, carcinogens and cytotoxic
compounds.

## Other Uses of Subcellular Fractions in Xenobiotic Metabolism Studies

A relatively recent use of subcellular fractions is in bacterial test systems for mutagenicity of the type developed by Ames and coworkers (144). The fraction commonly used is a 9000 g fraction (S-9 fraction) from the livers of rats treated with an Arachlor (to induce microsomal enzymes). Its role in the test system is the provision of a mammalian metabolism capability for the (possible) activation of intrinsically inactive compounds. This may not commonly be seen as a use in metabolism studies; but if the bacteria are regarded as a bioassay technique for the detection of mutagens, the system is a useful addition to the techniques used for the study of metabolism in vitro. The main component of the bioactivation system is regarded as being the microsomal mono-oxygenase (hence the use of inducers to prepare a more 'potent' S-9 fraction). However, it will be clear from the various reactions discussed above that some of the type II reactions effect the bioactivation of certain metabolites. They also effect the deactivation of many compounds and their metabolites. The potentially great predictive value of these test systems has led to their widespread, but often uncritical use. The importance of a standardised preparation containing active microsomal mono-oxygenase is appreciated but the role of the many other enzymes in the S-9 fraction has been largely ignored.

The widespread use and enthusiastic reception gained by this simple, quick and potentially very useful system has led to a reaction from certain quarters and a heated debate is currently being conducted. There is clearly a need to define the reactions occurring in the test system. The balance between activation and deactivation is critical to its relevance to the in vivo situation. The state of the various enzymes in the S-9 fraction and the concentrations of the various cofactors (many of which are described above) requires measurement and control. Species variations are important. For example it is possible that 2-aminoanthracene (mutagenic in the presence of S-9 from rat liver) would not give a positive response if dog liver S-9 fractions were used. The first step in its bioactivation (N-acetylation, see Figures 9 and 10) is inoperative. Glutathione-dependent deactivation is largely inoperative in standard S-9 fraction because, although the glutathione S-transferases are present, glutathione itself is largely destroyed by catabolism, dilution and oxidation (145). A study of the various enzyme activities and cofactor concentrations in human liver fraction (prepared as S-9) would also prove very useful in the interpretation of results of the Ames test.

## Literature Cited

1.  Brodie, B. B., Gillette, J. R. and LaDu, B. N.
    Ann. Rev. Biochem. (1958), 27, 427.
2.  Gillette, J. R. Prog. in Drug Res. (1963), 6, 11.
3.  Wright, A. S., Potter, D., Wooder, M. F., Donninger, C. and
    Greenland, R. D. Food Cosmet. Toxicol. (1972), 10, 311.
4.  Crawford, M. J., Hutson, D. H. and King, P. A. Xenobiotica
    (1976), 6, 745.
5.  Lowry, O. H., Rosebrough, N. J., Farr, A. L. and
    Randall, R. J. J. Biol. Chem. (1951), 193, 265.
6.  Robinson, H. W. and Hogden, C. G. J. Biol. Chem. (1940),
    135, 727.
7.  Fry, J. R. and Bridges, J. W. Biochem. Soc. Trans. (1974),
    2, 600.
8.  Kamath, S. and Rubin, E. Biochem. Biophys. Res. Comm.
    (1972), 49, 52.
9.  Kupfer, D. and Levin, E. Biochem. Biophys. Res. Comm.
    (1972), 47, 611.
10. Cinti, D. L., Moldeus, P. and Schenkman, J. B.
    Biochem. Pharmacol. (1972), 21, 3249.
11. Litterst, C. L., Mimnaugh, E. G., Reagan, R. L. and
    Gram, T. L. Life Sci. (1975), 17, 813.
12. Tangen, O., Jonsson, J. and Orrenius, S. IUB Ninth Int.
    Congr., Stockholm (1973), p. 34. Abstract (1e 24).
13. Capdevila, J., Jakobsson, S. W., Jernström, B., Helia, O.
    and Orrenius, S. Cancer Res. (1975), 35, 2820.
14. Dutton, G. J., Wishart, G. J., Leakey, J. E. A. and
    Goheer, M. A. in 'Drug Metabolism - from Microbes to Man',
    Eds. Parke, D. V. and Smith, R. L. Taylor and Francis,
    London (1977), p. 71.
15. Dutton, G. J. and Burchall, B. Prog. Drug Metab. (1977),
    2, 1.
16. Ziegler, J. M., Lisboa, B. P., Batt, A. M. and Siest, G.
    Biochem. Pharmacol. (1975), 24, 1291.
17. Mulder, G. J. and van Doorn, B. D. Biochem. J. (1975),
    151, 131.
18. Tredger, J. M. and Chhabra, R. S. Drug Metab. Disposit.
    (1976), 4, 451.
19. Burchell, B. Biochem. J. (1977), 161, 543.
20. Dell Villar, E., Sanchez, E., Autor, A. P. and Tephly, T. R.
    Mol. Pharmacol. (1975), 11, 236.
21. Dingell, J. V. and Sossi, N. Drug Metab. Disposit.
    (1977), 5, 397.
22. Bedford, C. T., Harrod, R. K., Hoadley, E. C. and
    Hutson, D. H. Xenobiotica (1975), 5, 485.
23. Litterst, C. L., Gram, T. E., Mimnaugh, E. G., Leber, P.,
    Emmerling, D. and Freudenthal, R. I. Drug Metab. Disposit.
    (1976), 4, 203.

24.  Millburn, P. Biochem. Soc. Trans. (1974), 2, 1182.
25.  Jansen, P. L. M. and Henderson, P. Th. Biochem. Pharmacol. (1972), 21, 2457.
26.  Lech, J. J. Biochem. Pharmacol. (1974), 23, 2403.
27.  Dutton, G. J. and Montgomery, J. P. Biochem. J. (1958), 70, 17P.
28.  Salseduc, M. M. Biochem. Pharmacol. (1968), 17, 1163.
29.  Aitio, A. Xenobiotica (1973), 3, 13.
30.  Aitio, A. Int. J. Biochem. (1974), 5, 325.
31.  El-Shourbagy, N. A. and Dorough, H. W. J. Econ. Entomol. (1974), 67, 344.
32.  Bock, K. W., van Ackeren, G., Lorch, F. and Birke, F. W. Biochem. Pharmacol. (1976), 25, 2351.
33.  Mulder, G. J., Hinson, J. A. and Gillette, J. R. Biochem. Pharmacol. (1977), 26, 189.
34.  Hutson, D. H. Food Cosmet. Toxicol. (1976), 14, 577.
35.  von Bahr, C. and Bertilsson, L. Xenobiotica (1971), 1, 205.
36.  Dodgson, K. S. in 'Drug Metabolism from Microbes to Man', Eds. D. V. Parke and R. L. Smith, Taylor and Francis, London, 1977, p. 91.
37.  Armstrong, L. M. and Carroll, J. Biochem. Soc. Trans. (1974), 2, 743.
38.  Wu, S. G. and Straub, K. D. J. Biol. Chem. (1976), 251, 6529.
39.  Irving, C. C., Jones, D. H. and Russell, L. T. Cancer Res. (1971), 31, 387.
40.  van Kemper, G. M. J. and Jansen, G. S. I. M. Anal. Biochem. (1972), 46, 438.
41.  Mulder, G. J. and Hagedoorn, A. H. Biochem. Pharmacol. (1974), 23, 2101.
42.  Mulder, G. J. Anal. Biochem. (1975), 64, 350.
43.  Mulder, G. J. and Scholtens, E. Biochem. J. (1977), 165, 553.
44.  Hook, G. E. R. and Bend, J. R. Life Sci. (1976), 18, 279.
45.  Gram, T. E., Litterest, C. L. and Mimnaugh, E. G. Drug Metab. Disposit. (1974), 2, 254.
46.  Schneider, P. J. and Dingell, J. V. Pharmacologist (1975), 17, 184.
47.  Irving, C. C. in "Biological Oxidation of Nitrogen in Organic Molecules", Eds. J. W. Bridges, J. W. Gorrod and D. V. Parke, Taylor and Francis, London, 1972, p. 75.
48.  DeBaun, J. R., Miller, E. C. and Miller, J. A., Cancer Res. (1970), 30, 577.
49.  DeBaun, J. R., Smith, J. Y. R., Miller, E. C. and Miller, J. A. Science (1970), 167, 184.
50.  Hinson, J. A., Mitchell, J. R. and Jollow, D. J. Mol. Pharmac. (1975), 11, 462.
51.  Hinson, J. A. and Mitchell, J. E. Pharmacologist (1975), 17, 217.

52. Boyland, E., Kinder, C. H. and Mansen, D. Biochem. J. (1961), 78, 175.

53. Lotlikar, P. D. and Wasserman, M. B. Biochem. J. (1970), 120, 661.

54. Capel, I. D., Millburn, P. and Williams, R. T. Biochem. Soc. Trans. (1974), 2, 305.

55. Willetts, A. Biochem. Biophys. Acta (1974), 362, 448.

56. Weber, W. in "Metabolic Conjugation and Metabolic Hydrolysis", Ed. W. H. Fishman, Academic Press, New York, 1973, Vol. 3, p. 249.

57. Steinberg, M. S., Cohen, S. N. and Weber, W. W. Biochem. Biophys. Acta (1971), 235, 89.

58. Weber, W. W., Miceli, J. N., Hearse, D. J. and Drummond, D. J. Drug Metab. Disposit. (1976), 4, 94.

59. Green, R. M. and Elce, J. S. Biochem. J. (1975), 147, 283.

60. Weber, W. W. and Cohen, S. N. Mol. Pharmacol. (1967), 3, 266.

61. Glinsukon, T., Benjamin, T., Grantham, P. H., Lewis, N. L. and Weisburger, E. K. Biochem. Pharmacol. (1976), 25, 95.

62. Glinsukon, T., Benjamin, T., Grantham, P. H., Weisburger, E. K. and Roller, P. R. Xenobiotica (1975), 5, 475.

63. Hearse, D. J. and Weber, W. W. Biochem. J. (1973), 132, 519.

64. Lower, G. M. and Bryan, G. T. Biochem. Pharmacol. (1973), 22, 1581.

65. Mitchell, J. R., Thorgeirsson, U. P., Black, M., Timbrell, J. A., Snodgrass, W. R., Potter, W. Z., Jollow, D. J. and Keiser, H. R. Clin. Pharmacol. Therap. (1975), 18, 70.

66. Guldberg, H. C. and Marsden, C. A. Pharmacol. Rev. (1975), 27, 135.

67. Creveling, C. R., Morris, N., Shimizu, H., Ong, H. H. and Daly, J. Mol. Pharmacol. (1972), 8, 398.

68. Axelrod, J. and Daly, J. Biochem. Biophys. Acta (1968), 159, 472.

69. Gulliver, P. A. and Tipton, K. F. Biochem. Pharmacol. (1978), 27, 773.

70. Fujita, T. and Suzuoki, Z. J. Biochem. (Japan) (1973), 74, 717.

71. McBain, J. B. and Menn, J. J. Biochem. Pharmacol. (1969), 18, 2282.

72. Grunewald, G. L., Grindel, J. M. and Vincek, W. C. Mol. Pharmacol. (1975), 11, 694.

73. Climie, I. J. G. and Hutson, D. H. in "Proceedings of the Fourth International Meeting on Pesticide Chemistry (IUPAC) Zurich, 1978, Pergamon Press, Oxford.

74. Mahler, H. R., Wakil, S. J. and Bock, R. M. J. Biol. Chem. (1953), 204, 453.

75.  Garland, P. B., Yates, D. W. and Haddock, B. A. Biochem. J.
     (1970), 119, 553.
76.  Schachter, D. and Taggart, J. V. J. Biol. Chem. (1954),
     208, 263.
77.  Bartlett, K. and Gompertz, D. Biochem. Med. (1974), 10, 15.
78.  Gatley, S. J., Sherratt, H.S.A.
     Biochem. Soc. Trans. (1976), 4, 525.
79.  Osmundsen, H. and Sherratt, H. S. A. FEBS Lett. (1975), 55,
     38.
80.  Halling, P. J., Brand, M. D. and Chappell, J. B. FEBS Lett.
     (1975), 34, 169.
81.  Yousef, I. M. and Fisher, M. M. Can. J. Phsyiol. Pharmacol.
     (1975), 53, 880.
82.  Vessey, D. A. and Zakim, D. Biochem. J. (1977), 163, 357.
83.  Siperstein, M. D. and Murray, A. W. Science (1955), 123,
     377.
84.  Bremer, J. Acta Chem. Scand. (1956), 10, 56.
85.  Elliott, W. H. Biochem. J. (1956), 62, 433.
86.  Schersten, T. Biochim. Biophys. Acta (1967), 141, 144.
87.  Vessey, D. A., Crissey, M. H. and Zakim, D. A. Biochem. J.
     (1977), 163, 181.
88.  Killenberg, P. G. and Jordan, J. T. J. Biol. Chem. (1978),
     253, 1005.
89.  Schachter, D. and Taggart, J. V. J. Biol. Chem. (1953),
     203, 925.
90.  James, M. O. and Bend, J. R. Biochem. J. (1978), 172, 285.
91.  Killenberg, P. G. and Dukes, D. F. J. Lipid Res. (1976),
     17, 451.
92.  James, M. O. and Bend, J. R. Biochem. J. (1978), 172, 293.
93.  Caldwell, J., Moffatt, J. R. and Smith, R. L. Xenobiotica
     (1976), 6, 275.
94.  Irjala, K. Ann. Acad. Sci. Fenn., Ser. A. (1972), V, 154.
95.  Hirom, P. C., Idle, J. R. and Millburn, P. in "Drug
     Metabolism from Microbes to Man", Eds. D. V. Parke and
     R. L. Smith, Taylor and Francis, London, 1976, p. 299.
96.  Emudiaghe, T. S., Caldwell, J. and Smith, R. L. Biochem.
     Soc. Trans. (1977), 5, 1006.
97.  Gaughan, L. C., Unai, T. and Casida, J. E. J. Agric. Fd.
     Chem. (1977), 25, 9; Gaughan, L. C., Ackerman, M. E.,
     Unai, T. and Casida, J. E. J. Agric. Fd. Chem. (1978),
     26, 613.
98.  Hutson, D. H. and Casida, J. E. Xenobiotica, in press.
99.  Crawford, M. J., Crayford, J. V., Croucher, A. and
     Hutson, D. H. Unpublished work.
100. Dixon, P. A. F., Caldwell, J. and Smith, R. L.
     Xenobiotica (1977), 7, 727.
101. James, M. O., Smith, R.L.,Williams,R.T. and Reidenberg,M.M.
     Proc. Roy. Soc. Lond. B. (1972), 182, 25.

102.   James, M. O., Smith, R. L. and Williams, R. T.
       Xenobiotica (1972), 2, 499.
103.   Dixon, P. A. F., Uwaifo, A., Caldwell, J. and Smith, R. L.
       Biochem. Soc. Trans. (1974), 2, 879.
104.   Dixon, P. A. F., Caldwell, J. and Smith, R. L.
       Xenobiotica (1977), 7, 695.
105.   Dixon, P. A. F., Caldwell, J. and Smith, R. L.
       Xenobiotica (1977), 7, 707.
106.   Dixon, P. A. F., Caldwell, J. and Smith, R. L.
       Xenobiotica (1977 ), 7, 717.
107.   Hughey, R. P., Rankin, B. B., Elce, J. S. and Curthoys,
       N. P. Arch. Biochem. Biophys. (1978), 186, 211.
108.   Suga, T., Kumaoka, H. and Akagi, M. J. Biochem. (Tokyo)
       (1966), 60, 133.
109.   Chasseaud, L. F. in "Glutathione: Proceedings of the 16th
       Conference of the German Society of Biological Chemistry,
       Tübingen, 1973", Eds. L. Flohé, H. Ch. Benöhr, H. Sies,
       H. D. Waller and A. Wendel. G. Thieme, Stuttgart 1974,
       p. 90.
110.   Chasseaud, L. F. Drug Metab. Rev. (1974), 2, 185.
111.   Hutson, D. H. ACS Symposium Series, No. 29 (1976), 103.
112.   Habig, W. H., Pabst, M. J. and Jakoby, W. B.
       J. Biol. Chem. (1974), 249, 7130.
113.   Jakoby, W. B. Adv. Enzymol. (1978), 46, 383.
114.   Ketley, J. N., Habig, W. H. and Jakoby, W. B. J. Biol. Chem.
       (1975), 250, 8670.
115.   Jakoby, W. B., Habig, W. H., Keen, J. H., Ketley, J. N.
       and Pabst, M. J. in "Glutathione: Metabolism and Function",
       Eds. I. M. Arias and W. B. Jakoby, Raven Press, New York,
       1976, p. 189.
116.   Hutson, D. H., Pickering, B. A. and Donninger, C.
       Biochem. J. (1972), 127, 285.
117.   Usui, K., Shishido, T. and Fukami, J. Agric. Biol. Chem.
       (1977), 41, 2491.
118.   Hutson, D. H. Chem. Biol. Interact. (1977), 16, 315.
119.   Lawrence, R. A., Baker, P. R. and Cuschieri, A. Agenda
       Papers of 575th Meeting of the Biochemical Society,
       Glasgow, 1978, p. 10.
120.   Grahnen, A. and Sjoholm, I. Eur. J. Biochem. (1977), 80,
       573.
121.   Clarke, A. G., Cropp, P. L., Smith, J. N., Speir, T. W.
       and Tan, B. J. Pest. Biochem. Physiol. (1976), 6, 126.
122.   Hayakawa, T., LeMahieu, R. A. and Udenfriend, S.
       Arch. Biochem. Biophys. (1974), 162, 223.
123.   Buckpitt, A. R., Rollins, D. E., Nelson, S. D.,
       Franklin, R. B. and Mitchell, J. R. Analyt. Biochem.
       (1977), 83, 168.
124.   Bedford, C. T., Crawford, M. J. and Hutson, D. H.
       Chemosphere (1975), 4, 311.

125.  Hubell, J. P. and Casida, J. E. <u>J. Agric. Fd. Chem.</u>
      (1977), <u>25</u>, 404.
126.  Akhtar, M. H. and Foster, T. S. <u>J. Agric. Fd. Chem.</u>
      (1977), <u>25</u>, 1017.
127.  Shishido, T., Usui, K., Sato, M. and Fukami, J.
      <u>Pest. Biochem. Physiol</u>. (1972), <u>2</u>, 51.
128.  Kraus, P. <u>Arch. Pharmacol</u>. (1976), <u>296</u>, 67.
129.  Lamoureux, G. L. and Davison, K. L. <u>Pest. Biochem. Physiol</u>.
      (1975), <u>5</u>, 497.
130.  Habig, W. H., Keen, J. H. and Jakoby, W. B.
      <u>Biochem. Biophys. Res. Comm</u>. (1975), <u>64</u>, 501.
131.  Ohkawa, H., Ohkawa, R., Yamamoto, I. and Casida, J. E.
      <u>Pest. Biochem. Physiol</u>. (1972), <u>2</u>, 95.
132.  Crayford, J. V. and Hutson, D. H. <u>Pest. Biochem. Physiol</u>.
      (1972), <u>2</u>, 295.
133.  Hutson, D. H., Holmes, D. S. and Crawford, M. J.
      <u>Chemosphere</u> (1976), <u>5</u>, 79.
134.  Asaoka, K., Ito, H. and Takahashi, K. J.
      <u>J. Biochem. (Tokyo)</u> (1977), <u>82</u>, 973.
135.  Asaoka, K. and Takahashi,K.J.<u>J. Biochem. (Tokyo)</u> (1977),
      <u>82</u>, 1313.
136.  Hayakawa, T., Udenfriend, S., Yagi, H. and Jerina, D. M.
      <u>Arch. Biochem. Biophys</u>. (1975), <u>170</u>, 438.
137.  Habig, W. H., Kamisaka, K., Ketley, J. N., Pabst, M. J.,
      Arias, I.M. and Jakoby, W. B. in "Glutathione: Metabolism
      and Function", Eds. I. M. Arias and W. B. Jakoby, Raven
      Press, New York, 1976, p. 225.
138.  Clifton, G. and Kaplowitz, N. <u>Cancer Res</u>. (1977), <u>37</u>, 788.
139.  Pinkus, L. M., Ketley, J. N. and Jakoby, W. B.
      <u>Biochem. Pharmacol</u>. (1977), <u>26</u>, 2359.
140.  Kaplowitz, N., Spina, C., Graham, M. and Kuhlenkamp, J.
      <u>Biochem. J</u>. (1978), <u>169</u>, 465.
141.  Baines, P. J., Bray, H. G. and James, S. P. <u>Xenobiotica</u>
      (1977), <u>7</u>, 653.
142.  Hales, B. F. and Neims, A. H. <u>Biochem. J</u>. (1976), <u>160</u>,
      231.
143.  DePierre, J. W. and Ernster, L. <u>Biochim. Biophys. Acta</u>
      (1978), <u>473</u>, 149.
144.  Ames, B. N., McCann, J. and Yamasaki, E. <u>Mutat. Res</u>.
      (1975), <u>31</u>, 347.
145.  Dean, B. J., Hutson, D. H. and Wright, A. S. Joint
      meeting of the American Society of Experimental
      Therapeutics and the Society of Toxicology, Houston,
      Texas, August, 1978.

RECEIVED December 20, 1978.

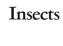

Insects

# Methods for the Study of Metabolism of Xenobiotics in Insect Cell and Organ Cultures

EDWIN P. MARKS

Metabolism and Radiation Research Laboratory, Agricultural Research, Science and Education Administration, U.S. Department of Agriculture, Fargo, ND 58102

MALCOLM J. THOMPSON and WILLIAM E. ROBBINS

Insect Physiology Laboratory, Agricultural Research, Science and Education Administration, U.S. Department of Agriculture, Beltsville, MD 20705

Although insect organ and cell culture methodologies have been used for several years in the study of insect endocrinology and development (1,2,3), little use has been made of these techniques in studying the metabolism of xenobiotics in insect tissues. However, as our knowledge of insect biochemistry and the necessity for environmentally compatible pesticides increase, the use of such methodologies will grow.

The physiological studies that have been done with insect organ cultures so far have shown us that when experiments are carried out using appropriate techniques and carefully defined conditions, cultured tissues can be induced to behave much the same way as they do in whole insects (1). To date, studies have included such diverse processes as the biosynthesis and secretion of hormones (4,5), the production and deposition of cuticle (6,7), the biosynthesis of yolk materials (8,9), the regeneration of nerve tissues (10), and the differentiation of epidermal cells into setae (11). In all these studies, acceptable approximations of what is known to occur in vivo have also been demonstrated in vitro. Thus, it seems reasonable that cell and organ culture systems could be used to advantage for studying the metabolism of xenobiotics in insects, particularly as it relates to mode of action. The questions, then, are what can be gained from the use of tissue culture methodology and whether the advantages justify the additional effort and expense.

## Organ Culture Systems

Most of the physiological and biochemical studies on insect cell and organ cultures to date have been done with organ culture systems. Organ culture differs from other in vitro techniques in that an organ must be cultured for more than 24 hours under aseptic conditions and in medium that contains an adequate energy source. In such a culture, the

architecture of the organ remains intact, and some degree of
organotypic activity can be anticipated (12).  Under these
conditions the tissues are often viable for several weeks or
even months.  For example, processes such as nerve regeneration
or cuticle deposition may begin weeks after the tissue is
explanted and may continue for as long as 90 days (10,11).
In organ cultures the problems encountered with short-term
incubations, such as surgical trauma and microbial contamination, are no longer a factor in interpreting the results.

## Advantages of Organ Culture Techniques

One of the main advantages of organ culture is the
experimental flexibility.  The investigator can add or remove
tissues, substrates, and products at any time during the
incubation period; can select or exclude any tissues or
substrates; and can include tissues from different insects in
the same culture.  Also, the medium can be sampled at intervals,
and substrate levels can be controlled and by-products removed
without seriously disturbing the system.  This experimental
flexibility is demonstrated by the use of a hanging drop
preparation to show that the release of peptide neurohormones
synthesized by cultured brains could be induced by adding
cultured cardiaca, which, in turn, sequestered and stored the
neurohormones released into the medium (13).

A second advantage of the organ culture methodology is
that a larger quantity of metabolites can be obtained from a
given amount of tissue because of the prolonged incubation.
Also, feedback inhibition can be prevented by frequent renewal
of the medium.  Isolation and purification of metabolites are
frequently easier from the relatively clean medium than from
whole body extracts.  These advantages have been discussed
previously (14).

Additional advantages include the exclusion of unwanted
tissue from the cultures and the preservation of intact cell
membranes in the living cells.  Thus, when one is working
with whole animals, it has been virtually impossible to
determine whether or not $\alpha$-ecdysone in itself has any activity
since it is readily converted by adjacent tissues to 20-
hydroxyecdysone in quantities sufficient to produce an
endocrine response (15).  With homogenates, although tissue
specificity is maintained, the cell membranes are destroyed
and endogenous inhibitors and other intracellular products
that are normally retained by the cells are released, and
these in turn induce a variety of uncontrolled reactions.
Thus, organ cultures, in which the integrity of the cells is
maintained, provide a biochemical specificity that is difficult
to obtain in other kinds of in vitro systems.

Finally, a most important advantage of the organ culture
approach is that the investigator can include both the
metabolizing and the target tissues in the same system.  This

permits study of the interrelationship or interaction between the metabolism of the test compound and the mode or site of action. This is illustrated by our work on the metabolism of 22,25-dideoxyecdysone (16,17).

## Disadvantages of Organ Culture Techniques

The disadvantages of organ culture are as numerous and as apparent as the advantages. For example, isolated tissues may lack substrates or cofactors normally present in the intact animal, which may, in turn, cause minor pathways to assume a dominant role, and thereby confuse the true picture (18). Thus, in vitro results must be compared carefully with what is known from in vivo studies.

Some tissues do not survive well in vitro and thus cannot be used successfully in organ culture studies; for example mature muscle frequently dies shortly after explantation. Another difficulty lies in obtaining uncontaminated tissues for culture. With holometabolous pupae or eggs, this is not a problem (19) but in some other stages of the life cycle, it may be extremely difficult (20). The problem of contaminated tissue also puts a practical limit on the number of explants that can be placed in a single culture. For example, if one explant out of four is contaminated, 75% success may be expected in cultures containing one explant per culture, less than 45% success would be expected in cultures containing 3 explants and there is only a 17% chance of success in cultures containing six explants and contamination is a virtual certainty. Thus, when large amounts of tissue are needed, the explants must be cultured separately or in small groups, an arduous task. Even with large numbers of cultures, the amounts of metabolites are often vanishingly small, so microchemical methods must be used (4).

Finally, organ culture is expensive, both in time and materials, and should be used only when less laborious methods are not available.

## Metabolism of 22,25-Dideoxyecdysone (Triol) in Organ Culture

Having discussed the use of organ culture in the abstract, we would now like to discuss in some detail a study of the metabolism of the ecdysteroid 22,25-dideoxyecdysone (triol, Fig. 1). In different species of insects, or at different times or stages during the development of the same species of insect, this interesting ecdysteroid may either enter the major pathway(s) of molting hormone metabolism and serve as a precursor for the biosynthesis of the insect molting hormones (21,22) or it may be treated as a xenobiotic and metabolized to a complex mixture of hydroxylated steroids (22,23). The same dual role is reflected in the biological or physiological activity and the action of 22,25-dideoxyecdysone: In certain insects or biological test systems, it has molting hormone

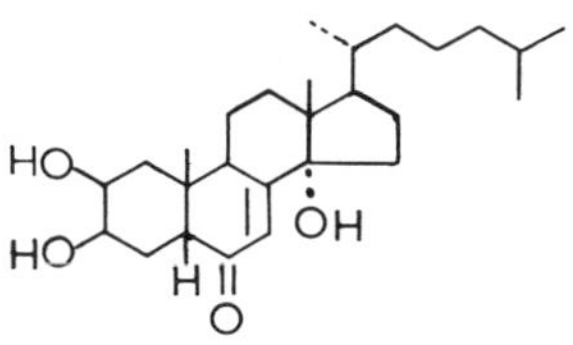

22,25-Dideoxyecdysone
(Triol)

*Figure 1*

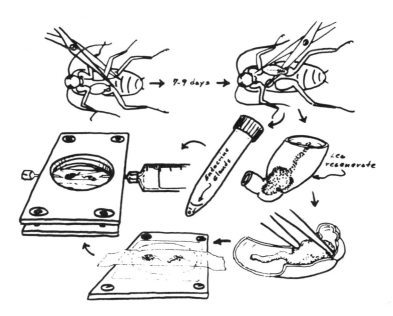

*Figure 2.    Schematic of leg regenerate–Rose chamber technique.*

*The mesothoracic legs are removed from freshly molted, late instar cockroach nymphs.*
*After 28 days the coxal stump is removed and the leg regenerate is dissected out.  The*
*test tissues are placed under the dialysis strip and the chamber is assembled and filled*
*with medium.  The test compound(s) are placed under the dialysis strip with a micro-*
*syringe.*

activity (21,24,25); in a number of other insect species it
is a potent in vivo inhibitor of development, metamorphosis,
and reproduction (24,25,26).

   Our initial studies with the triol were carried out in
Rose multipurpose tissue chambers. These chambers, which we
have found to be extremely useful for many kinds of experiments,
consist of a silicone gasket that is held between two coverslips
by a pair of metal plates. With a strip of dialysis membrane
to hold the leg regenerate tissue in place, (Fig. 2) the Rose
chamber permits experimental flexibility combined with a high
quality optical image for visual evaluation of the tissue
with a compound microscope (27). Also, the soft silicone
gaskets permit the use of a microsyringe to place the
experimental compound in direct contact with the tissue. In
chambers containing a threshold concentration of 20-hydroxy-
ecdysone (0.05 µg/ml), cuticle appeared on explanted cockroach
leg regenerates between 10 and 14 days after the molting
hormone is added (10).

   When the triol was tested against cultured leg regenerates
of the cockroach Leucophaea maderae (F.), it produced cuticle
formation in only 27% of the regenerates and gave erratic
results even at high doses (28) (Table I). The experimental
results obtained were not readily understood, especially
since the responses that did occur were not concentration-
dependent. Only when the triol was looked upon as a substrate
that could be converted to biologically active ecdysteroids
by peripheral tissues such as blood or fat body, did the
results become meaningful. When we tested this hypothesis by
co-culturing fat body and leg regenerates, the incidence of

Table I.  Induction of cuticle formation in cockroach leg
          regenerates by certain ecdysteroids when tested in
          the presence or absence of fat body.

| Ecdysteroids[a] | Cuticle Formation | | | |
| | Leg Regenerates | | Leg Regenerates + Fatbody | |
| | N | % | N | % |
| --- | --- | --- | --- | --- |
| Control | 10 | 10 | 10 | 0 |
| 20-Hydroxyecdysone | 14 | 93 | – | – |
| α-Ecdysone | 17 | 82 | – | – |
| 22,25-Dideoxyecdysone | 22 | 27 | 22 | 93 |
| 22-Isoecdysone | 12 | 8 | 10 | 0 |

[a] All ecdysteroids tested at 10 µg per chamber.

To confirm these findings, we made a second series of
experiments in which we separately cultured cockroach fat
bodies and leg regenerates with [14]C-labeled triol for 6 days
in 1 ml of M20S medium in clean, sterile glass scintillation
vials.  Two volumes of methanol were added, and the cultures
were worked up and then analyzed for radiolabeled steroids by
thin-layer radiochromatography.  The cultures containing only
leg regenerate tissue and triol produced no additional
steroidal compounds.  They contained only the unmetabolized
triol.  However, the fat body cultures showed chromatographic
peaks for tetraols, pentaols, and conjugates as well as the
triol (Fig. 3), evidence that the metabolism of the triol had
proceeded via hydroxylation and conjugation (17).  Thus, our
initial hypotheses were confirmed:  the triol acts as a
precursor rather than as an active hormone, and the leg
regenerate and fat body have quite different biochemical
capabilities.

Table II.  Effect of certain azasteroids and nonsteroidal
           amines and an amide in inhibiting the activity of
           22,25-dideoxyecdysone (triol) in cockroach leg
           regenerate-fat body cultures.

| Compound[a] | Cuticle Formation % | Inhibition % |
|---|---|---|
| Control | 93 | 0 |
| I | 0 | 100 |
| II | 16 | 83 |
| III | 50 | 46 |
| IV | 50 | 46 |
| V | 70 | 25 |
| VI | 80 | 14 |

[a] All coumpounds tested at 10 µg per chamber.

From this point, the work proceeded in two directions.
One thrust was concerned with a group of compounds consisting
of certain 25-azasteroids and nonsteroidal amines and amides
(Fig. 4) that disrupt steroid metabolism and molting and
metamorphosis in insects (29,30); these were tested for
inhibition of the activity of the triol in inducing cuticle
deposition in cockroach leg regenerate-fat body cultures
(16).  The results obtained with several of these compounds
indicated significant inhibition of metabolism of the triol
to an active ecdysteroid by the cultured tissue (Table II).
Subsequent metabolic studies with three of the more active

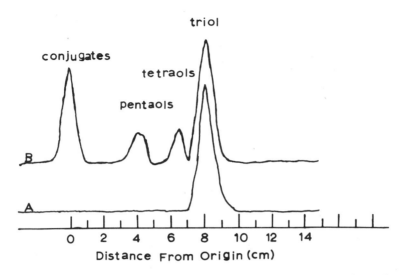

Figure 3. *Radiochromatograms of 4-C¹⁴-ecdysteroids extracted from the medium of cockroach tissue cultures incubated with 4-¹⁴C-22,25-dideoxyecdysone (triol): (A) from cultures containing leg regenerates; (B) from cultures containing leg regenerates plus fat body.*

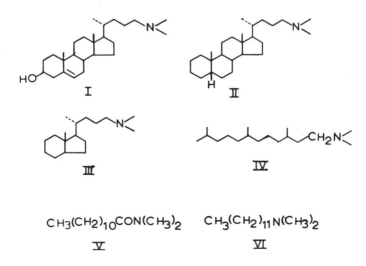

Figure 4. *Azasteroids, nonsteroidal amines, and an amide*

inhibitors (17) demonstrated that they have a pronounced
effect on the metabolism of the triol in cockroach fat body
cultures (Table III).  Taken together, these two studies
provided the first in vitro physiological data and first
biochemical evidence that certain of the inhibitory azasteroids
and nonsteroidal amines represent a new class of insect
hormonal chemicals with a novel mode of action—they interfere
with the metabolism of the endogenous molting hormones of
insects.

Table III.   The effects of an azasteroid and nonsteroidal
             amines on the metabolism of $4-^{14}C-22,25$-dideoxy-
             ecdysone (triol) in cockroach fat body cultures
             during an incubation period of 6 days.

| Inhibitory Compounds[a] | % Unmetabolized 22,25-Dideoxyecdysone[b] | % Metabolites[b] | | |
|---|---|---|---|---|
| | | Conjugates | Pentaols | Tetraols |
| Control | 45.5 | 35.6 | 11.3 | 7.6 |
| II | 6.0 | 55.0 | 0.0 | 39.0 |
| III | 15.9 | 40.8 | 5.6 | 37.8 |
| IV | 18.7 | 34.7 | 5.2 | 41.5 |

[a] The concentrations of the inhibitory compounds and of $4-^{14}C-$
22,25-dideoxyecdysone were 10 µg each per culture flask.

[b] Determined by radio TLC analyses.

     The second thrust, which is perhaps more germane to the
metabolism of xenobiotics, involved over 100 cultures of fat
body that were incubated with triol.  The principal pathways
of metabolism of triol in the fat body cultures turned out to
be hydroxylation and conjugation, as they are in vivo.
Interestingly, enzymic hydrolysis of the conjugate fraction
showed no unmetabolized triol.  The major tetraol metabolite
was 22-deoxyecdysone, and other tetraol and pentaol metabolites
were hydroxylated at the 25, 26, or 20 positions (17)(Fig. 5).
Most of the metabolites found had been previously isolated
from the frass of triol-fed larvae of the tobacco hornworm
Manduca sexta (L.) (23).  In this respect, the metabolic
pathways for triol in cultured cockroach fat body resembled
the pathways that occur in hornworm larvae.  Also, in both
cases the mechanism for hydroxylation of the triol at C-22
appears to be lacking.  When samples of the tetraol and
pentaol fractions were tested against cultured leg regenerates,

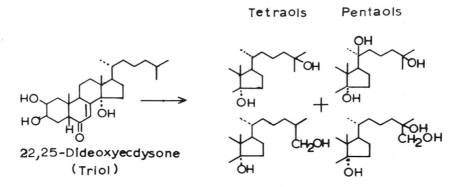

Figure 5. *Hydroxylation of 22,25-dideoxyecdysone (triol) by cockroach fat body cultures*

both fractions induced cuticle formation (Table IV). Since
the leg regenerates cannot metabolically activate the triol
directly, they are probably unable to efficiently hydroxylate
the C-25 position. In addition, assuming that 22-deoxyecdysone,
like α-ecdysone, is effective in the leg regenerate system
only after metabolic conversion (31), then further metabolism
of the tetraol and pentaol metabolites by the leg regenerates
may also occur. Thus, both fat body and leg regenerate
tissue may be necessary to traverse the entire pathway from
triol to an ecdysteroid(s) with molting hormone activity in
the leg regenerate system.

Table IV.  Effect of metabolite fractions isolated from
           cockroach fat body tissue cultures incubated with
           22,25-dideoxyecdysone (triol) on cuticle formation
           by cultured cockroach leg regenerates.

| Metabolite Fractions[a] | N | Cuticle Formation | |
|---|---|---|---|
| | | % | $\bar{X}$ days |
| Control | 4 | 0 | − |
| Tetraol | 5 | 62 | 10.8 |
| Pentaol | 4 | 80 | 11.3 |

[a] Tested at 10 µg equivalents as determined by UV analyses.

This study is still in progress, and a number of questions
remain unanswered. One of these concerns the biological
activity of the various tetraol and pentaol metabolites of
the triol that are produced in fat body cultures. Other
questions involve the site and mode of action of certain of
the inhibitory azasteroids and nonsteroidal amines.
     During the course of this work, we learned certain
things that may be of use to investigators who use similar
techniques: One of these is that the use of antibiotics to
control contamination must be approached with extreme caution.
We found that the presence of gentamicin, an antibiotic
commonly used in tissue cultures, interfered with the metabolism
of the triol in fat body cultures. It was also observed that
the amount of substrate and/or the length of incubation
produce changes in the ratios of the metabolic products
formed (17).
     The purpose of discussing the work on the metabolism of
22,25-dideoxyecdysone has been to show how organ culture
methodology has been applied to the study of this ecdysteroid
that often behaves as a xenobiotic. Our results obtained by
using organ culture techniques so far agree quite well with

what has been learned by using in vivo methods. However, the usefulness of this methodology is limited somewhat by the expense in both time and materials compared with the use of live insects. In general, these in vitro methods would appear to be more useful for the in-depth investigation of critical problem areas rather than for general usage.

## Cell Culture Systems for Metabolic Studies

The use of insect cell culture systems for the study of the metabolism of xenobiotics has not, to our knowledge, been attempted to date. The peripheral literature consists of only a few papers on the effects of pesticides (32,33) and insect growth regulators (34,35) on insect cell lines and a series of studies on the effects of various ecdysteroids on the morphology of cultured cells (36,37,38). However, we would like to discuss briefly some of the possibilities for using insect cell lines for the study of the metabolism of xenobiotics.

Cell cultures differ from organ cultures primarily in that they consist of populations of dividing individual cells rather than highly organized tissues from a single organism. As a result, the life of an organ culture is finite, while the life of cell cultures is potentially infinite (12). Primary cultures that are derived directly from the donor may or may not develop into self replicating established cell lines. Monolayer cultures of fat body cells from pupae of large insects such as the tobacco hornworm and embryonic cells from the oothecae of grasshoppers and cockroaches have been successfully prepared in sufficient quantities for experimental work (19) (Fig. 6). However, because such small amounts of tissue are available from most insects and the contamination problems arising from the use of large numbers of tissue donors are so severe, the use of primary cultures of insect cells for experimental purposes offers few advantages over organ cultures. The number of established lines of insect cells is rapidly increasing, and many of these are available for experimental purposes (39).

## Advantages of Cell Culture Systems

The use of cell lines for metabolic studies has a number of inherent advantages and disadvantages (40). Perhaps the most obvious advantage is that large amounts of uniform material are available for experimentation. Large-scale replication is possible and there is good sample uniformity when spinner flasks (41) and roller bottles are used (42). The problems of surgical shock and microbiological contamination can be virtually eliminated; and automatic devices for handling and counting cells are available to keep labor at a minimum. Cell lines are available from a number of major dipteran, lepidopteran, and homopteran pests, although to

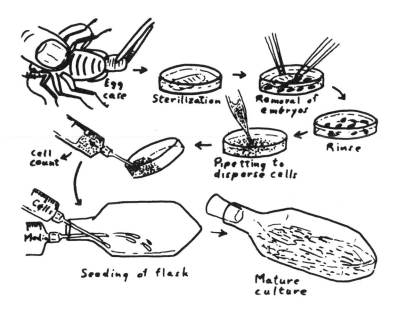

*Figure 6.    Schematic of technique for preparing primary cell cultures from pre-dorsal closure cockroach embryos.  In preparing primary cultures of fat body cells, trypsinization is required to disperse the cells.*

date, none are available from coleopteran or hymenopteran species (39).

## Disadvantages of Cell Culture Systems

At the present time, only a limited number of cell lines for which the tissue of origin can be identified is available. Even for these lines, the evidence for identity is weak (3). Skillful and determined efforts will be necessary to develop new lines from known tissues such as fat body or to identify the tissue of origin for present lines.  Another problem is that while organ cultures can be related back to individual insects, cell lines reflect the dynamics of large populations of individuals kept under constant selection pressure.  The cells must therefore be frequently cloned and kept as frozen stocks to maintain stability and prevent shifts in the biochemical characteristics of the population (40,43).  As yet, very little is known about the metabolic capabilities of existing insect cell lines and much remains to be done before such cell lines can be considered useful tools for the study of metabolism.

At the present time we are working with a cell line (MRRL-CH-2) derived from embryos of the tobacco hornworm (44).  These cells respond with a change in morphology to the presence of 20-hydroxyecdysone at physiological concentrations and are capable of hydroxylating the C-20 position of α-ecdysone (43) (Table V).  Other biochemical parameters of this cell line are currently under investigation.

Table V.   α-Ecdysone and 20-hydroxyecdysone present in cell
           cultures during incubation of tobacco hornworm
           embryonic cell line with 30 μg of α-ecdysone.

| Incubation Days | α-Ecdysone μg | 20-Hydroxyecdysone μg |
|---|---|---|
| 0 | 26.2 | 0.0 |
| 1 | 25.9 | 0.0 |
| 3 | 15.5 | 0.1 |
| 5 | 20.0 | 0.1 |
| 7 | 18.0 | 0.2 |

## Cell Cultures as a Source of Subcellular Components

We have recently been using another tobacco hornworm embryonic cell line (MRRL-CH-1) as a source of cell membrane for studies of membrane transport systems.  As a result of this work it has become apparent to us that cell lines have

some unique advantages as a source of subcellular components
for various types of metabolism studies. We found that cell
cultures can be subjected to bioassay and indeed to some
biochemical procedures in the same medium in which they were
grown (45). Thus, several of the hazards involved in tissue
preparation such as osmotic shock and contamination with
microorganisms are eliminated. Furthermore, large amounts of
highly uniform material are available. Mammalian and plant
tissue cultures are being used for such purposes (46,47), but
few examples of such work with insect tissue cultures have
been reported. (48).

## Concluding Remarks

Insect organ cultures have proved to be extremely useful
tools for studies of the metabolism of the ecdysteroid 22,25-
dideoxyecdysone. The experimental flexibility of this
methodology and its use for the confirmation and extension of
information obtained from in vivo studies make organ culture
the method of choice for certain types of studies. The use
of insect cell cultures for studying the metabolism of
xenobiotics is still only in the early stages of development.
Much work will have to be done before cell cultures can be
considered useful tools for such studies. However, insect
cell cultures are presently being used successfully to
provide a highly uniform source of subcellular components for
metabolic studies.

## Literature Cited

1. Marks, E. P., "Invertebrate Tissue Culture, Research
         Applications", (1976), Academic Press, NY, 177.
2. Agui, N., "Invertebrate Tissue Culture, Research
         Applications", (1976), Academic Press, NY, 133.
3. Landureau, C., "Invertebrate Tissue Culture, Applications
         in Medicine, Biology and Agriculture", (1976),
         Academic Press, NY, 101.
4. Judy, K., Schooley, D., Dunhanm L., Hall, M., Bergot,
         J., and Siddall, J., Proc. Natl. Acad. Sci. U.
         S. A., (1973) 70: 1509.
5. King, D., Bollenbacher, W., Borst, D., Vedeckis, W.,
         O'Conner, J., Ittycheriah, P., and Gilbert, L.,
         Proc. Natl. Acad. Sci. U. S. A., (1974) 71: 973.
6. Marks, E. P., Biol. Bull., (1971) 73: 83.
7. Agui, N., Appl. Entomol. Zool., (1974) 9: 256.
8. Wyatt, G. R., Chen, T., and Couble, T., "Invertebrate
         Tissue Culture, Applications in Medicine, Biology
         and Agriculture", (1976), Academic Press, NY, 195.
9. Koeppe, J., and Offengand, J., "Invertebrate Tissue
         Culture, Applications in Medicine, Biology and
         Agriculture", (1976), Academic Press, NY, 185.

10. Marks, E. P., Biol. Bull., (1973) 145: 171.
11. Marks, E. P., Biol. Bull., (1968) 135: 520.
12. Federoff, S., In Vitro, (1966) 2: 155.
13. Marks, E. P., and Holman, G., J. Insect. Physiol., (1974) 20: 2087.
14. Schooley, D., Judy, K., Bergot, J., Hall, M., and Siddall, J., Proc. Natl. Acad. Sci. U. S. A., (1973) 70: 2921.
15. King. D. S., and Marks, E. P., Life Sci., (1974) 15: 147.
16. Marks, E. P., Robbins, W. E., and Thompson, M. J., Lipids, (1978) 13: 259.
17. Thompson, M. J., Marks, E. P., Robbins, W. E., Dutky, S. R., Finegold, H., and Filipi, P., Lipids, in press.
18. Müller, P., Masner, K., Trautman, K., and Maag, R., Life Sci. (1974) 15: 915.
19. Marks, E. P., "Tissue Culture, Methods and Applications", (1973), Academic Press, NY, 153.
20. Judy, K. and Marks, E. P., Gen. Comp. Endocrinol., (1971) 17: 351.
21. Kaplanis, J. N., Robbins, W. E., Thompson, M. J., and Baumhover, A., H., Science, (1969) 166: 1540.
22. Kaplanis, J. N., Dutky, S. R., Robbins, W. E., and Thompson, M. J., "Invertebrate Endocrinology and Hormonal Heterophylly", (1974), Springer-Verlag, NY, 161.
23. Kaplanis, J. N., Thompson, M. J., Dutky, S. R., Robbins, W. E., and Lindquist, E., Steroids, (1972) 20: 105.
24. Robbins, W. E., Kaplanis, J. N., Thompson, M. J., Shortino, T. J., and Joyner, S. C., Steroids, (1970) 16: 105.
25. Robbins, W. E., Kaplanis, J. N., Thompson, M. J., Shortino, T. J., Cohen, C. F., and Joyner, S. C., Science, (1968) 161: 1158.
26. Earle, N., Padovani, I., Thompson, M. J., and Robbins, W. E., J. Econ. Entomol., (1970) 63: 1064.
27. Rose, G., Pomerat, C., Shindler, T., and Trunnel, J., J. Biophys. Biochem. Cytol., (1958) 4: 761.
28. Marks, E. P., "Invertebrate Tissue Culture, Applications in Medicine, Biology and Agriculture", (1976) Academic Press, NY, 223.
29. Svoboda, J. A., Thompson, M. J., and Robbins, W. E., Lipids, (1972) 7: 553.
30. Robbins, W. E., Thompson, M. J., Svoboda, J. A., Shortino, T. J., Cohen, C. F., Dutky, S. R., and Duncan, O., Lipids, (1975) 10: 35.
31. Marks, E. P., Gen. Comp. Endocrinol., (1973) 21: 472.
32. Grace, T. D. C. and Mitsuhashi, J., "Arthropod Cell Cultures and Their Application to the Study of Viruses", (1971), Springer-Verlag, NY, 108.

33. Mitsuhashi, J., Grace, T. D. C., and Waterhouse, D.,
    Entomol. Exp. Appl., (1970) 13: 327.
34. Cohen, E. and Gilbert, L., J. Insect Physiol. (1973) 19:
    1857.
35. Wyss, C., Experientia, (1976) 32: 1272.
36. Courgeon, A. M., Exp. Cell Res., (1972) 75: 327.
37. Best-Belpomme and Courgeon, A. M., C. R. Acad. Sci.,
    (1976) 283: 155.
38. Cherbas, P., Cherbas, L., and Williams, C. M., Science,
    (1977) 197: 275.
39. Hink, W. F., "Invertebrate Tissue Culture, Research
    Applications", (1976), Academic Press, NY, 319.
40. Fry, J. R. and Bridges, J. W., "Progress in Drug
    Metabolism", (1977), John Wiley & Sons, NY, 71.
41. Thayer, P. S., "Tissue Culture, Methods and Applications",
    (1973), Academic Press, NY, 345.
42. Whittle, W. and Kruse, P., "Tissue Culture, Methods and
    Applications", (1973), Academic Press, NY, 327.
43. Marks, E. P. and Holman, G. M., In Vitro, (1978) in
    press.
44. Eide, P., Caldwell, J., and Marks, E. P., In Vitro,
    (1975) 11: 395.
45. Marks, E. P., In Vitro, (1978) 14: 374.
46. Gregor, H. D., Protoplasma, (1977) 91: 201.
47. North, H. and Menzer, R., Pestic. Biochem. Physiol.,
    (1972) 2: 278.
48. Davis, J. and Hartig, W., Insect Biochem., (1977) 7: 77.

RECEIVED December 20, 1978.

# The Use of Insect Subcellular Components for Studying the Metabolism of Xenobiotics

C. F. WILKINSON

Department of Entomology, Cornell University, Ithaca, NY 14853

Our ability to use to maximum advantage and in relative safety the vast number of drugs, pesticides and other lipophilic xenobiotics currently at our disposal is dependent to a large extent on our ability to establish their metabolic fate in living organisms. Metabolic studies in mammals are essential in assessing the efficacy and safety of new drugs and data on the nature and toxicological properties of pesticide metabolites are mandatory in evaluating the potential hazard to man of residues of these materials in food or in the environment. Comparative studies with fish, birds and other species are important in determining the hazards posed to these animals by a large variety of environmental pollutants.

In addition to their direct importance in safety/hazard evaluation metabolic studies are basic to our understanding of the mode of action of biologically active materials. They often yield important information on enzymatic activation and detoxication processes and frequently provide a mechanistic explanation of cases of selective toxicity. It is in the quest to obtain a better understanding of these processes and to utilize this information in the design of more effective and safer insecticides that has stimulated interest in metabolic studies in insects.

As is obvious from the presentations in this symposium, metabolic studies may be carried out in vivo in the living organism or in vitro in a variety of preparations consisting of isolated organs, tissues, cells or subcellular components. In vivo investigations provide quantitative information on the overall rate of metabolism and on the nature of the terminal metabolites; they seldom provide data on the nature of the metabolic intermediates or on the enzymatic mechanisms by which they are formed. In vitro experiments on the other hand permit the identification and study of individual reaction mechanisms and products but are usually of only limited use in explaining the rate and pattern of metabolism in the intact organism. Clearly any complete metabolic study has to include both in vivo and in vitro components; the situation is analogous to a puzzle where the

0-8412-0486-1/79/47-097-249$09.00/0

in vivo studies provide the pieces to the puzzle and the in vitro
studies yield the clues which enable the pieces to be put together
in a meaningful way.

This chapter will address itself to the use of insect subcellular components in in vitro studies of the metabolism of
xenobiotics. Since most of the advantages and disadvantages of
in vitro studies are of a general nature and largely independent
of the species employed, emphasis will be given to discussing
some of the major problems encountered in developing suitable
in vitro systems and techniques with insect species. It is not
the objective of this chapter to conduct a comprehensive survey
of metabolic reactions with individual compounds or to discuss in
detail the characteristics of the various enzymes involved in
xenobiotic metabolism. Those interested in these areas are
referred to some of the recent books or review articles which are
available (1-10), and the many references contained therein.

## Historical development

The capacity of insects to metabolize synthetic organic
chemicals in vivo was first recognized during the late 1940s
when it was discovered that metabolic dehydrochlorination of DDT
to the relatively nontoxic DDE was a major causative factor in
the development of insect resistance to this insecticide. In the
years immediately following this discovery in vivo investigations
with other insecticides including the cyclodienes, the organophosphorus compounds and the carbamates revealed that almost all
groups of compounds were susceptible to metabolic attack by both
insects and a variety of non-target organisms and that this was
often the dominant factor in determining the degree and duration
of their toxic action. Recognition of the critical role of
metabolism in relation to selective toxicity and insect resistance
to insecticides gave further impetus to metabolic studies and the
intense activity of agro chemical industry during the 1950s
provided a steady flow of new compounds with which to work. As a
result, in vivo metabolic studies with insects, mammals and other
organisms assumed an ever important position in insecticide
research and were aided considerably by improved technology,
particularly the use of radioactive tracers and the introduction
of more sophisticated instrumentation for the resolution,
detection and identification of small amounts of metabolites.
Since almost all of the early studies with insects were
conducted in vivo only the end products of metabolism were
observed. In most cases these were water soluble secondary conjugates which were difficult to identify and which provided little
or no information on the structures of the primary or intermediate
metabolites from which they were derived or on the nature of the
enzyme systems effecting the initial attack on the parent compound. Indeed in most of the early work these conjugates were
simply classified as "water solubles" and no further attempt was

made to identify them.  In spite of these problems the importance
of several primary metabolic reactions was well established and it
was known that these could catalyze both the activation and
detoxication of the parent compound.  Dehydrochlorination was
known to constitute a major metabolic pathway for DDT and its
derivatives and hydrolysis and desulfuration were well recognized
reactions with a variety of organophosphorus compounds.  In addition the probable involvement of enzymatic oxidation was strongly
indicated by the identification of metabolites such as epoxides,
sulfoxides and sulfones from several compounds although the full
extent of this involvement was not obvious.  This then was the
general situation which pertained in insect metabolic studies up
to and during the early 1950s.

Somewhere around this time there occurred a rather sudden
realization that the nature of the metabolites produced by insects
and mammals were essentially similar and that presumably this
reflected a basic similarity in the enzymatic mechanisms involved.
This tended to open up new and improved lines of communication
between individuals conducting metabolic studies in insects and
those working with mammals.  The use of a variety of in vitro
systems such as liver slices, homogenates and subcellular fractions had already proved useful in mammalian studies and it was
not long before the first attempts were made to develop similar
systems from insects.

Early in vitro studies in insects usually employed intact
tissues or crude minces and homogenates.  Although several organophosphorus esters were found to be hydrolyzed by the "aromatic
esterase" of the bee (Apis mellifera) abdomen (11) and malaoxon
and acethion were shown to be degraded slowly by carboxylesterase
action in cockroach (Periplaneta americana) minces and whole guts
(12), homogenates of other insects proved generally inactive
towards a variety of organophosphorus insecticides (13).  Somewhat
earlier than this, intact insect tissues especially the gut had
been found capable of activating schradan (14) and catalyzing the
oxidative activation (desulfuration) of phosphorothionates such
as parathion (15).  Fenwick (16,17) was the first to demonstrate
phosphoramidate activation in a subcellular preparation from
locust (Schistocerca gregaria) fat body.  He reported that 84% of
the schradan oxidizing activity of a fat body homogenate was in
the upper layer of a heterogeneous 14,000g centrifugal sediment
(referred to somewhat questionably as the microsomal fraction) and
that activity required the addition of either the supernatant or
exogenous NADPH.  It is interesting that as a result of these and
related studies Fenwick (17) as late as 1958 found it worthwhile
to note that the locust fat body homogenate contained ". . . (at
least) two distinct types of particles which resemble mammalian
liver mitochondria and microsomes."

By the late 1950s it was well established that in mammals
the primary metabolic attack on a large number of lipophilic
drugs and xenobiotics was effected by a series of oxidative

reactions associated with hepatic microsomes (18). The first in vitro demonstration of microsomal enzyme activity in insects was that of Agosin et al. (19) who showed that NADPH-fortified microsomes prepared from whole german cockroaches (Blattella germanica) and other species catalyzed the hydroxylation of DDT. This represented a milestone of sorts since it provided the first real indication that insects contained an active microsomal oxidase system similar to that in mammalian liver and also that in vitro metabolic systems could be developed to reproduce the reactions occurring in the living insect.

Since this time in vitro studies employing subcellular fractions derived from whole insects or insect tissues have become almost routine practice in many laboratories. As a result a great deal of information has been obtained on the types of metabolic reactions which take place in insect tissues and on the general biochemical characteristics of the enzymes catalyzing these reactions (1,6-10). It has become clear that as in mammals, xenobiotic metabolism in insects is accomplished by relatively few general types of reactions. The importance of ester cleavage by a series of hydrolases (phosphatases, carboxylesterases, amidases, etc.) has been demonstrated with various substrates (20) and glutathione transferases are known to play important roles in primary reactions such as dealkylation and dearylation (21,22), dechlorination (22,23,24) and thiocyanate metabolism (22,25). Epoxide hydratase activity is known to be widely distributed in insects (20,26) and conjugating enzymes are known to catalyze numerous secondary reactions such as glucosidation and sulfation (22). But perhaps most important of all is clear recognition of the dominance of the cytochrome P-450 mediated system in insects and its ability to catalyze the primary metabolic attack on a large number of lipophilic xenobiotics through reactions such as epoxidation, hydroxylation, N- and O-dealkylation thioether oxidation and desulfuration (1,8,9,10,27). What is now emerging from comparative studies is a picture of remarkable functional unity with respect to the reactions of xenobiotic metabolism. There are of course some differences between species as will be discussed later in this symposium by Dr. Terriere but in spite of the dramatic variations in size, morphology, nutrition, ecological habitat and general life style between say mammals and insects, one cannot help but be impressed by the basic similarities which exist at the subcellular level. At the present time, however, the picture is still out of focus and much remains to be done, particularly at the in vitro level, before a more complete understanding can be achieved.

## General considerations relating to in vitro studies

The first major decisions which have to be made in initiating an in vitro study are the species and life stage of the insect to be employed. This will be dictated largely by the purpose of the proposed study.

In vitro metabolic studies are usually directed towards
providing information either on the products of a particular
reaction(s) or on the biochemical character and mechanism of the
enzyme which catalyzes the reaction.  In the former case, the
in vitro system is used as a tool to produce primary or intermediary metabolites of a particular xenobiotic which may be
required to confirm the identity of trace metabolites or metabolic
pathways suggested from corresponding in vivo studies; in the
latter case selected xenobiotics are used as tools to characterize
the system which can then be employed as a source of more quantitative metabolic data or in comparative studies.

If the proposed investigation is concerned with establishing
the primary metabolites of some insecticide in a specific insect
pest then clearly the species to be employed is already determined and the life stages of most interest (egg, larva, nymph or
adult) are presumably those at which the insecticide is directed
in the field, i.e. those causing the most economic damage.  The
major requirement here is to develop an in vitro system that will
reproduce metabolites observed in vivo.  In this type of study a
detailed knowledge of the system is not of primary importance and,
indeed, in many cases the use of intact tissues or crude homogenates may be more useful than individual subcellular components.

If on the other hand the objective of the study is to characterize the enzymatic system responsible for a certain type of
metabolic reaction, it is usually desirable to work with more
homogeneous, purified fractions and to give greater emphasis to
obtaining quantitative information.  For studies of this type
there is considerably more leeway in the selection of the species
to be employed and in view of the estimated existence of 2-10
million species of insects, the theoretical possibilities are
enormous.

In practice, however, the choice of species is usually
determined by a series of convenience factors which relate mainly
to the amount of biomass available for study.  This is probably
the major limiting factor in most studies on insect biochemistry.
Consequently, wherever possible a relatively large insect species
should be selected.  In many cases the life cycles of large
insects are quite long so that it is often necessary to reach a
compromise between size and turnover time (i.e. length of generation).  The species selected for study should be readily amenable
to mass rearing under laboratory conditions (the availability of
a satisfactory artificial diet is advantageous) and should be
available on a year-round basis.  Clearly a species with only one
generation per year or one with an obligative period of diapause
would not be convenient for continuous study.  It is as a result
of requirements of this type that to date in vitro studies have
been limited to perhaps 30-40 insect species very few of which
can be considered serious pests of agriculture or public health.

## Tissue sources

Having selected an appropriate insect species and life stage with which to work the next step is to decide on the tissue source to be employed as a starting point for subcellular fractionation.

Because of obvious limitations on the amount of tissue usually available, most of the early metabolic studies were conducted with homogenates or subcellular fractions derived from whole insects. The use of whole-insect preparations is still common in several laboratories and can frequently provide useful qualitative information on xenobiotic metabolism. More often than not, however, enzyme activity in such preparations, particularly that associated with the microsomal fraction, is very low or non-existent and usually bears little resemblance to the true enzymatic capability of the insect under investigation. Indeed, in view of the heterogeneous mixture of materials they contain it is really quite surprizing that such whole-insect preparations exhibit any enzyme activity at all. Clearly, the homogenization of whole insects causes a total disruption of tissue and cellular organization and results in the release of a large number of endogenous materials with potential inhibitory effects on the enzyme under investigation.

Several different types of endogenous inhibitors have been encountered and identified in the course of studies with insect microsomes (8,10) and there is no doubt that they often represent a serious practical problem in in vitro investigations.

The insect eye pigment, xanthommatin has been established as an important inhibitory factor in preparations from whole house flies (28,29), fruit flies (Drosophila melanogaster) and honey bees (Apis mellifera) (30). It causes substantial inhibition of house fly epoxidase activity at concentrations as low as $5 \times 10^{-7}M$ and inhibitory activity is accompanied by a marked increase in NADPH oxidation (28,29). Studies on the mode of action of xanthommatin have shown that it accepts electrons from the flavin, NADPH cytochrome c reductase, of the microsomal electron transport chain thereby acting as an electron sink to impede the flow of reducing equivalents to cytochrome P-450 (Figure 1) (28,29). The ability of dihydroxanthommatin to undergo autoxidation and to be oxidized in the presence of cytochrome c or tyrosinase suggests the rapid regeneration of xanthommatin and a consequent enhancement in its inhibitory potential. Since xanthommmatin is widely distributed as an insect eye pigment this type of inhibition is of potential importance in almost all preparations from whole insects.

What may be a similar type of inhibition has also been encountered in attempts to measure microsomal oxidation in preparations from whole last-instar lepidopterous larvae just prior to pupation (31,32). In this case, inhibition is associated with soluble products (a variety of quinones) of the melanization or darkening process which involves the tyrosinase-mediated oxidation

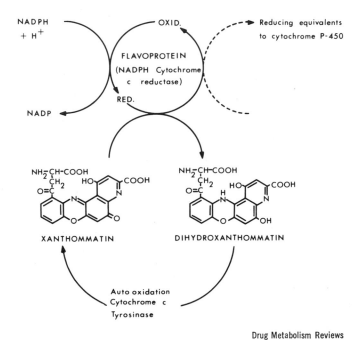

Drug Metabolism Reviews

*Figure 1.   Inhibition of microsomal oxidation by xanthommatin (8)*

of a variety of ortho-dihydroxy compounds (e.g. DOPA) and their subsequent incorporation into the insect cuticle. In lepidopterous larvae, this type of inhibition appears to be important only during late larval development when the tyrosinase system is activated in preparation for formation of the pupal coat. It can be counteracted by the addition of 1-phenyl-2-thiourea to the preparations to inhibit tyrosinase activity (31,32). A similar type of inhibition has also been implicated in the instability of mixed-function oxidase activity in house fly microsomes where the addition of cyanide (also a tyrosinase inhibitor) has a marked stabilizing effect (33). In theory, quinones may be formed whenever catechols are brought into contact with tyrosinase and since both are common in insects, workers should beware of preparations which become progressively darker on exposure to air.

Another major group of endogenous inhibitors which can seriously impede in vitro studies in whole-insect preparations are those associated with the insect gut contents. Potent inhibitors of microsomal oxidations have been reported in the gut contents of several insect species including several lepidopterous larvae (34,35), a caddisfly larva (Limnephilus sp.) (37), a sawfly larva (Macremphytus varianus) (38) and the house cricket (Acheta domesticus) (38,39). The inhibitory factors in the gut contents of the southern armyworm (Spodoptera eridania) (40) and the house cricket (39) have been partially purified and characterized as proteolytic enzymes with molecular weights of 26,000 and 16,500 respectively. They are both undoubtedly naturally occurring digestive proteinases quite similar to trypsin and like trypsin their inhibitory action results from a direct proteolytic attack on the microsomal protein (39,41). The effect of these proteases on the microsomes is quite specific in that they cause the solubilization of the flavoprotein, NADPH cytochrome c reductase, and consequently disrupt electron flow to cytochrome P-450 (39,41) (Figure 2). There appears to be no effect on cytochrome $b_5$ of P-450 and no effect on substrate binding to the latter (41) so it appears that the flavoprotein is the major target, possibly due to its vulnerable location on the outer surface of the membrane. Although similar in their overall effect on the microsomes, the armyworm and cricket gut content materials exhibit properties indicating they are not identical (Table 1). Thus in contrast to the armyworm material which shows a similar inhibitory effect on insect and mammalian liver microsomes the cricket material is much less active towards the latter and while both appear to be serine proteinases susceptible to inhibition by phenylmethanesulfonyl fluoride (PMSF) the cricket but not the armyworm material is sensitive to soy trypsin inhibitor. Bovine serum albumin (BSA) has a marked protective effect on microsomes in the presence of the armyworm gut inhibitor whereas this is observed with the cricket material only at high levels of BSA (39). The protective action of BSA against at least some of these proteolytic enzymes undoubtedly accounts for the enhanced microsomal enzyme activity

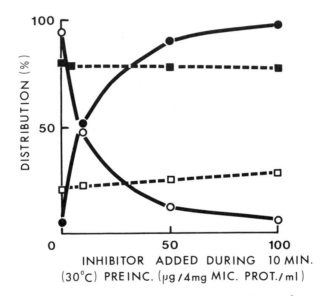

Figure 2.   *Solubilization of NADPH–Cytochrome c reductase by gut contents inhibitor of southern armyworm* (S. eridania) (41).

TABLE I

Properties of gut content inhibitors from
<u>S</u>. <u>eridania</u> and <u>A</u>. <u>domesticus</u>[a]

|  | Source of inhibitor | |
| Property | <u>S</u>. <u>eridania</u> | <u>A</u>. <u>domesticus</u> |
| --- | --- | --- |
| Molecular weight | 26,000 | 16,500 |
| <u>Proteolytic activity</u> (casein) | Yes | Yes |
| $Mg^{2+}$, $Ca^{2+}$ (mM) | Stimulates ($F_2$) | No effect ($F_1$) |
| Soy trypsin inhibitor (1mg/inc.) | No effect ($F_2$) | Inhibition ($F_1$) |
| PMSF | Inhibition | Inhibition |
| <u>Inhibition epoxidase</u> ($I_{50}$, mg/inc.) | | |
| Armyworm midgut | 0.97 ($F_1$) | 0.17 ($F_1$) |
| Mammalian liver | ∿2.0 ($F_1$) (mouse) | 7.0 ($F_1$) (rat) |
| <u>Reversal of microsomal inhibition</u> | | |
| BSA | Yes | No (slight) |
| PMSF (0.5–1.0mM) | Yes | Yes |
| Soy trypsin inhibitor (1mg/inc.) | --- | Yes |

[a] Data from Krieger and Wilkinson (<u>40</u>) and Brattsten and
Wilkinson (<u>39</u>). $F_1$ is crude freeze-dried gut contents soluble
fraction; $F_2$ is freeze-dried material after passage through
Sephadex G-50 or G-100.

observed following addition of this material to homogenates of
whole house flies (<u>42</u>). Caseinolytic activity has been reported
in whole insect homogenates of several species (<u>40</u>) and it is
likely that proteolytic enzymes of this type are of broad general
significance in <u>in vitro</u> studies in insects.

It should be obvious from this discussion that a variety of
endogenous inhibitors liberated during homogenization make whole
insects a generally poor tissue source for <u>in vitro</u> studies
particularly those concerned with the biochemical characterization

of the enzymes involved in metabolism.

In some cases, however, due to factors such as very small size (e.g. mosquitoes or aphids) or limited availability of the species in question the use of whole insect preparations is unavoidable and can often be useful in gross metabolic studies. In this case compromises must be made. The chances of encountering endogenous inhibitors are, of course, considerably decreased when specific body regions of the insect are employed. Thus the use of house fly abdomens has proved advantageous over whole house flies (8,9,43) (since it immediately avoids the problems associated with xanthommatin) and ingenious methods have been developed for the mass separation of insect body segments. Further improvement may be achieved by the addition of BSA (39), cyanide (33) or other protective agents to the preparations although care must be taken to ascertain that such materials are not having other effects on the system.

In general, the clear message is that wherever the size of the insect permits, individual tissues or organs should be employed as a tissue source for homogenization and subcellular fractionation. Unfortunately, tissue dissection is often a tedious process and there is usually no way to avoid the individual handling of large numbers of insects. The most convenient procedures for this vary considerably from one species to another.

As a result of considerable work in recent years, it has been established that the patterns of tissue distribution of microsomal oxidase activity vary considerably both between different orders of insects and between species in a single order. In general, however, the tissues found to be most active are various portions of the alimentary tract, the fat body or the Malpighian tubules (Figure 3) (8).

In lepidopterous larvae maximum oxidase activity is associated with the gut tissues, particularly those of the midgut (Figure 4) (34). This distribution pattern has been demonstrated with approximately 40 different species (44,45) the only exception to date being the cabbage looper (Trichoplusia ni) where preparations from the fat body are more active than those from the gut (35). High titers of microsomal oxidase activity have also been reported in the gut tissues of various other insects (8) although in many cases this is associated with a much broader pattern of tissue distribution as in various orthopteran species. In several species of cockroach epoxidation and hydroxylation activity occur in various tissues including the gut, fat body and Malpighian tubules the relative activity of each varying with the species (Figure 4B,C) (8). In the house cricket (Acheta domesticus) maximum activity is found in the Malpighian tubules (Figure 4D) (38).

As in mammals, therefore, microsomal oxidase activity in insects is found in several different tissues and the observed patterns may reflect a strategic localization linked with the major portals of entry of xenobiotics into the organism (8,27).

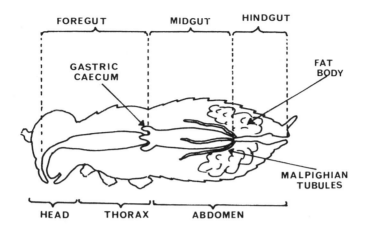

*Figure 3.  Insect tissues involved in microsomal oxidation*

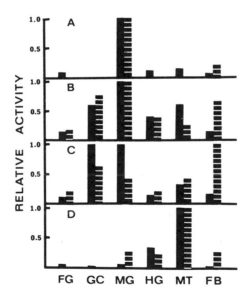

*Figure 4.  Distribution of microsomal epoxidase activity in insect tissues: (A) southern armyworm (S. eridania) (34); (B) Madagascar cockroach (G. portentosa) (C) American cockroach (P. americanum) (48); (D) house cricket (A. domesticus) (38).  Solid bars represent specific activity (per mg protein); striped bars represent activity per insect.*

Thus the gut tissues may constitute the major site for metabolism
of xenobiotics ingested in the food whereas the fat body and/or
Malpighian tubules possibly play a greater role in the metabolism
of materials entering the insect by direct integumental penetration.  This can be viewed as analogous to the distribution of
microsomal oxidation in the skin, lung, gut and liver of mammals
where they appear to be strategically located to act as the first
line of defense against xenobiotics.

In assessing the relative metabolic importance of a given
tissue to the intact insect, it is important to consider not only
the specific activity of the enzyme in a homogenate or subcellular
fraction (i.e. activity/mg protein) but also the relative biomass
of the various tissues.  Consequently, a tissue of large biomass
but low specific oxidase activity may be more important in its
overall metabolic capacity than one of small biomass and high
specific activity.  This can be clearly seen by comparing the
patterns of distribution of oxidase activity based on measurements
of specific activity with those calculated on a per insect basis
(Figure 4).

Even when working with individual tissues, it is important to
be aware of the possibility of encountering endogenous enzyme
inhibitors.  These can often be detected by combining homogenates
of different tissues and examining the activity data for inhibitory effects.  As shown in Table 2, the total activities of
combinations of homogenates of various armyworm tissues are equal
to the sum of their individual activities and, therefore, can be
assumed to be free of inhibitory factors.  In other cases, the

TABLE 2

Epoxidase activities of armyworm midgut homogenate alone
and in presence of homogenates of other tissues

| Tissue | Protein (mg/incubation) | Epoxidase activity (nmoles/10 min) | |
|---|---|---|---|
| | | Observed | Calculated |
| Midgut (MG) | 2.1 | 14.8 | |
| Foregut | 1.0 | 0.5 | |
| Foregut + MG | 3.1 | 15.1 | 15.3 |
| Hindgut | 1.2 | 0.6 | |
| Hindgut + MG | 3.3 | 15.6 | 15.4 |
| Fat body | 6.6 | 3.3 | |
| Fat body + MG | 8.7 | 17.8 | 18.1 |
| Malpighian tubules | 1.0 | 2.2 | |
| Malpighian tubules + MG | 3.1 | 16.8 | 17.0 |

activities of homogenates or subcellular fractions of tissues can
be compared with that of the intact tissue.  In the case of adult
worker honey bees, epoxidase activity of intact midguts was
decreased approximately 90% simply by opening the gut by longi-
tudinal incision and was totally lost following homogenization of
the tissue (Table 3) (46).  Subsequently a potent intracellular
inhibitory factor was isolated and partially purified from the
soluble fraction of the gut (47).  Inhibition was associated with
the nucleic acid (RNA) moiety of a macromolecule (possibly a
nucleoprotein) with a molecular weight of approximately 19,000 and
could be reversed by digestion with ribonuclease (RNase $T_1$ of

TABLE 3

Epoxidase activity in intact and homogenized

honey bee (adult worker) midgut tissues

| Midgut treatment | Epoxidase activity pmole/min/mg wet. wt. |
|---|---|
| Intact | 1.31 |
| Opened | 0.14 |
| Homogenized | Not detectable |

Data from Gilbert and Wilkinson (46)

pancreatic RNase) (Table 4).  Following this finding, it was discovered that several commercially available nucleic acids
including core and transfer RNA from baker's yeast and transfer
RNA from Torula yeast also inhibited insect (armyworm gut) microsomal oxidases but had little or no effect on those from mammalian
liver (47).  Although to date this is the only inhibitor of this
type reported, it is possible that others will be found in various
insect preparations.
     Another important parameter which has to be considered in the
selection of a suitable source of tissue for in vitro investigation is the age or life stage of the insect to be used.  It is now
well established that the activity of the enzymes involved in
xenobiotic metabolism change dramatically with age and stage of
development in various insect species (8).  This is clearly
illustrated by the patterns of microsomal oxidase activity shown
in Figure 5.  In general, microsomal oxidase activity is only
found in actively feeding life stages of the insect.  Thus maximum
activity is usually associated with the larval or nymphal stages
of development and in the adults where these feed; insect eggs and
pupae are usually devoid of oxidase activity.  In southern armyworm larvae, microsomal oxidation activity (specific activity) in

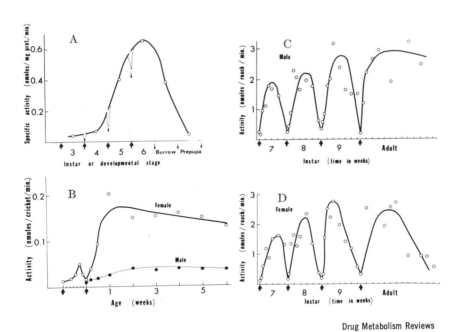

Drug Metabolism Reviews

*Figure 5.    Age–activity profiles of microsomal epoxidation in (A) southern army-worm* (S. eridania) *(34); (B) house cricket* (A. domesticus) *(38); and (C and D) Madagascar cockroach* (G. portentosa) *(48).*

TABLE 4

Effect of RNase T$_1$ and pancreatic RNase on activity

of the honey bee midgut inhibitor

| Enzyme (unit) | | Reversal of inhibition (%) |
|---|---|---|
| RNase T$_1$ | (5) | 0 |
| | (260) | 24 |
| | (2800) | 100 |
| Pancreatic RNase | (0.072) | 14 |
| | (0.144) | 22 |
| | (0.216) | 28 |
| | (0.360) | 50 |

Data from Gilbert and Wilkinson (47)

the gut increases about 30-fold during development from the fourth
to sixth larval instar (Figure 5A) and shows an equally dramatic
decline as the larvae terminate feeding and prepare for pupation
(34); a similar pattern has been observed with several other
species (44). The increase in activity does not occur in a
continuous manner, however, but shows a marked decrease during
each larval molt (dotted lines Figure 5A).

Studies with other insect species have emphasized the
remarkable patterns of oxidase activity which occur during insect
development particularly those occurring during the larval or
nymphal molts. Thus aldrin epoxidation activity in the Malpighian
tubules of the house cricket is low during the molts from 8th to
9th nymphal instar and from the 9th instar to the adult and then
increases as the adult matures (Figure 5B) (38). This rhythmic
developmental cycle becomes much clearer in the midgut-caeca
preparation from the Madagascar cockroach (Figure 5C and D) where
it is quite evident that oxidase activity is low during the molt
and passes through a maximum about midway through each instar
(48). The results of these and other investigations strongly
suggest that microsomal oxidase activity is under strict metabolic
control and that this is closely linked with the process of
metamorphosis.

From a practical viewpoint these rapid and dramatic changes
in enzyme activity can provide a real headache in in vitro
studies. Researchers in this field would be well advised to
either establish the activity patterns in the insect species with
which they are working or to avoid working with insects close to
the molt. In some types of investigations (e.g. enzyme induction
studies) where comparisons between treated and control groups are
required, it is essential to use groups of insects closely matched

(+2h) with respect to age (49).

Procedures for obtaining insect subcellular components

As with other tissues, the preparation of subcellular components from insects is effected by two successive steps:
homogenization and fractionation.  In general, the methods which
have been employed are based on procedures which have proved
successful for mammalian tissues.  However, due to large variations in the nature and morphological heterogeneity of the insect
tissues employed, numerous modifications have been made in
attempts to optimize the procedures.  These have been discussed at
some length in previous reviews (8,9,10).
    Various procedures have been described for the homogenization
of whole insects, insect body regions or individual insect tissues
and usually the method of choice can only be determined by a
process of trial and error for any given tissue source.  Homogenization is usually achieved with either a mechanical blender, a
hand-operated or motor-driven tissue grinder or a mortar and
pestle (8,9,10).  There is a general concensus of opinion that
the procedure should be as gentle as possible and yet sufficiently
drastic to satisfactorily disrupt cells in heterogeneous tissues
often containing sclerotized cuticle, muscle fibers, etc.  All
operations should be carried out at 0-2°C.
    Mechanical blenders (Waring blender, Omni-mixer, etc.) have
been used for large batches of whole insects or insect body
regions (e.g. house flies or house fly abdomens) but in general,
oxidase activity in microsomal fractions derived from such homogenates is considerably lower than in those from homogenates
prepared with a Potter Elvehjem tissue grinder (43,50) or by a
gentle pounding action in a mortar (10,51).  This loss of enzyme
activity may result in part from denaturation through excessive
abrasive action of hard chitinous portions of the insect or by the
more efficient release of endogenous inhibitors.  Violent mechanical blending undoubtedly aids in the release of the sparingly-
soluble xanthominatin in preparations containing insect heads and
there are reports that microsomes from blended whole house flies
contain a b-type cytochrome (probably cytochrome oxidase) which is
associated with thoracic sarcosomes or sarcosomal fragments and
which interferes with spectral determination of microsomal
cytochrome P-450 (10,51,52).  The latter is not observed in house
fly homogenates prepared by the so-called "mortar" procedure
(10,51).  The degree or duration of homogenization of whole
insects or body regions is also important even when a tissue
grinder is employed.  Usually only a few passes of the plunger are
required and better results are achieved by use of a relatively
loose-fitting pestle of Teflon or smooth glass.
    The homogenization of individual tissues usually presents
fewer problems and here a variety of hand-operated or motor-
driven tissue grinders provide the best results.  The small

amounts of tissue available as well as the heterogenous often
"stringy" nature of the tissue (e.g. armyworm gut) usually make
mechanical blenders quite ineffective for homogenization purposes.
Homogenization with a tissue grinder should be as gentle and brief
as possible and again Teflon or smooth glass pestles are preferable to those of ground glass.

Several different types of homogenization media have been
employed by various workers and obviously can have an effect on
the final enzymatic activity of the preparation. Although there
are reports that the ionic strength of the medium may be important
(43) the most commonly used media are 0.15 M KCl or 0.25 M sucrose
which may or may not be buffered at various pH levels (8,9,10).
Occasionally BSA (1-2% w/v) or other materials such as cyanide,
phenylmethanesulfonyl fluoride, etc. may be added to at least
partially counteract the effects of endogenous inhibitors
(8,42,43).

Subcellular fractionation of homogenates of whole insects or
insect tissues is usually achieved by the technique of differential centrifugation, first pioneered by Albert Claude with mammalian liver cells and subsequently widely applied to many other
tissues (53). Briefly the technique involves centrifuging the
initial homogenate at about 1,000xg for 10 minutes to remove
nuclei and larger cell debris followed by a 9,000-12,000xg
centrifugation for 10-30 minutes to sediment mitochondria and
other intermediate sized particles and cell organelles. Further
centrifugation of the postmitochondrial supernatant for 60 minutes
at 100,000-200,000xg yields the so-called microsomal fraction and
a "soluble" supernatant. With insect tissues this general procedure is often modified and the actual centrifugal conditions
(force, time) usually vary somewhat between different laboratories. The procedure may also include filtration of the original
brei through cheese cloth, cotton or glass wool to remove the
often substantial amounts of chitinous debris and lipids released
during homogenization.

The application of this technique to the subcellular fractionation of insect tissue homogenates is based on the largely
unproven assumption that the subcellular organelles and membrane
particles derived from insect tissues exhibit similar sedimentation characteristics to those from mammalian liver cells. In view
of the highly heterogeneous nature of most of the insect tissue
courses used for studies of xenobiotic metabolism this is a
dangerous assumption which should be only made with extreme care.
Moreover the procedures found satisfactory for one tissue may not
be applicable to another.

Subcellular fractions can be classified morphologically by
means of light or electron microscopy as containing nuclei,
mitochondria, microsomal particles (from the membranous endoplasmic reticulum) etc. In addition, the discovery that certain types
of enzymes are usually associated with a single class of particles
has led to the development of a series of "marker" enzymes which

can be used to classify the various subcellular fractions in biochemical terms. Few attempts have yet been made to characterize
insect subcellular fractions either morphologically or biochemically and most workers in this field still seem content to
associate their enzyme activities with subcellular fractions
defined only by values obtained from the ultracentrifuge. Little
attention is also given to calculating a complete balance sheet of
the total enzyme activity and protein concentration in each fraction and comparing these with values for the original homogenate.
Thus in the absence of total protein concentration the high
specific activity of an enzyme in some subcellular fraction yields
little information with regard to its overall distribution and a
meaningful discussion of subcellular fractionation is difficult.

From the studies which have been conducted, it is reasonable
to conclude that as in mammals, the enzymes involved in xenobiotic
metabolism in insects are almost all located in either the soluble
or the microsomal fractions of the cell. Although it is possible
that problems could be encountered by the adsorbance of soluble
enzymes onto larger cell organelles, the preparation of satisfactory soluble enzyme fractions does not appear to have been a
serious problem to date. Most attention has been focussed on
subcellular fractionation procedures to obtain satisfactory
microsomal fractions from insect tissues.

In several cases, microsomal fractions exhibiting high levels
of drug and insecticide oxidizing activity can be prepared by a
differential centrifugation procedure similar to that used for
mammalian liver. Thus in the case of the armyworm (Spodoptera
eridania) larval gut preparation, the microsomal fraction
(100,000xg, 60 minutes) is clearly the major intracellular location of the enzymes catalyzing epoxidation and N-demethylation
(Figure 6A and B respectively) and Figure 6B shows that the
distribution pattern for N-demethylase activity is essentially
identical to that for NADPH-cytochrome c reductase a recognized
microsomal marker enzyme (54); that this fraction is derived
mainly from the endoplasmic reticulum has been obtained by
electron microscopy (55).

In other cases, however, the preparation of insect microsomes
by differential centrifugation has proved much more difficult.
One of the most common problems which is encountered is that most
of the xenobiotic oxidizing activity associated with the microsomal fraction is sedimented at unexpectedly low g-forces (8).
This has been reported for fat body preparations from the American
cockroach (Periplaneta americana) (56,57), and blowfly larva
(Calliphora erythrocephala) (58) and homogenates of cricket
(Acheta domesticus) Malpighian tubules (38) and Madagascar cockroach (Gromphadorhina portentosa) gut-caeca tissues (48). Thus
in the latter example approximately 48% of the aldrin epoxidase
activity was sedimented during a 15 minute spin at 12,000xg
(Figure 6C) using the typical differential centrifugation procedure. If, instead the crude homogenate (in 0.25M sucrose

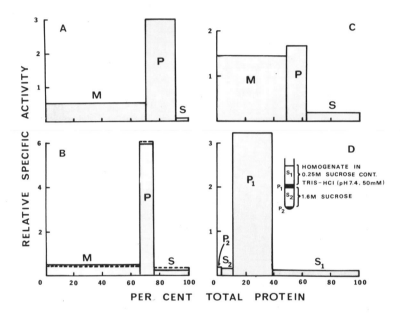

*Figure 6.  Subcellular fractionation of microsomal oxidase activity from insect tissues.*

*A and B are epoxidation (34) and N-demethylation (54) activities, respectively, in southern armyworm midgut tissues; dotted line in B is NADPH–cytochrome c reductase activity.  M is 10,000–12,000 g × 10–15 min pellet, P is 105,000 g × 60–90 min pellet, S is supernatant.  C and D are epoxidation activity from midgut caeca tissue of Madagascar cockroach (48).*

containing 50mM Tris-HCl, pH 7.4) is layered over 1.6M sucrose and
centrifuged for 45 minutes at 150,000xg in a swinging bucket rotor
two major particulate fractions are obtained a dense pellet ($P_2$)
which sediments to the bottom of the tube and a light protein band
($P_1$) at the sucrose interface. The latter which represents about
28% of the total protein contains 90.4% of the total epoxidase
activity (Figure 6D) has been shown by electron microscopy to
consist largely of membranous vesicles from the endoplasmic
reticulum. A similar procedure involving sucrose density gradient
centrifugation has been found useful in preparing microsomal
fractions from cricket Malpighian tubules (38) and honey bee
larval gut tissues (46).

It therefore appears that under certain conditions, the
microsomal particles in homogenates of some insect tissues either
aggregate or become adsorbed to the surfaces of larger particles
such as mitochondria. Workers in the field should be aware of
this possibility and where necessary modify their procedures
accordingly. The suspension medium may have some effect on this
behavior since it can modify the physicochemical forces involved.
It is interesting to note that in the case of microsomes from the
southern armyworm midgut, the morphological appearance of the
membrane vesicles prepared in 0.25M sucrose and 0.15M KCl are
quite distinct; thus although both fractions exhibit essentially
identical levels of microsomal oxidase activity the vesicles
prepared in sucrose are relatively smooth and rounded compared
with the angular appearance of those prepared in KCl.

As a result of the sometimes broad distribution of microsomal
oxidase activity in several subcellular fractions, the activity
measured in the microsomal fraction per se may be a poor indicator
of the total enzyme capability of a given insect tissue. In
comparative studies, therefore, where a measure of total metabolic
capacity is often required, it may be more appropriate to measure
the activity in less homogeneous fractions such as the 10 000xg
supernatant or even in crude homogenates. Indeed, such preparations are probably most convenient in many metabolic studies since
their use significantly decreases the time of preparation.

The stability of enzyme activity in homogenates and subcellular fractions from insect tissues varies considerably depending on
the tissue source, the method of preparation and the storage
conditions employed (8,9,10). As a general rule they should be
used without delay after preparation. Oxidase activity in
preparations from whole house flies or house fly abdomens usually
is rapidly lost on storage at 0-2°C (8,10,31,43) but may be
retained for several weeks under certain conditions (8,10,31).
Freezing of these microsomes has been reported to be deleterious
(8,10,51). However, microsomes from armyworm gut may be stored
for up to a month as well-drained pellets at -15°C (59) (Table 5)
and microsomal suspensions from cricket Malpighian tubules lost
only about 15% of their initial epoxidation activity after 3 weeks
at the same temperature (38).

TABLE 5

Effect of freezing on oxidase activity and cytochrome P-450

content in armyworm midgut microsomal preparations

| Storage (weeks) | Oxidase activity (nmoles/mg protein/min) $(x10^3)$ | | Cytochrome P-450 (nmoles/mg protein) |
|---|---|---|---|
| | Epoxidation | Hydroxylation | |
| 0 | 92.5 | 46.5 | 1.37 |
| 1 | 92.5 | 54.2 | 1.30 |
| 2 | 88.0 | 46.0 | 1.37 |
| 3 | 94.6 | 48.4 | 1.48 |
| 4 | 98.2 | 51.4 | 1.42 |

Data from Krieger and Wilkinson (59)
Microsomes were stored as well-drained pellets at -15°C

## Measurement of enzymatic activity

Following preparation of a suitable subcellular fraction with which to work the next step is to measure its enzymatic activity towards an appropriate substrate. The incubation mixture and conditions to be used will clearly depend on the nature of the enzyme, subcellular fraction and substrate under investigation and, of course, the purpose of the study. The optimization of incubation and assay conditions is extremely important and can in itself provide a great deal of information on the nature and mech- anism of the enzyme concerned. Unfortunately it is often over- looked or given minimal attention where the subcellular fractions are being used primarily as biochemical tools to generate metabolites.

The procedures employed to optimize conditions for measuring enzyme reactions in insect subcellular fractions are essentially those pertaining to mammalian systems. Major parameters which should be evaluated are the type, strength and pH of the buffer, the temperature under which the incubations are conducted and the addition of appropriate cofactors or other materials.

Phosphate or Tris buffers of varying pH (7.0-8.5) and ionic strength usually prove adequate for most in vitro studies on xenobiotic metabolism (8,9,10). Although most of the early in vitro studies were carried out at 37°C it is now generally agreed that insect enzymes seem to function more satisfactorily at a temperature of about 30°C (8) and in many cases optimum values of 20-25°C have been reported (35,36). Since enzyme activity in many insect preparations is less stable than that in corresponding mammalian fractions, linearity of the reaction with respect to both time and protein concentration should be ascertained.

The addition of cofactors is usually necessary to obtain maximal in vitro activity and the nature of these clearly depends

on the type of enzyme under study.  For the enzymes involved in
xenobiotic metabolism there are only a few major types of
cofactors.

Microsomal oxidation activity is dependent primarily on the
addition of NADPH or an appropriate generating system, the latter
often proving preferable by extending the time linearity of the
reaction (8).  Incubations must be conducted aerobically as oxygen
is a requirement for oxidase activity.  Although materials such as
EDTA and/or nicotinamide are often added to enhance microsomal
activity in mammalian microsomes where they stabilize NADPH
through blocking lipid peroxidation and pyridine nucleotidase
activity respectively, their inclusion in insect microsomes
appears to have little or no beneficial effect on oxidase activity
(8).  This is also generally true of most metal ions (8).  BSA
(1-2% w/v) is sometimes added to the incubation medium to counteract the actions of residual proteinase inhibitors but care must be
taken that this or other additions do not have other deleterious
effects on enzyme activity.

Soluble enzymes of importance in xenobiotic metabolism
include a variety of hydrolases (phosphatases, carboxyesterases,
amidases and pyrethroid hydrolases) (20), several glutathione
(GSH) requiring enzymes (alkyl and aryl transferases, DDT-
dehydrochlorinase and organothiocyanate metabolizing enzymes)
(21,22) and numerous other conjugating enzymes (glucosyl transferase, sulphotransferase, etc.) (22).  The properties and in
vitro requirements, many of these enzymes have already been
discussed in this symposium.

Perhaps a few words should be added at this point with
respect to the substrate employed in in vitro studies.  Unfortunately most of the substrates which are used in xenobiotic studies
are of necessity highly lipophilic materials and their addition to
an aqueous incubation medium often presents a problem.  Usually
this can be achieved by dissolving the substrate in a small volume
of ethanol, acetone or other organic solvent (care should be taken
to ensure that this does not inhibit the enzyme) but even then it
can often be observed to precipitate out of the incubation medium.
This raises serious questions about the actual concentration of
substrate in the incubation mixture and how this should be
expressed.  Studies with microsomal preparations from mammalian
liver and armyworm midgut have shown that in the presence of a
constant amount of microsomal protein, the amount of aldrin
epoxidized to dieldrin is independent of the total volume of the
reaction mixture and related only to the absolute amount of aldrin
added (Table 6) (60,61).  This suggests that the true concentration of substrate available for enzyme conversion is not that
expressed by the molar concentration calculated from the total
incubation volume but is probably the unknown concentration
existing in the lipid phase of the microsomes.  There are, therefore, problems inherent in expressing the concentrations of
lipophilic substrates in molar terms and $K_m$ values and other

TABLE 6

Effect of aldrin solubility on epoxidation in pig liver microsomes

| Incubation Medium | | Aldrin added (μg) | Dieldrin produced (μg) | Aldrin Concentration | |
|---|---|---|---|---|---|
| Total vol. (ml) | Microsomal suspension (ml) | | | (μg/ml) | (μM)[a] |
| 1 | 0.2 | 50 | 9.2 | 50 | 137 |
| 2 | 0.2 | 50 | 9.3 | 25 | 68.5 |
| 3 | 0.2 | 50 | 9.4 | 12.5 | 45.7 |
| 4 | 0.2 | 50 | 10.2 | 10 | 34.3 |

Data from Lewis et al. (60)

[a] Based on total volume of incubation medium

kinetic parameters reported in this way should be accepted with
reservation. Perhaps the best way of expressing substrate concentration is in terms of the absolute amount added to the reaction
medium since the actual concentration is directly related to this
value.

Particularly in the case of the microsomal oxidase system,
the choice of substrates for in vitro studies is large and many
excellent and sensitive assays are currently available. Initial
studies to optimize the conditions for some reaction or to characterize a given subcellular fraction are often facilitated by using
a model substrate which yields a single metabolic product. Having
thus established the characteristics of the system these can
usually be applied directly to studies with more complex drug or
insecticide substrates which may have several sites at which
enzyme attack can occur and which consequently produce several
different metabolites.

## Application of in vitro studies

To date, the major application of in vitro studies with
insect subcellular fractions has been to complement in vivo
studies on the metabolic fate and pathways of insecticide chemicals. In vivo studies are often complicated by the fact that the
terminal metabolic products (conjugates) are the ones commonly
observed and these often provide little information on the nature
of primary or intermediary metabolites which may exist at trace
levels or be of a transient nature. In insects the situation is
compounded by the fact that with highly toxic materials only very
small doses of material can be applied without killing the insect.
With in vitro systems toxicity does not have to be considered and
high concentrations of toxicants can be employed. Furthermore,
the use of various subcellular fractions permits the individual

study of isolated components of the overall metabolic machinery in a relatively concentrated form without the complications arising from the presence of other metabolic components. Thus using a suitably fortified microsomal fraction the nature of the primary oxidative metabolites can be studied in the absence of the type II conjugating systems found largely in the soluble fraction.

Early in vivo metabolic studies with the carbamates, for example, showed that these insecticides were rapidly metabolized by insects to water soluble products and many of which were conjugates of primary hydroxylated metabolites (5) (Figure 7). Subsequent in vitro studies using isolated microsomal and soluble fractions have enabled these primary and secondary products to be more readily identified and the appropriate enzyme systems better characterized.

Of particular significance to the utility of subcellular components in in vitro metabolism studies is the potential which exists for manipulating the system by the omission or addition of specific cofactors or inhibitors. Thus the requirement of a certain subcellular fraction for a particular cofactor to produce a certain metabolite often provides a fairly clear picture of the type of enzyme which is involved in the conversion. This type of experiment is especially informative where a compound may be metabolized to the same product by two different enzyme systems. The data shown in Table 7 were obtained during the course of a study of diazinon and diazoxon metabolism in house flies (62).

TABLE 7

Effect of reduced glutathione and NADPH on the degradation of diazinon and diazoxon by house fly subcellular fractions in vitro

| Enzyme source[a] | Cofactors | Degradation (mμmoles/hr/g ♀ abdomen) | |
| --- | --- | --- | --- |
| | | Diazinon | Diazoxon |
| Microsomes: | None | 0 | 0 |
| | GSH | 3.2 | 0 |
| | NADPH | 122.1 | 23.2 |
| | NADPH + GSH | 164.3 | 27.0 |
| Soluble fraction: | None | 52.3 | 5.2 |
| | GSH | 259.0 | 80.6 |
| | NADPH | 47.0 | 1.5 |
| | NADPH + GSH | 251.0 | 78.4 |

Data from Yang et al. (62)

[a] Microsomes and soluble fractions equivalent to 35 and 10 ♀ house fly abdomens respectively

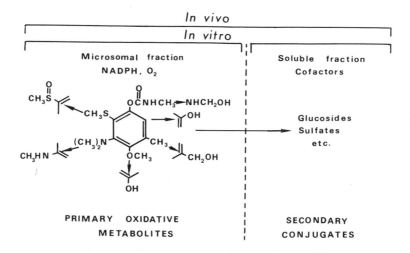

Figure 7.  *Metabolism of carbamate insecticides by microsomal and soluble fractions*

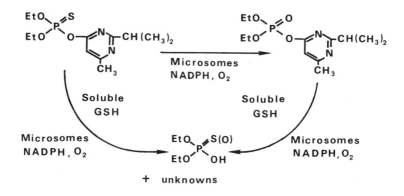

Figure 8.  *Metabolism of diazinon and diazoxon (62)*

These clearly show that because of the requirement for NADPH the
microsomal degradation of diazinon and diazoxon is primarily
oxidative in nature.  In contrast the soluble fraction contains
an efficient GSH-dependent enzyme capable of degrading both
compounds.  The results of these studies combined with an analysis
of the metabolites found in the in vitro incubations indicated
that diazinon could be either oxidatively activated (desulfuration) to diazoxon or could be degraded by microsomal oxidation or
soluble GSH-transferase to diethyl phosphorothioic acid.  Diazoxon
was likewise susceptible to the two degradation pathways to yield
diethyl phosphoric acid (Figure 8).

Several groups of compounds are known to act as inhibitors of
the enzymes involved in xenobiotic metabolism and some of these
have value as insecticide synergists which enhance the insecticidal potency of various materials in vivo (63).  Inhibitors of
microsomal oxidation include many methylenedioxyphenyl derivatives, aryl-2-propynyl ethers, 1,2,3-benzothiadiazoles and a large
number of substituted imidazoles (63).  Many of the soluble
hydrolases such as carboxylesterase and the pyrethroid metabolizing esterases are effectively blocked by phosphates such as tetraethylpyrophosphate and tri-o-cresyl phosphate (20,64) or
carbamates such as 1-naphthyl N-propylcarbamate (65) and many GSH-
transferases are blocked by compounds such as p-chloromercuri-
benzoate (21).  Like the various cofactors previously discussed
such inhibitors can be extremely useful in pinpointing the enzymes
involved in certain reactions.

For example in some cases a xenobiotic may be metabolized by
more than one type of enzyme system in the same subcellular
fraction.  In this case specific enzyme inhibitors can be
employed to discriminate between the two enzymes.  To illustrate
how this technique can be applied in vitro we will use the results
from a mammalian study.  It has been known for some time that many
of the modern pyrethroids are metabolized in mammals by both
esterases and mixed-function oxidases in liver microsomes (66).
Recent in vitro studies have established structure-biodegradabil-
ity relationships with a series of 44 pyrethroids and model
compounds and have clearly shown the comparative role of esterases
and oxidases in their metabolism.  Each of the test compounds was
incubated with microsomes alone (esterase activity) with
microsomes + NADPH (esterase plus oxidase activity) and with
microsomes + NADPH + tetraethylpyrophosphate, an esterase
inhibitor (oxidase activity).  The results shown in Table 8 for
the isomers of phenothrin and cyanophenothrin typify the results
obtained with all compounds tested.  Thus the primary alcohol
esters of IR, trans-substituted cyclopropane carboxylic acids
(e.g. phenothrin) were most rapidly metabolized by both esterase
and oxidase attack, the corresponding IR, cis isomers were
degraded mainly by oxidase action and were quite resistant to
esterase attack and the α-cyano compounds were resistant to the
degradative action of both types of enzymes.

TABLE 8

Effect of structure on in vitro metabolism of 3-phenoxybenzyl
chrysanthemum esters by mouse liver microsomes

Structure (IR, trans isomer)

| Compound and isomer | Percent metabolism rate relative to [IR, trans]-resmethrin[a/] | | | |
| | Esterase | Oxidase | Esterase + found | Oxidase calc. |
|---|---|---|---|---|
| Phenothrin (R = H) | | | | |
|    IR, trans | 59 + 3 | 27 + 2 | 78 + 7 | 86 |
|    IR, cis | <4 | 37 + 5 | 37 + 3 | 37 |
| Cyanophenothrin (R = CN) | | | | |
|    IR, trans, α-RS | 3 + 1 | 5 + 1 | 11 + 2 | 8 |
|    IR, cis, α-RS | <3 | 8 + 1 | 12 + 1 | 8 |

[a/]Esterase + oxidase activity with IR, trans resmethrin is 100 and
its $t_{1/2}$ is 3.3 + 0.8 min.

Data from Soderlund and Casida (64)

In addition to showing how specific enzyme inhibitors can be
used in vitro to more clearly identify the metabolic role of other
enzymes in the same system, the results of this study illustrates
another important application of in vitro studies, i.e. to establish relationships between chemical structure and biodegradability
in large series of structurally related compounds.  This type of
information is of considerable importance in the development of
new drugs, insecticides and other biologically active compounds.
    Other examples of the use of in vitro systems in structure-
activity studies are those employed in the search for new and
potentially more active insecticide synergists.  It is now well
established that most known synergists act in vivo by virtue of
their ability to block microsomal oxidation (63).  Consequently
measurement of their ability to inhibit microsomal mixed-function
oxidation in vitro provides a rapid and effective way of assessing
their synergistic potential in vivo and of establishing the

structural requirements or physicochemical parameters on which
their activity depends.  Regression analysis of data on the
potencies of twenty 5-, 6- and 5,6-substituted 1,2,3-benzothiadia-
zoles as inhibitors of epoxidation in armyworm midgut preparations
revealed that inhibition could be satisfactorily described by the
following equation in terms of hydrophobic ($\pi^2$ and $\pi$) and
electronic ($\sigma$) parameters (67).  Similar structure-activity
studies have been conducted with selected series of substituted
imidazoles.

$$pI_{50} = -0.249\pi^2 + 0.761\pi - 0.457\sigma + 3.834$$

[negative log. $I_{50}$(M)]                     $n = 20$; $r = 0.942$; $s = 0.212$

    In the same way that a given *in vitro* system can provide use-
ful qualitative and quantitative information on the biological
activity or ease of degradation of a series of chemicals, a single
model compound (or type of reaction) can be employed as an
indicator for comparing enzymatic activity in a series of different strains or species of organisms.  Comparative studies of this
type where the emphasis is on establishing the biochemical
similarities or differences between different species or strains
of resistant insects are extremely important in the design of
compounds which exhibit some degree of selectivity in their
biological activity.  Since the comparative aspects of this
subject will be covered by Dr. Terriere in the next presentation
it will not be given further consideration here.

## Relationship between *in vitro* and *in vivo* studies

    In the process of conducting *in vitro* studies with subcellu-
lar fractions we have essentially dismantled the insect in an
attempt to simplify the system and understand more clearly the
properties and functions of some of its component parts.  The
study of an isolated enzyme *in vitro* is clearly a highly unphysio-
logical situation since we have totally destroyed the morphological and functional integrity of the system and the complex and
delicate interrelationships on which the intact animal depends.
In interpreting the results of such studies, we must be aware of
the possibility of artifacts.  Nonetheless one of the requirements
of any *in vitro* study is that it should have some relevance to the
intact animal and an attempt should always be made to evaluate
this.
    Although it is quite clear that the *in vivo* toxicity of many
compounds to insects is often related directly to metabolism,
correlations between the results of *in vitro* metabolic studies and
*in vivo* toxicity are rather few and far between and to date are
only of a qualitative nature.  We are still a long way from being
able to approximate in quantitative terms the *in vivo* metabolic
capability of an intact organism from the sum of the individual

metabolic capacities of its individual organs.  Indeed in view of
the large number of factors which have to be taken into consideration (penetration barriers, binding to inert tissues, etc.) in the
living animal, it is unlikely that this will be accomplished in
the near future.

The best qualitative in vitro/in vivo correlations can be
made in those cases where relatively large changes in metabolic
activity occur within a single species.  This situation exists in
the dramatic age-related variations in microsomal oxidase activity
which occur in several insect species and also where microsomal
oxidase activity can be enhanced by treatment of the insects with
various inducing agents.

In the house cricket (Acheta domesticus) microsomal enzyme
activity is located primarily in the Malpighian tubules; it
increases dramatically during the first one to two weeks of adult
life and thereafter decreases through weeks two to six.  The
in vivo importance of the Malpighian tubules in insecticide
detoxication is strongly suggested by the fact that these changes
in the toxicity of carbaryl and its synergism by piperonyl
butoxide to crickets of different age and sex (Figure 9) (68).

A good correlation has also been observed in the toxicity of
carbaryl to control and induced armyworm larvae (Table 9) (49).
Thus armyworms with microsomal activity in the gut tissues
enhanced 3-fold as a result of a 3-day dietary exposure to penta-
methylbenzene (2,000 ppm) showed a remarkable 11-fold increase in
tolerance to orally administered carbaryl; a good correlation was
also observed with the less effective inducing agent hexamethyl-
benzene.

TABLE 9

Effect of induction on in vitro microsomal oxidase activity and in

vivo tolerance of armyworm larvae to orally administered carbaryl

| Inducer treatment | Percent control activity | | $LD_{50}$ Carbaryl $(\mu g/g)$ |
|---|---|---|---|
| | Epoxidase | Cytochrome P-450 | |
| Control | 100 | 100 | 30 |
| Hexamethylbenzene (2,000 ppm in diet) | 225 | 219 | 67 |
| Pentamethylbenzene (2,000 ppm in diet) | 314 | 299 | 350 |

Data from Brattsten and Wilkinson (49)

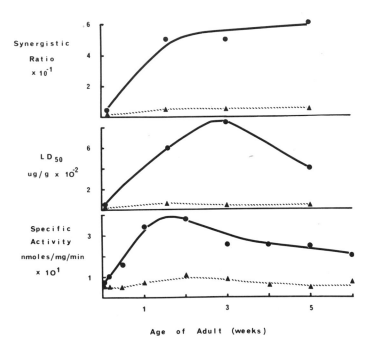

*Figure 9.   Relationship between epoxidation activity in Malpighian tubules, susceptibility to carbaryl, and degree of synergism of carbaryl by piperonyl butoxide in adult crickets (A. domesticus) of different age and sex: (———), females; (– – –), males (68).*

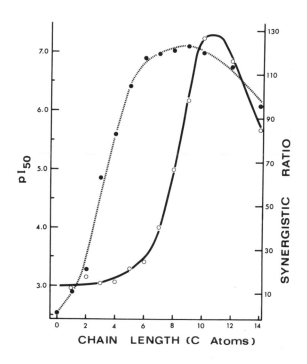

*Figure 10.* *Activity of 1-alkylimidazoles in insects in vitro and in vivo:* (●---●),
$pI_{50}$ *aldrin epoxidase activity in armyworm gut preparation;* (○ — ○), *synergistic
ratio with carbaryl to house flies (69).*

Finally, the in vitro potency of many inhibitors of microsomal oxidation in insects is often reflected in their ability to
synergize insecticidal activity in vivo.  This is evident from
Figure 10 which shows that the activity of a series of 1-alkyl-
imidazoles as inhibitors of microsomal aldrin epoxidation in armyworm midgut preparations closely parallels their in vivo activity
as synergists for carbaryl in house flies.

## Conclusion

Although numerous problems are encountered in in vitro
studies with insect subcellular fractions, it is apparent that
such studies can and will provide a great deal of valuable information concerning the metabolism of xenobiotics.  Substantial
progress has already been made in developing satisfactory methodology for the preparation of appropriate subcellular fractions from
insects and in establishing the biochemical characteristics of the
many of the enzymes concerned.  Indeed, within the constraints
imposed by the limited availability of insect tissues there is no
reason to suppose that insect subcellular fractions and purified
enzyme components cannot be used in exactly similar ways to those
from mammalian tissues.

## Abstract

In vitro studies employing subcellular components from whole
insects or insect organs can provide valuable information on the
structure of primary metabolites likely to be encountered in in
vivo studies and the use of specific cofactors or inhibitors can
prove useful in pinpointing reaction mechanisms and indicating
qualitative differences in metabolite patterns between species or
strains.  There are, however, several problems which require
special attention in conducting in vitro studies with insect
subcellular components and little can be assumed in moving from
one species to another.  Particularly in the case of microsomal
oxidation, the presence of a variety of endogenous inhibitors in
homogenates from whole insects can have serious effects on enzyme
activity and the stability of the preparation and the patterns of
organ localization change in different species.  Even in preparations derived from specific organs, optimal preparatory procedures
must be established and anomalous centrifugal sedimentation
characteristics of subcellular fractions are often observed.
Furthermore, in vitro enzyme activity in subcellular components
changes dramatically with physiological factors such as age and
stage of development and is highly susceptible to the presence of
inducing agents in the diet.  Data so far obtained emphasize the
basic similarities which exist in the enzymatic composition and
metabolic function of insect and mammalian subcellular components.

## Literature Cited

1.  Brooks, G. T., in "Environmental Quality and Safety" (eds. Coulston, F. and Korte, F.) vol. 1, p. 106. Thieme, Stuttgart, Academic Press, N.Y., 1972.
2.  Fukuto, T. R. and Sims, J. J., in Pesticides in the Environment (ed. White-Stevens, R.) p. 145. Marcel Dekker, Inc., N.Y., 1971.
3.  Brooks, G. T. "Chlorinated Insecticides", Vols. 1 and 2, CRC Press, Cleveland, Ohio, 1974.
4.  Eto, M. "Organophosphorus Pesticides: Organic and Biological Chemistry", CRC Press, Cleveland, Ohio, 1974.
5.  Kuhr, R. J. and Dorough, H. W., "Carbamate Insecticides: Chemistry, Biochemistry and Toxicology", CRC Press, Cleveland, Ohio, 1976.
6.  Wilkinson, C. F. (ed.), "Insecticide Biochemistry and Physiology", Plenum Press, N.Y., 1976.
7.  Kuhr, R. J., in "Mechanism of Pesticide Action", (ed. Kohn, G. K.), p. 39. ACS Symposium Series 2, American Chemical Soc., Washington, D.C., 1974.
8.  Wilkinson, C. F. and Brattsten, L. B., Drug Metab. Rev. (1972), $\underline{1}$, 153.
9.  Hodgson, E. and Plapp, F. W. Jr. J. Agr. Food Chem. (1970), $\underline{18}$, 1048.
10. Agosin, M. and Perry, A. S., in "The Physiology of Insecta", (ed. Rockstein, M.), 2nd edition, Vol. V, p. 537. Academic Press, N.Y., 1974.
11. Metcalf, R. L., Maxon, M., Fukuto, T. R. and March, R. B., Ann. Entomol. Soc. Am. (1956), $\underline{49}$, 274.
12. O'Brien, R. D., J. Econ. Entomol. (1957), $\underline{50}$, 159.
13. O'Brien, R. D. and Wolfe, L. S., J. Econ. Entomol. (1959), $\underline{52}$, 692.
14. O'Brien, R. D. and Spencer, E. Y. J. Agr. Food Chem. (1953), $\underline{1}$, 1946.
15. Metcalf, R. L. and March, R. B. Ann. Entomol. Soc. Am. (1953), $\underline{46}$, 63.
16. Fenwick, M. L. Biochem. J. (1958), $\underline{70}$, 373.
17. Fenwick, M. L. Nature (1958), $\underline{182}$, 607.
18. Brodie, B. B., Gillette, J. R. and LaDu, B. N. Ann. Rev. Biochem. (1958), $\underline{27}$, 427.
19. Agosin, M., Michaeli, D., Miskus, R., Nakasawa, S. and Hoskins, W. M. J. Econ. Entomol. (1961), $\underline{54}$, 340.
20. Dauterman, W. C., in "Insecticide Biochemistry and Physiology" (ed. Wilkinson, C.) p. 149. Plenum Press, N.Y., 1976.
21. Shishido, T., Kenji, U., Sato, M. and Fukami, J. Pestic. Biochem. Physiol. (1972), $\underline{2}$, 51.
22. Yang, R. S. H., in "Insecticide Biochemistry and Physiology" (ed. Wilkinson, C.) p. 177. Plenum Press, N.Y., 1976.

23. Ishida, M. and Kahm, P. A.  J. Econ. Entomol. (1965), 58, 383.
24. Lipke, H. and Kearns, C. W.  Advan. Pest Control Res. (1960), 3, 253.
25. Ohkawa, H., Ohkawa, R., Yamamoto, I. and Casida, J. E. Pestic. Biochem. Physiol. (1972), 2, 95.
26. Brooks, G. T.  Gen. Pharmac. (1977), 8, 221.
27. Nakatsugawa, T. and Morelli, M. A., in "Insecticide Biochemistry and Physiology" (ed. Wilkinson, C.) p. 61. Plenum Press, N.Y., 1976.
28. Schonbrod, R. D. and Terriere, L. C.  Pestic. Biochem. Physiol. (1971), 1, 409.
29. Wilson, T. G. and Hodgson, E.  Pestic. Biochem. Physiol. (1972), 2, 64.
30. Nakatsugawa, T.  Personal communication.
31. Williamson, R. L. and Schechter, M. S.  Biochem. Pharmac. (1970), 19, 1719.
32. Krieger, R. I. and Wilkinson, C. F.  Biochem. Pharmac. (1971), 20, 2907.
33. Crankshaw, D. L., Zabik, M. and Aust, S. D.  Pestic. Biochem. Physiol. (1977), 7, 564.
34. Krieger, R. I. and Wilkinson, C. F.  Biochem. Pharmac. (1969), 18, 1403.
35. Kuhr, R. J.  J. Agr. Food Chem. (1970), 18, 1023.
36. Krieger, R. I. and Lee, P. W.  J. Econ. Entomol. (1973), 66, 1.
37. Krieger, R. I., Gilbert, M. D. and Wilkinson, C. F.  J. Econ. Entomol. (1970), 63, 1322.
38. Benke, G. M. and Wilkinson, C. F.  Pestic. Biochem. Physiol. (1971), 1, 19.
39. Brattsten, L. B. and Wilkinson, C. F.  Comp. Biochem. Physiol. (1973), 45B, 59.
40. Krieger, R. I. and Wilkinson, C. F.  Biochem. J. (1970), 116, 781.
41. Orrenius, S., Berggren, M., Moldeus, P. and Krieger, R. I. Biochem. J. (1971), 124, 427.
42. Tsukamoto, M. and Casida, J. E.  Nature (1967), 213, 49.
43. Hansen, L. G. and Hodgson, E.  Biochem. Pharmac. (1971), 20, 1569.
44. Krieger, R. I. and Wilkinson, C. F., Hicks, L. J. and Taschenberg, E. F.  J. Econ. Entomol. (1976), 69, 1.
45. Krieger, R. I., Feeny, P. P. and Wilkinson, C. F.  Science (1971), 172, 579.
46. Gilbert, M. D. and Wilkinson, C. F.  Pestic. Biochem. Physiol. (1974), 4, 56.
47. Gilbert, M. D. and Wilkinson, C. F.  Comp. Biochem. Physiol. (1975), 50B, 613.
48. Benke, G. M., Wilkinson, C. F. and Telford, J. N.  J. Econ. Entomol. (1972), 65, 1221.

49. Brattsten, L. B. and Wilkinson, C. F.   Pestic. Biochem.
    Physiol. (1973), 3, 393.
50. Schonbrod, R. D. and Terriere, L. C.   J. Econ. Entomol.
    (1966), 59, 1411.
51. Morello, A., Bleecker, W. and Agosin, M.   Biochem. J. (1971),
    124, 199.
52. Philpot, R. M. and Hodgson, E.   Chem.-Biol. Inter. (1972),
    4, 399.
53. DeDuve, C.   J. Theoret. Biol. (1964), 6, 33.
54. Crankshaw, D. L., Hetnarski, K. and Wilkinson, C. F.   J.
    Insect Biochem. (1978).   In press.
55. Cassidy, J. D., Smith, E. and Hodgson, E.   J. Insect Physiol.
    (1969), 15, 1573.
56. Nakatsugawa, T. and Dahm, P. A.   J. Econ. Entomol. (1965),
    58, 500.
57. Brindley, W. A. and Dahm, P. A.   J. Econ. Entomol. (1970),
    63, 31.
58. Price, G. M. and Kuhr, R. J.   Biochem. J. (1971), 112, 133.
59. Krieger, R. I. and Wilkinson, C. F.   J. Econ. Entomol.
    (1970), 63, 1343.
60. Lewis, S. E., Wilkinson, C. F. and Ray, J. W.   Biochem.
    Pharmac. (1967), 16, 1195.
61. Krieger, R. I.   (1970).   Ph.D. dissertation, Cornell
    University, Ithaca, N.Y.
62. Yang, R. S. H., Hodgson, E. and Dauterman, W. C.   J. Agr.
    Food Chem. (1971), 19, 14.
63. Wilkinson, C. F. in "Insecticides for the Future:  Needs and
    Prospects" (eds. Metcalf, R. L. and McKelvey, J. J., Jr.)
    p. 195.   John Wiley and Sons, Inc., N.Y., 1976.
64. Soderlund, D. M. and Casida, J. E.   Pestic. Biochem. Physiol.
    (1977), 7, 391.
65. Jao, L. T. and Casida, J. E.   Pestic. Biochem. Physiol.
    (1974), 4, 456.
66. Casida, J. E., Ueda, K., Gaughan, L. C., Jao, L. T. and
    Soderlund, D. M.   Arch. Envir. Contam. Toxicol. (1975/76),
    3, 491.
67. Gil, D. L. and Wilkinson, C. F.   Pestic. Biochem. Physiol.
    (1977), 7, 183.
68. Benke, G. M. and Wilkinson, C. F.   J. Econ. Entomol. (1971),
    64, 1032.
69. Wilkinson, C. F., Hetnarski, K., Cantwell, G. P. and
    DiCarlo, F. J.   Biochem. Pharmac. (1974), 23, 2377.

RECEIVED December 20, 1978.

# The Use of In Vitro Techniques to Study the Comparative Metabolism of Xenobiotics

L. C. TERRIERE

Department of Entomology, Oregon State University, Corvallis, OR 97331

The underlying motive of all biochemical comparisons, in vivo or in vitro, of different species of plants and animals is the search for differences. The discovery of such differences can be useful in many ways--the improvement of drugs and pesticides, the protection of beneficial species and of man, the understanding of evolution, and the development of new principles. Indeed, some reflection about past accomplishments will show that species comparisons have led to some of our most important discoveries in biochemistry.

Gillette (1) has described the many ways in which species may differ in their metabolic disposition of foreign compounds and why it is difficult to interpret such differences on the basis of urinary excretion or the plasma level of these compounds or their metabolites. Of the several major parameters which can cause species differences, he considers the quantity and quality of the enzymes and their interactions with endogenous and exogenous compounds to be the most important. Since the in vitro method is well suited to the study of the kinetics, substrate specificities, and metabolites of single as well as multiple enzyme systems, it would appear that a full understanding of species differences in metabolism cannot be gained without this tool.

Some of the more common uses of the in vitro method to study species differences include: 1) comparisons of enzymes and enzyme systems, 2) correlation of enzyme activity with toxicity or other biological response, 3) study of the selectivity of drugs and pesticides, 4) evolutionary comparisons, i.e. association of detoxication activity with habitat or feeding habits, 5) mode of action studies, 6) environmental studies, i.e. the detoxication capacity of non-target species, and 7) development of the technique to replace in vivo methods. In search of such

0-8412-0486-1/79/47-097-285$09.50/0

information birds have been compared with mammals, insects
have been compared with fish and mammals, fish with crusta-
ceans, and reptiles with amphibians, fish, birds, mammals, and
insects, just to mention a few of the more unusual combinations.

In vitro methods offer the same advantages in comparative
biochemistry as in other fields but, because of the inherent differences in physiology, morphology, genetics, and behavior of
species, their use is more uncertain. The investigator who uses
in vitro methods in this way should be aware of the potential for
error in the design of experiments and in the interpretation of
results. The purpose of this review is to critically examine
current practices in the use of these methods in species comparisons, to suggest some procedures for conducting such studies,
and to mention problems in need of further study.

Due to their importance in the metabolism of drugs, pesticides, and other xenobiotics by plant and animal species, the
enzymes of the microsomal oxidase system have been the subject
of most comparisons in vitro. This has resulted in more information about methods and problems and is the reason for their
prominence in this review. However, the ideas discussed here
should apply equally well to other metabolic systems.

## Historical

Quinn et al (2) appear to be the first to use the newly discovered microsomal oxidase assay to explain species differences
in response to a drug. They obtained a good correlation between
hexabarbital sleeping time and the in vitro metabolism of this
drug in the mouse, rabbit, rat, and dog. Similar results were
reported by Brodie et al. (3) who, in addition, noted a sex difference in hexabarbital metabolism in rats and were able to
explain this on the basis of microsomal oxidase activity.

An interest in the evolution of detoxication mechanisms led
Brodie and Maickel (4) to compare the microsomal metabolism
of several drugs in mammals, birds, reptiles, amphibians,
fishes, and invertebrates (crab, lobster, and cricket). Although
some of their conclusions were not supported by later work, they
stimulated much interest and many similar comparisons began to
appear in the late 1960's and have continued to this time.
Apparently the first species comparison, in vitro, involving
aquatic species, was that of Potter and O'Brien (5) who studied
the conversion of the insecticide, parathion, to its more toxic
product, paraoxon.

The in vitro method was used to compare the azo and nitro-reductase activity of the five major classes of vertebrates (6), showing that the fishes were much less active in such metabolism than the birds and mammals. An important contribution of this work was the demonstration that the species varied in their temperature optima for maximum enzyme activity, aquatic species requiring lower temperatures (21-26°C) while the reductases of the birds were more active at 40°C). In the case of the turtle, nitroreductase activity was 20 times greater at 21°C than at 37°C.

Early evidence that the substrate specificity of the microsomal oxidases might vary with the species was obtained by Creaven et al. (7) who studied the in vitro hydroxylation of biphenyl by 11 species. Some species hydroxylated this compound in both the 2 and 4 position while others favored one but not the other of these positions. This was probably one of the earlier indications that cytochrome P-450 exists in more than one form.

An early attempt to use in vitro techniques to compare the metabolism of xenobiotics in insects was that of Chakraborty and Smith (8) but their in vitro tests were unsuccessful in detecting the expected metabolic activity. This was probably due to the presence of natural inhibitors released during preparation of the homogenates. Another early use of the in vitro method in the study of insect species was that of Schonbrod et al. (9). The microsomal hydroxylation of naphthalene was shown to correlate fairly well with naphthalene toxicity to resistant and susceptible house flies and to blow flies.

## The Reliability of in vitro Methods in Species Comparisons

If in vitro methods are to be used in predicting or explaining species differences in the metabolism of xenobiotics, their reliability must be established. This is done most readily by comparing results from appropriate experiments in vitro and in vivo on the same species. Not many investigators do this, however, so it is necessary to use other criteria such as agreement between laboratories studying the same species. In such cases a reliable method of enzyme assay should result in the same relative activity for the species studied. Another test of reliability is whether the patterns and products of metabolism revealed by in vitro techniques agree with those of the intact organism. This is, of course, very necessary in the use of

in vitro methods to relate or extrapolate between man and
experimental animals.

A good example of such comparisons is the report of
Chipman et al. (10) who studied the in vivo and in vitro metabolism of the dieldrin analog, 1, 2, 3, 4, 9, 9-hexachloro-exo-5, 6-
epoxy-1, 4, 4a, 5, 6, 7, 8, 8a-octahydro-1, 4-methano-naphthalene
(HCE) in rats, rabbits, pigeons, and Japanese quail. Their in
vivo method included the use of a re-entry bile cannula with pro-
visions for the routine collection of samples. The nature and
quantity of metabolites collected with the bile, as well as the
urine, were compared with those found after a 30 minute incubation of HCE with liver microsomes (in vitro at 37°C for mammals, 42°C for birds). The in vivo metabolites (bile and urine)
which were largely conjugates were converted to the primary
compounds prior to measurement.

As shown in Figure 1, HCE undergoes two routes of metabolism, epoxide hydration to the trans-diol, a minor product in the
species studied, and hydroxylation of the epoxide to HHC, the
major metabolites in all four species. This is followed by
epimerization and further hydroxylation to the dihydroxy epoxide,
DHHC.

The results of Chipman et al. are summarized in Table I
and Figure 2. It will be seen that the failure of the pigeon to
convert the epoxide, HCE, to its trans-diol was correctly predicted by the microsomal studies, Table I. Also, the in vitro
experiments confirmed the relative order of importance of the
oxidative metabolites HHC, endo-HHC, and DHHC (Table I) in
the pigeon, quail, and rabbit, and reversing only the endo-HHC
and DHHC in the rat. The two methods disagree on the relative
importance of epoxide hydration in the rabbit.

Figure 2 shows that time is an important variable in such
comparisons. Only in the short tests (20 minutes in vitro, 1 day
in vivo) do the two methods agree that HHC is the major metabolite. After 2 days in vivo the order, most to least, is DHHC,
HHC, and endo-HHC and after 80 minutes in vitro it is endo-HHC,
DHHC, and HHC, although the differences here are much less.
This disagreement is probably due to the availability, in vivo, of
additional enzymes, the conjugases, which alter the levels of
HHC and endo-HHC.

Sullivan et al. (11) have developed a tissue maintenance
technique for the comparative study of drug metabolism. The
method involves the incubation of small pieces (e.g. 2mm
cubes) of fresh tissue for up to 18 hrs with the radioactive drug.
The incubation medium is then extracted and the metabolic

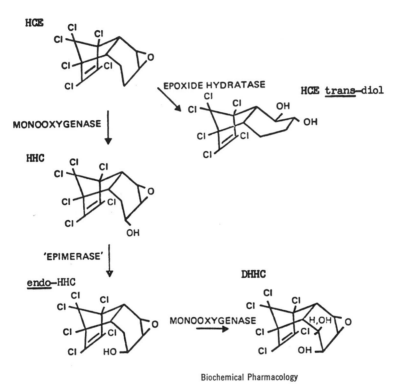

Biochemical Pharmacology

*Figure 1. Metabolism of HCE (10)*

Table I. HCE Metabolites Found in vitro and in vivo.

**(a) in vivo**

| Species | $^{14}C$, % extractable | Metabolites, % of Total | | | | | |
|---|---|---|---|---|---|---|---|
| | | HHC | endo-HHC | DHHC | HCE trans diol | X | Others |
| in bile[a] | | | | | | | |
| rat (7) | 89 | 61 | 7 | 14 | 4 | 8 | 6 |
| pigeon (4) | 91 | 50 | 46 | 4 | 0 | 0 | |
| Jap. quail (4) | 57 | 63 | 19 | 5 | 0 | 13 | |
| in urine[b] | | | | | | | |
| rabbit (3) | 87 | 68 | 10 | 19 | 3 | | |
| pigeon (4) | 95 | 89 | 6.4 | 4.6 | 0 | | |

**(b) in vitro (microsomes)[c]**

| Species | % Substrate converted | g Liver represented/ incubation | Individual metabolites as % of total metabolites | | | | |
|---|---|---|---|---|---|---|---|
| | | | HHC | endo-HHC | DHHC | HCE trans diol | Other |
| rat (6) | 60 | 1.5 | 41 | 33 | 20 | 5 | 0 |
| rabbit (3) | 75 | 0.8 | 41 | 4 | 10 | 30 | 15 |
| pigeon (3) | 55 | 1.0 | 45 | 31 | 20 | 0 | 4 |
| Jap. quail (3) | 25 | 1.0 | 70 | 12 | 8 | 7 | 0 |

[a] Only traces of radioactivity were found in rat urine and rabbit bile. All urine and bile collections were made during the first 2 hours following dosing (15 mg kg$^{-1}$ $^{14}$C-HCE). Urine samples were adjusted to 2 M HCl before incubating for 30 min. at 75°C to break down conjugates.

[c] Microsomes incubated 30 min. at 37° C or 42° C (birds). Five milliliters of incubation medium contained 40 µg HCE.

Data from Chipman et al. (10).

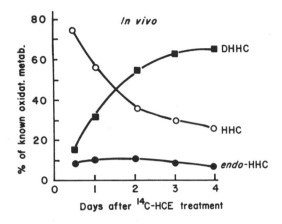

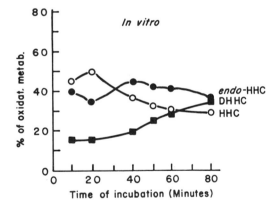

Biochemical Pharmacology

*Figure 2.   Pattern of HCE oxidative metabolism observed in the rat with respect to time.  In vivo: metabolites found in bile with intermittent collections; in vitro: metabolism by hepatic microsomes reinforced with NADPH and $O_2$ (10).*

products resolved by DEAE cellulose chromatography. Using [14]C-carbaryl, ring and N-methyl labelled, as a model, they were able to obtain good agreement in the number and nature of metabolites produced, with those previously found in in vivo studies. The comparisons were made with liver explants of rat, dog, guinea pig, and man. Their results also have some quantitative value, indicating major and minor metabolites in the four species. Some typical results from their study are shown in Figures 3 and 4.

In a further demonstration of their method, Chin et al. (12) compared carbaryl metabolism in several human tissues. This study also illustrated another useful aspect of the method, the ability to compare various organs and tissues of the same species with respect to the metabolic capabilities of each.

It is clear from the results of Sullivan et al. and of Chin et al. that the tissue explants exhibit most, if not all, of the primary and secondary metabolic processes expected of the organ in vivo. In addition to the oxidase and conjugase systems observed in the metabolism of carbaryl, (N-demethylation, epoxidation, ring hydroxylation, epoxide hydration, glucuronidation, and sulfation), the authors claim to have observed nitroreduction and sulfoxidation. All this was attained without added co-factors.

In seeking an explanation for the 1000-fold greater oral toxicity of the insecticide chlorfenvinphos to rats than to dogs, Hutson and Hathway (13) found several differences in the two species. Rat brain acetylcholinesterase was about 10 times more sensitive to inhibition by chlorfenvinphos, rat erythrocytes absorbed the toxicant more readily from plasma (difference about 3-fold) and there was a greater uptake of chlorfenvinphos by rat brain. There was about 15-fold less toxicant in the blood of the dogs, probably due to a combination of absorption and metabolic differences.

The metabolism of chlorfenvinphos by liver slices from the rat, mouse, rabbit, and dog was studied in a further investigation of species differences in the toxicity of this insecticide (14). The liver slices were incubated with the [14]C-labelled compound for 1-2 hrs at 37°C. The metabolism was shown to be due to a microsomal mono-oxygenase, resulting in the elimination of one of the ethyl groups. This had already been shown to be the major in vivo reaction in both rats and dogs. Initial reaction rates for the de-ethylation, calculated from the curves shown in Figure 5, place the four species in the order 1, 8, 24, 88 (rat, mouse, rabbit, dog). In comparison, the acute, oral $LD_{50}$'s (mg/kg) of

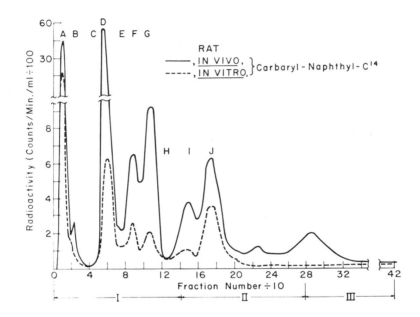

*Figure 3.   DEAE–cedlulose chromatogram of in vivo and in vitro rat metabolites of carbaryl-naphthyl-¹⁴C. Gradient elution program: (I) 0.01M Tris · HCl buffer, pH 7.5 to 0.05M Tris · HCl buffer, pH 7.5; (II) 0.05M Tris · HCl buffer, pH 7.5 to 0.1M Tris · HCl buffer, pH 7.5; (III) 0.1M Tris · HCl buffer, pH 7.5 to 0.5M Tris · HCl buffer, pH 7.5 (11).*

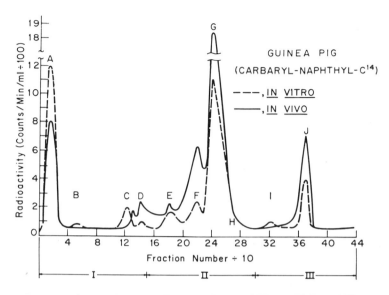

Toxicology and Applied Pharmacology

*Figure 4. DEAE–cellulose chromatogram of in vivo and in vitro guinea pig metabolites of carbaryl-naphthyl-*$^{14}C$. *Gradient elution program as in Figure 3 (11).*

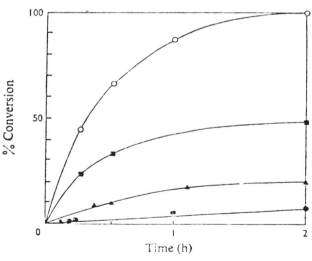

Biochemical Journal

*Figure 5. Relative rates of dealkylation of chlorfenvinphos in liver slices: (●), rat; (▲), mouse; (■), rabbit; (○), dog (14).*

chlofenvinphos in these species is 10 (rat), 100 (mouse), 500 (rabbit), and >1200 (dog). Thus the in vitro experiments would have correctly predicted the order of acute toxicity in the four species.

Only two in vitro studies could be found in which the same species and the same drugs were compared. These were the reports of Chhabra et al. (15) who compared the microsomal oxidase activities of liver and intestine against four compounds in five species (hamster, guinea pig, rat, mouse, rabbit) and Litterst et al. (16) who used some of the same drugs to compare microsomal metabolism in lung, liver, and kidney of the same species. Table II shows that they found very little difference in cytochrome P-450 content, the rabbit, hamster, and guinea pig having higher P-450 levels but with considerable overlap. Both studies agree in ranking the rat as the lowest of the five species and in the narrow range, less than 2-fold, of cytochrome P-450 concentration.

Table II. A Comparison of Hepatic Cytochrome P-450 in
Five Species

| Litterst et al. (16) | | Chhabra et al. (15) | |
|---|---|---|---|
| Species | $\Delta A$ 490-450 /mg protein/ml | Species | nmoles /mg protein |
| rabbit | 0.177 ± 0.038[a] | guinea pig | 1.45 ± 0.16[b] |
| hamster | 0.140 ± 0.023 | hamster | 1.26 ± 0.07 |
| guinea pig | 0.125 ± 0.038 | rabbit | 1.1 ± 0.32 |
| mouse | 0.108 ± 0.022 | mouse | 1.1 ± 0.07 |
| rat | 0.098 ± 0.025 | rat | 0.84 ± 0.07 |

[a] ± S. D.                    [b] ± S. E.

There was reasonable agreement in the ranking of the five species according to their microsomal analine hydroxylase activities, Table III, the hamster and mouse being highest in both studies, and both showing the rabbit and guinea pig as the lowest. The activities differed about 4-fold in the Litterst et al. study. In the case of biphenyl hydroxylase, Table IV, the two studies agree on the rat as lowest in liver hydroxylase activity but there is little agreement in the ranking of the other species. The mean activities for the biphenyl hydroxylase varied about 3-fold in both studies.

From this limited review of results from two laboratories, it appears that the technique is reasonably reliable in the ranking

Table III.  A Comparison of Hepatic Analine Hydroxylase in
Five Species

| Litterst et al. (16) | | Chhabra et al. (15) | |
| --- | --- | --- | --- |
| | Activity | | Activity |
| Species | nmoles/mg protein/min | Species | nmoles/mg protein/15 min |
| hamster | $2.7 \pm 0.9$ [a] | mouse | $24.1 \pm 1.9$ [b] |
| mouse | $1.5 \pm 0.3$ | hamster | $19.1 \pm 1.3$ |
| rat | $0.8 \pm 0.4$ | rat | $15.0 \pm 0.9$ |
| guinea pig | $0.8 \pm 0.4$ | guinea pig | $10.6 \pm 1.0$ |
| rabbit | $0.6 \pm 0.4$ | rabbit | $9.8 \pm 2.3$ |

[a] $\pm$ S. D.                                [b] $\pm$ S. E.


Table IV.  A Comparison of Hepatic Biphenyl Hydroxylase in
Five Species

| Litterst et al. (16) | | Chhabra et al. (15) | |
| --- | --- | --- | --- |
| | Activity | | Activity |
| Species | nmoles/mg protein/min | Species | nmoles/mg protein/15 min |
| guinea pig | $4.1 \pm 3.1$ [a] | mouse | $95.3 \pm 10.0$ [b] |
| hamster | $3.4 \pm 1.3$ | guinea pig | $77.9 \pm 1.8$ |
| mouse | $2.8 \pm 0.6$ | rabbit | $58.1 \pm 1.6$ |
| rabbit | $1.7 \pm 0.5$ | hamster | $47.4 \pm 3.0$ |
| rat | $1.6 \pm 0.4$ | rat | $34.4 \pm 1.4$ |

[a] $\pm$ S. D.                                [b] $\pm$ S. E.

of microsomal oxidase activity if the differences between species are at least 2-fold.

In comparing the enzyme activities of Table III and IV with the cytochrome P-450 concentrations shown in Table II, it will be seen that there is often little correlation between the two parameters even though cytochrome P-450 is known to be the key enzyme in these oxidase systems. This has also been observed in studies of single species. Indeed, in view of our present understanding of this important hemoprotein, a direct relationship on the basis of cytochrome P-450 content alone would be surprising since this enzyme is known to exist in several forms with different substrate specificities.

A careful study of the liver enzyme (oxidases and esterases) involved in the activation and degradation of parathion in nine species failed to provide an explanation for the differing toxicities of parathion (17). This in spite of the fact that there were large differences, 20-fold in paraoxon formation and 8-fold in paraoxon degradation, among the species studied. The authors concluded that organs or tissues other than the liver must be involved in protecting the animal against such toxicants. Of course it is also possible that the target of the toxicant, the acetylcholinesterase system, also varied in sensitivity among the nine species.

The agreement between in vitro metabolism and toxicity in five mammalian and three avian species was also unsatisfactory in a study of the insecticide, diazinon (18). Only with the sheep, which can tolerate 2-50 times more diazinon than pigs, guinea pigs, cows, rats, turkeys, chickens, and ducks, was the toxicity relatively well correlated with in vitro metabolism. The authors concluded that extra hepatic metabolism was more important than liver metabolism.

## Factors Affecting Comparisons--Sources of Error

There are several biological, experimental, and even environmental factors which can affect the performance of in vitro systems. Some examples which are to be found in the current literature include:

1. Sex and age effects: DeWaide (19) found that the variation in aminopyrine N-demethylase and aniline hydroxylase activity between individuals in four species of fish obscured any possible sex differences in the activities of these enzymes. Sex differences in microsomal oxidase activity are well known, however. For example, the rat and mouse exhibit sex

differences in kinetic constants ($K_m$ and $V_{max}$) but the guinea pig, rabbit, and monkey do not (20). Another example is seen in the report of Whitehouse et al. (17) who found a sex difference in the desulfuration of parathion in two of nine species tested, guinea pig and rat, and in its hydrolysis in only one, the rat.

Differences in the rate of enzyme development are well known from studies of the common laboratory animals, hence similar characteristics should be expected in other species. Some investigators fail to take this into account in comparisons of invertebrates or of wild vertebrates, however, perhaps because they have no choice or because they are unaware of the possible effects of age differences. Extreme variations in microsomal oxidase activity can occur in insects of different stages of development as data from the author's laboratory (Figures 6, 7, 8) show. Similar observations have been made with the esterases which metabolize juvenile hormone analogs (21, 22) and with epoxide hydrase which metabolizes the juvenile hormone (23). Age dependent fluctuations in microsomal oxidase activity have also been seen in the house cricket (24) and the cockroach (25).

Species differences in the rate of development have been observed with the glucuronidation system (26). Chick embryos were almost as active in the glucuronidation of O-aminophenol at 12 days as in 6 week-old cockrels whereas the liver of the 16 day-old mouse fetus was negative and even the 10-day infant liver contained only 50% of the adult activity.

2. Source of enzymes: DeWaide (19) measured the apparent $V_{max}$ and $K_m$ for the p-hydroxylation of aniline of eight tissues, liver, kidney, heart, lung, gut, muscle, blood, and spleen in pigeon, rat, trout, roach, and crab (substituting hepatopancreas for liver in the latter). In the crab, trout, and roach, he also included the gill in these measurements. The liver was the most active source of enzyme in the four vertebrates, but the crab gill was considerably more active than its hepatopancreas. The kidney was nearly as active as the liver in the case of the trout and both the kidney and lung were important sources of the enzyme in the pigeon.

Pohl et al. (27) also found differences in the distribution of enzyme activity among the organs of different species. In the little skate, for example, the liver and kidney had approximately the same activity, per mg of microsomal protein, while in the winter flounder the liver was approximately 20 times as active as the kidney.

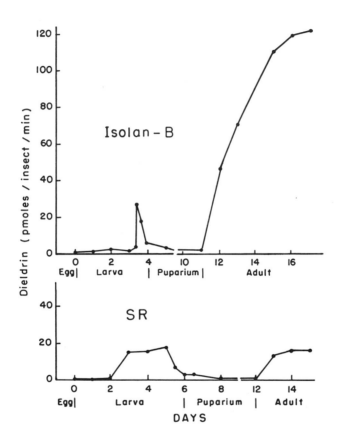

*Figure 6. Microsomal aldrin epoxidases activity in the developmental stages of Isolan-B and SR house flies*

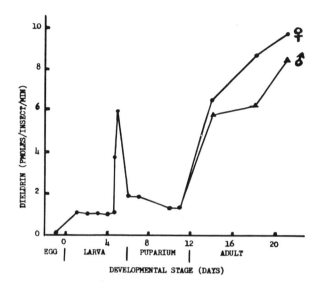

*Figure 7.   Microsomal aldrin epoxidase activity in developmental stages of the blow fly (39)*

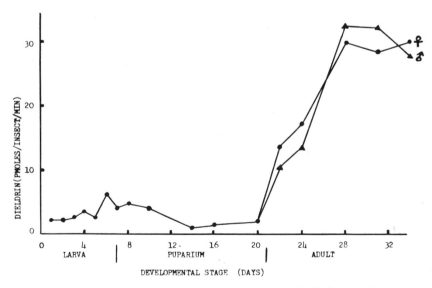

*Figure 8.   Microsomal aldrin epoxidase activity in developmental stages of the flesh fly (39)*

There is considerable uncertainty about the site of mfo activity in invertebrate animals. Pohl et al. (27) were unable to detect hydroxylase or dealkylase activity in the hepatopancreas of the lobster or crab while Burns (28) did find some drug metabolizing activity in this tissue in the crab but found more in gill and in claw muscle tissue. DeWaide (19) also found more activity in the gill tissue of the crab than in the hepatopancreas.

Elmamlouk and Gessner (29) were also unable to detect hydroxylase or demethylase activity in the microsomal fraction of the hepatopancreas of the lobster but they did find some aniline hydroxylase and nitroreductase activity in the soluble fraction.

An interesting result in Burns' (28) study of aldrin epoxidase activity in various tissues of the fiddler crab was the high activity of claw muscle. In terms of specific activity, the gill microsomes were considerably more active than those of hepatopancreas or claw muscle but the total capacity of the muscle system was higher than that of gill and hepatopancreas combined, 3.6 nmoles per hour compared to 1.3 and 1.2 nmoles per hour for gill and hepatopancreas.

3. Cell fraction: In comparing the usual centrifugal fractions of liver homogenates of the rat and the trout, DeWaide (19) found that trout microsomes contained only 47% of the N-demethylase activity of the homogenate whereas the rat liver microsomes contained 79% of the activity. Even the process of centrifuging the 9000 xG fraction (containing microsomes and soluble fraction) at 100,000 xG for 1 hour, then remixing with a tissue grinder, resulted in a 31% loss of activity by the trout system compared to a negligible loss by the rat system. These results led DeWaide to use the 9000 xG fraction in his species comparisons. As he points out, this not only reduces errors due to the differential loss of activity in tests involving different species and tissues, but it simplifies the procedures by shortening the time involved and eliminating other opportunities for loss of activity.

Other observations support the use of the more inclusive intermediate fraction of tissue homogenates (e.g. the 9000 xG fraction, etc.). Buhler and Rasmussen (30) found that the nitroreductase activity of several species of fish was almost entirely in the soluble fraction while in mammalian species it is equally distributed between the microsomal and soluble fraction (31). Other examples of this kind are the report by Elmamlouk and Gessner (29) who observed that the aniline hydroxylase activity

of lobster hepatopancreas homogenates was in the soluble fraction while nitroreductase activity was in both microsomal and
soluble fraction.

Eight species were studied in a direct comparison of microsomal and whole homogenate fractions of the liver as the enzyme
source for the desulfuration of parathion (17). The two systems
agreed in the relative positions of the first five species but
disagreed in the positions of the last three. The differences
among these three were only about 2-fold, however.

The insect esterases which hydrolyze the juvenile hormone
analogs are distributed between soluble fraction (20%) and microsomal fraction (40%) in the house fly (21) and flesh fly (22) while
the distribution in the case of the blow fly is soluble fraction
(60%) and microsomal fraction (20%) (22).

4. Enzyme stability: In comparisons between the rat and
the roach DeWaide (19) subjected the 9000 xG supernatant fraction to various treatments prior to incubation with the substrate.
When the enzymes were allowed to stand for 5 hrs at room
temperature prior to assay the N-demethylating system of the
roach lost 42% of its activity while that of the rat lost 14%.
Similar treatment of the whole homogenate (used in the assay of
p-nitrophenol glucuronidase) resulted in a 62% increase in the
activity of the roach and a 16% increase in that of the rat. Other
treatments (storage of the enzymes at -15°C for 15 hrs,
repeated freezing and thawing of the enzymes, and ultrasonica-
tion) affected the N-demethylase and hydroxylase systems of the
two species to approximately the same extent.

A difference in enzyme stability was also observed in a
study of the effect of temperature on microsomal aldrin epoxidase in eight strains of the house fly (32). Microsomal oxidases
of the World Health Organization Standard Reference Strain of
flies could be incubated at 47.5°C for 5 min and still retain 81%
of their maximum epoxidase activity whereas seven other strains
lost 62-90% of their maximum activity after such treatment.

5. Temperature of incubation: The error which can occur
by the use of the wrong temperature in incubations of microsomal
oxidase enzymes can be appreciated by a study of DeWaide's
results in which the temperature-activity curves were determined for eight species, Figure 9. In all cases the region of
maximum activity was narrow, about 5°C, dropping off sharply
at temperatures outside this range. DeWaide concluded, in
agreement with earlier studies by Adamson (6) and others, that
the liver demethylase of birds (based on studies with the pigeon)
should be incubated at 42°C, those of mammals at 37°C and

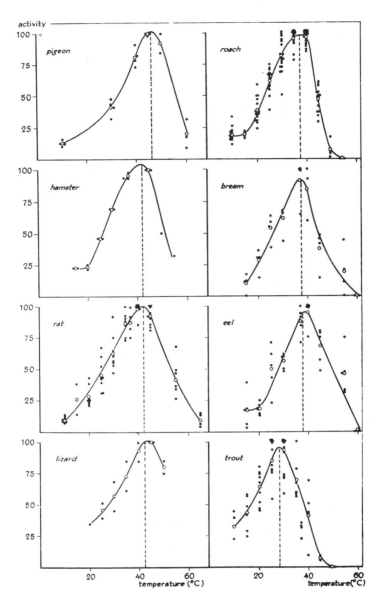

J. H. DeWaide (thesis)

*Figure 9.* N-demethylation of aminopyrine by 9000 g supernatants prepared from liver homogenates of various animal species. Activity was measured for 10 min at different temperatures. The values of each species were expressed in relation to the maximal value (numerically 100) (19).

those of fish at 25°C. These temperatures would not be optimum in every case, however, as was shown by further comparison of enzyme activities at these and at the specific temperature optima for each species. With some species the N-demethylase activity was as little as 46% that observed at the specific optimum. The differences were less in the p-hydroxylation of aniline where the operative temperature resulted in activities at least 64% of those obtained in the optimum range. Presumably it was not practical to conduct the incubations for each species at its optimum level.

Another example of a temperature effect during enzyme assay is mentioned by Bend (33). The liver O-dealkylase system of the little skate was much less active at both 41°C and 12°C than at 30°C.

Recent reports indicate that the choice of temperature for such studies is still open. Pohl et al. (27) incubated microsomes prepared from the livers of marine species or the hepatopancreas of crab and lobster at 30°C, while Burns (28) used temperatures of 14.5°C and 20°C for microsomes from the fiddler crab and Elmamlouk and Gessner (29, 34) incubated lobster hepatopancreas microsomes at 20°C. None of these authors provide data in support of their use of these temperatures.

DeWaide (19) also found a temperature differential in the stability of the N-demethylase system of rat and trout, the trout system remaining linear for a longer period (20-30 min) at incubation temperatures near its optimum, than that of the rat (5-10 min) when incubated at its optimum.

6. Kinetics: Aside from its value in characterizing enzymes, the kinetic constant $K_m$ is useful in the determination of the optimum level of substrate to be used in measuring enzyme activity. As a general practice substrate concentrations should be at least twice the $K_m$ to achieve maximum activity of the enzyme being measured. Frequently investigators comparing activity of an enzyme in different species use the same substrate concentration, apparently assuming that the $K_m$ for the enzyme is the same in all species or that the substrate concentration chosen will exceed even the highest $K_m$. DeWaide's study (Table V) shows that this assumption is not always justified. The $K_m$ values for N-demethylase varied 24-fold among the 16 species investigated (from 0.42 mM for the pigeon to 10 mM for the pike) and 200-fold for the hydroxylase system (0.05 mM for the rat to 10 mM for the white bream). The $K_m$ for the glucuronidase system, compared in 11 species, varied much less, from 0.32 mM for the mouse and lizard to 1.3 mM for the eel.

Table V. Apparent $K_m$-Values of Substrates for Hepatic Enzymes.[a]

| | N-demethylation of aminopyrine[b] | p-Hydroxylation of aniline[c] | Gluduronidation of p-nitrophenol[d] |
|---|---|---|---|
| hamster | 0.8 | 0.8 | 0.32 |
| mouse | 1.3 ± 0.5 | 0.29 ± 0.04 | 0.72 ± 0.10 |
| rat | 0.65 ± 0.20 | 0.05 ± 0.02 | |
| hen | 0.6 | | |
| pigeon | 0.42 ± 0.07 | 1.31 ± 0.34 | 0.64 ± 0.14 |
| lizard | 3.23 | 1.67 | 0.33 |
| frog | 3.0 ± 0.7 | 2.4 ± 0.3 | |
| bream | 6.1 | 4.5 | 0.47 |
| carp | 1.5 | 4.2 | 0.83 |
| tench | | 5.3 ± 1.3 | 0.53 |
| white bream | 7.6 ± 2.7 | 10 | |
| roach | 9.3 ± 0.6 | 2.4 ± 0.4 | 0.97 |
| rudd | 6.5 | 2.6 | |
| rainbow trout | 2.8 ± 0.5 | 0.48 ± 0.12 | 0.48 |
| eel | 3.5 ± 0.9 | 1.7 ± 0.3 | 1.3 ± 0.3 |
| pike | 10 | 4.0 | 0.67 |
| sea lamprey | 8.0 ± 3.5 | 5.5 ± 2.0 | |
| wool-handed crab[e] | | 0.3 | |

[a] $K_m$-values in mM; means of 2 or more determinations; for animals of which the apparent $K_m$-values are determined by 4-10 determinations the standard error of the mean is given.
[b] Range of aminopyrine concentration used: 1.5-35 mM.
[c] Range of aniline concentration used: 0.1-22 mM.
[d] Range of p-nitrophenol concentration used: 0.14-1.4 mM.
[e] Assayed with 9000 g supernatant of gill homogenate.

Data from DeWaide ([19]).

Knowledge of apparent $K_m$ and $V_{max}$ values is important in another way, the interpretation of in vitro data in terms of the in vivo conditions. This was discussed by Castro and Gillette (20) in their studies of the N-demethylation of ethylmorphine by microsomes of rat, mouse, rabbit, guinea pig, and monkey. As they state, the differences in substrate concentrations between the in vitro and in vivo situation could obscure a difference in enzyme activity in one case or the other if the $K_m$ is not taken into account.

7. Natural inhibitors of enzyme activity: Several of the early failures to detect enzyme activity in the tissues of insects were later found to be due to the presence of natural inhibitors which totally or partially inhibited the reactions. This is not too surprising since the small size of such animals prevents the use of specific organs or tissues. Thus the homogenizing of whole insects or major body segments might be expected to introduce catabolic enzymes into the subcellular fraction being assayed. This was the reason for low mfo activity in lepidopterous larvae (35), the house cricket (36), and the honey bee (37).

The inhibition of mfo activity in microsomes prepared from whole house flies was traced to eye pigments (38) and was corrected by removing the heads before homogenization. Such inhibitors are also present in the flesh fly and blow fly (39). Two natural inhibitors of house fly microsomal oxidases have been characterized by Jordan and Smith (40), one of these probably the eye pigment identified by Schonbrod and Terriere (38).

Another potential source of interference with microsomal oxidase activity in species comparisons is the lipid peroxidase system. A 15-fold difference in the activity of this system between rat liver and rabbit liver microsomes has been reported (41). This was sufficient to change the relative activity of the rat demethylase compared to that of the rabbit from 2.2 times (rat more than rabbit) to 3.4 times when the peroxidation was prevented by the addition of EDTA.

Pohl et al. (27) could not detect mfo activity in the hepatopancreas of lobster or crab, attributing this in part to the presence of digestive juices released during homogenization. These juices were found to be inhibitory of the hydroxylation of aniline and the N-demethylation of benzphetamine. However, the inhibitor had only a slight effect on the de-ethylation of 7-ethoxycoumarin. This observation could explain the failure of other workers (28, 29) to detect microsomal oxidase activity in the hepatopancreas of the crab and lobster.

8. Environmental effects: During his study of the drug metabolizing activity of liver microsomes from fish species obtained from the Rhine River and its tributaries, DeWaide (19, 42) observed a seasonal variation in enzyme activity. Further investigation revealed that the N-demethylase activity of the roach (Figure 10) and the rudd (Table VI) collected during the summer months was more than twice that of specimens collected in the winter. The difference was not explained on the basis of liver weight or protein content or on differences in water temperature. It was concluded that the presence of enzyme inducing chemicals in the fishes' environment during the summer months was the main cause of these differences in enzyme activity.

There is now considerable evidence that some marine species are induced by such pollutants as crude oil and the PCB's (43, 44, 45). Increases in aryl hydrocarbon hydroxylase activities (benzo-($\alpha$)-pyrene as substrate) up to 4-fold have been noted (46). However, not all species are affected nor are the effects on the xenobiotic metabolizing enzymes the same as noted by Payne (47). For example, the aryl hydrocarbon hydroxylase was induced in the trout but N-demethylase was not affected. Neither enzyme was induced in the crab and lobster.

Yawetz (48) also raised this question on finding both DDE and PCB's in the tissues of six species of birds in the in vitro study of aldrin epoxidation. Residue concentration in heart tissue (liver was not analyzed) were 0.1-1.2 ppm for the two inducers.

There may also be an effect on enzyme activity by the environmental temperature of the species under study. DeWaide (49) found that trout and roach held at $5^{\circ}$C for 2 weeks had liver hydroxylase and N-demethylase activities about twice those of fish held at $18^{\circ}$C. In similar experiments with the hamster and the rat (temperatures $5^{\circ}$C and $23^{\circ}$C) the differences were about 1.5-fold or less.

9. Basis of comparison: Nearly all investigators of xenobiotic metabolism report metabolic activity in terms of the protein content of the fraction being assayed. This is based on the assumption that the preparative methods used will result in constant and reproducible amounts of enzyme protein. In comparative studies a second assumption is required--that the tissues or organs of the different species will yield the same proportions of active protein if the methods used are the same. There are good reasons to doubt this, however, considering the possibilities for variation in tissue constituents, especially non-specific protein and in physical texture (thus altering grinding conditions). These

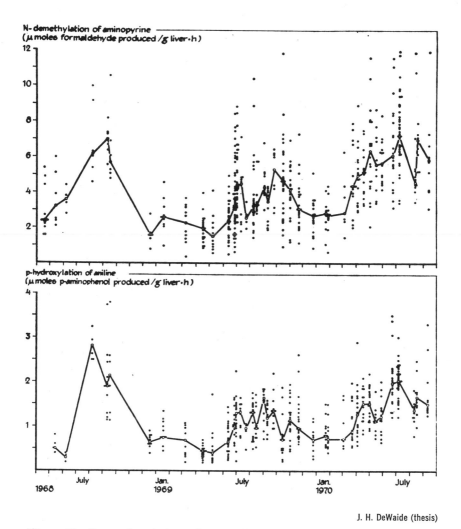

*Figure 10. Seasonal variation in hepatic drug-metabolizing capacity in the wild roach. Measurements were performed with 9000 g supernatants derived from liver homogenates. Curves are drawn through the median values of the samples (19).*

Table VI. Hepatic drug oxidation in the rudd at different times of the year

|  | Date of assay | |
|  | March 12, 1970 (n = 25) | June 29, 1970 (n = 11) |
|---|---|---|
| N-demethylation of aminopyrine activity per[a] | | |
| g fresh liver | 1.37 ± 0.52[b] | 3.60 ± 1.83 |
| mg liver protein | 0.0119 ± 0.0042 | 0.0379 ± 0.0197 |
| mg liver DNA | 0.63 ± 0.28 | 1.87 ± 0.89 |
| 100 g body-weight | 2.40 ± 0.86 | 10.8 ± 6.3 |
| p-Hydroxylation of aniline activity per[c] | | |
| g fresh liver | 0.41 ± 0.17 | 0.87 ± 0.45 |
| mg liver protein | 0.0035 ± 0.0015 | 0.0093 ± 0.0046 |
| mg liver DNA | 0.19 ± 0.09 | 0.47 ± 0.25 |
| 100 g body-weight | 0.72 ± 0.28 | 2.76 ± 1.67 |

[a] $\mu$moles formaldehyde produced per hour.

[b] Means with standard deviation. The corresponding values of the two dates are significantly different at $P < 0.01$ (Wilcoxon two-sided two-sample test).

[c] $\mu$moles p-aminophenol produced per hour.

Data from DeWaide (19).

factors could lead to differences in the amounts of specific and
non-specific protein in the fraction finally assayed. Inasmuch as
the methods used for protein determination do not distinguish
between active and inactive protein, the chances for error are
obvious.

The possible extent of the error can be seen in data from
Pohl et al. (27) who found a 6-fold variation in the yield of microsomal protein per gram of liver in 12 vertebrate species. A
variation in microsomal protein content is reported in a study of
six species of wild birds (7.0 ± 1.3 to 12.6 ± 2.5 mg protein per
g liver) (48) and for the rat, rabbit, mouse, hamster, and guinea
pig (24.0 ± 3.9 to 35.9 ± 10.3 mg protein per g liver ) (16).

DeWaide (19) compared the N-demethylation, hydroxylation,
and glucuronidation activity of the 27 species in his study on the
basis of liver weight, liver protein, liver DNA, and body weight.
As might be expected, the drug metabolizing activities of the
liver of the various species ranked differently when expressed in
different parameters. In the N-demethylation of aminopyrine,
the rat (average of 30 animals) was 14 times more active than
the trout (average of 30 animals) when compared on the basis of
liver weight, 10 times more active on the basis of liver protein,
12 times more active on the basis of liver DNA, and 35 times
more active on the basis of body weight. In the hydroxylation of
aniline, the multiples were 4, 3, 3, and 9 for comparisons on
the basis of liver weight, liver protein, liver DNA, and body
weight.

This problem has been discussed by Harper et al. (50).
They prefer to compare activities between species on the basis
of $V_{max}$ rather than specific activities and they also show comparisons on the basis of cytochrome P-450 content (catalytic
constant, $k_{cat}$). The benzene metabolism of liver and lung
enzymes from rat, rabbit, and hamster is ranked according to
these parameters in Table VII, compiled from their data. There
is no agreement between relative activities based on cytochrome
P-450 content and those based on protein content or $V_{max}$. The
reason for this is now understood as mentioned earlier in this
symposium.

Discussion

Three general conclusions emerge from the foregoing review
of the use of in vitro methodology in species comparisons:
1) most of the problems occur in studies with a quantitative
rather than a qualitative aspect; 2) the problems increase as the

Table VII. Microsomal Benzene Hydroxylase Activity of Rat, Rabbit, and Hamster Compared in Three Ways

| Microsomes from | Basis of Comparison | | |
|---|---|---|---|
| | $V_{max}$ [a] | Specific Activity [b] | $K_{cat}$ [c] |
| rat lung | 1.13 ± 0.29 | 0.49 ± 0.18 | - |
| hamster lung | 3.16 ± 0.35 | 2.41 ± 0.35 | 27 |
| rabbit lung | 10.36 ± 1.14 | 4.65 ± 0.44 | 18 |
| rat liver | 1.35 ± 0.55 | 1.09 ± 0.27 | 1.8 |
| hamster liver | 9.29 ± 4.03 | 4.26 ± 0.84 | 2.2 |
| rabbit liver | 3.86 ± 0.20 | 2.08 ± 0.29 | 1.8 |

[a] nmol/min/mg protein

[b] nmol/min/mg protein

[c] nmol/nmol cytochrome P-450/min

Data from Harper et al. (50)

systems become more highly defined; and 3) the problems are
more likely to occur in studies of invertebrates and wild vertebrates. It is also apparent that, in spite of the difficulties which
have been identified, the method has produced much useful
knowledge not available by other means, about species differences.

Much of the work which has been done so far in this area,
especially that involving non-laboratory animals, would have
been improved by more attention to the use of optimum conditions. A general recommendation for the future use of in vitro
methods in comparative studies is that none of the experimental
conditions or biological factors be taken for granted. This
includes the pH and temperature of incubation, activity of the
sub-cell fractions, substrate level, enzyme stability during
preparation, use, storage, and enzyme source, the possibility
of endogenous inhibitors, and the effect of age and sex. Some
suggestions for dealing with some of these problems are as
follows:

1. Choice of in vitro system: The choice of in vitro system
to be used in the comparisons will depend on the objectives of
the experiment. When metabolic activities are to be compared
quantitatively, the more complete systems such as tissue
explants and slices should be used. With these there is less
danger of losing important enzymes and co-factors and the
cellular organization of the constituents is preserved. A new
approach to such systems is the intact or whole cell, usually
prepared from the liver and thus known as the hepatocyte (51).
This technique appears to offer several advantages over the
liver slice or explant method, maintaining the organizational
integrity of the original tissue without the artifacts introduced by
mechanical injury to the cells and by abnormalities in the diffusion of substrate or oxygen. Some recent uses of this technique
are described below.

It is not possible to prepare such fractions from small
animals, either because methods are not known or because of the
size of the tissue or organ. In these cases there seems no
choice but to use a homogenate of the entire animal or a major
body segment followed by mild centrifugation. Although partially
disorganized, this system should contain all of the natural constituents required for the reactions under study. However, the
investigators should check the requirement for supplemental
co-factors such as NADPH.

More highly defined fractions such as microsomes or microsomal supernatant and subfractions of these are appropriate

when the objective of the experiments is more qualitative in
nature, such as the comparison of enzyme specificities,
structure-activity relationships, effect of inhibitors and activators, kinetic studies, etc. In these cases the investigator is
willing to sacrifice organization and completeness for better
control of experimental conditions.

   2.  Temperature of incubation:  The temperature for optimum metabolic activity should be determined for each of the
species being compared.  When this is not feasible, it is probably best to incubate enzymes from poikilothermic species at or
in the temperature range of their natural habitat.

   3.  Enzyme kinetics:  When the comparisons are being made
with specific sub-cellular fractions such as microsomes or
soluble fraction, it is important to determine the $K_m$ for the
substrate being studied in order that saturating concentrations
can be used in each incubation.  When tissue slices, tissue
explants, hepatocytes, etc., are used, $K_m$ determinations
will have little value, since, presumably, the substrate concentration within the cell will be determined by permeability and
diffusion properties characteristic of the tissues being studied.
In these cases, it is important to maintain the substrate level of
the medium at saturating conditions.

   4.  Age, sex, and source of animals:  Whenever possible
in vitro comparisons of metabolic activity should be made only
after the relationship between sex, age, and developmental stage
and enzyme activity have been determined.  The experiments
should then be designed to accommodate these variables.  In the
case of species obtained from the field, attention should be given
to environmental background, especially to such factors as temperature range of the habitat and the possibility of induction of
enzymes by environmental pollutants.

   5.  Endogenous inhibitors:  The presence of inhibitors which
prevent or reduce metabolic activity during in vitro assays
should be assumed in lieu of evidence to the contrary whenever
new species or new organs and tissues are being examined.
This is particularly important in studies of small invertebrates
where it is necessary to homogenize all or part of the animal
in order to perform the assay.  One method of detecting inhibition is to incubate the suspected fraction with one of known
activity for evidence of inhibition of the latter.

   6.  Basis of comparison:  The common practice of basing
metabolic activity on the protein content of the fraction being
assayed is probably the best which can be devised at present.
However, sufficient data should be provided to enable others to

make their own evaluation of the activity of the tissues and
organs chosen for study. This includes the yield of protein per
unit weight of tissue, the total weight of organ, tissue, or animal, and the protein method used. When the species being
compared are from different taxonomic groups at least one
additional method of expressing activities should be provided for
better cross-referencing between laboratories. With vertebrates and large invertebrates, activities should be related to
the fresh weight of the tissues being studied and for small
invertebrates, to the body weight.

It is regrettable that few investigators of the comparative
biochemistry of xenobiotics use the same substrates in their
studies. Often, of course, the special demands of the research
would not permit this, but there are many cases in which
"standard xenobiotics" could be used. Examples include effect
of inducers and inhibitors, sex and age dependency of enzyme
activity, relative enzyme activity, and the optimization of
experimental conditions. The use of such standard substrates
would greatly improve communication between laboratories and
thus contribute to the value of the in vitro approach.

Usefulness of the in vitro method in species comparisons.

All of the merits of in vitro methods which have been discussed in the previous chapters apply as well to their use in
species comparisons. These include improved control over
experimental conditions, elimination of variables, isolation and
study of specific systems, greater precision in measurements,
more flexibility in design of experiments, and economies of
time and labor. In addition, and in spite of the greater susceptibility to experimental error mentioned earlier in this
chapter, the method has some special advantages in species
comparisons. Some examples follow.

1. Studies of metabolism in wild species. In vitro methods
have already been of value in drawing attention to the lower
capacity of fish, reptiles, amphibians, and other wild species
for metabolizing foreign compounds (3, 6, 19, 27, 30, 33, 43).
It is not likely that this information could have been gathered so
quickly and on such a large scale by any other means.

The difficulties of collecting or rearing wild animal species
in sufficient numbers for in vivo studies and of treating such
species with chemicals without introducing various stresses,
almost eliminates the use of such methods of experimentation.
In addition, with aquatic species, there may be problems with

collecting excreted metabolites for identification.  Furthermore, these methods permit more use of the same animals since several metabolic systems could be studied with the same or different organs.

2.  Metabolism of xenobiotics by humans:   The in vitro method has obvious advantages in studies of the metabolism of foreign chemicals by humans.  Without the direct exposure of human subjects, these methods could provide urgently needed information about metabolic pathways, identity of metabolites, effect of inhibitors, detection of interactions between chemicals, location of sites of metabolism, and the detection of age and sex relationships.  Such information could be obtained only with difficulty by other means.  In connection with similar knowledge of laboratory animals, the translation of results from animal experiments into decisions about human safety could be done with greater precision than at present.

3.  Use in screening programs:  The author is unaware of the extent to which in vitro methods are being used at present by the drug and pesticide industries.  The techniques should be helpful in bridging gaps between synthesis of new compounds and their testing for efficacy with laboratory animals, insects, or plants.  It should also be useful in gathering information on environmental safety.  In vitro studies of metabolism by the experimental organisms might be helpful in determining the reasons for failures in toxicity, indicating whether this is due to inadequate uptake, lack of transport, or too rapid metabolism.  The method is also useful in detecting unexpected metabolites or in producing metabolites free of interfering compounds.

Research needs.

The greatest obstacle to the expanded use of in vitro methods is the lack of evidence of their reliability in explaining and predicting in vivo events.  This obstacle can be removed only by additional studies in which in vivo and in vitro methods are compared as in the experiments reported by Chipman et al. (10) and by Sullivan et al. (11, 12).  The greater use of common substrates and toxicants (i.e. standard chemicals) by different laboratories would help in achieving this goal.

More work is needed on enzyme systems other than the microsomal oxidases which are important in the metabolism of xenobiotics.  This includes the carboxyesterases which, along with the microsomal oxidases, account for most of the primary metabolism of drugs and pesticides.  More information is also needed on the glutathione-S transferases, epoxide hydrase, and other enzymes which are important in the secondary (Type 2) metabolism of xenobiotics. With knowledge of the distribution and properties of these enzymes in various species, the metabolism of xenobiotics can be conducted on a broader scale and thus improve the predictive value of the method.

Except for the common laboratory animals, there is a serious deficiency in our knowledge about the rate of development of xenobiotic metabolizing enzymes. It is quite likely that age and stage of development are important factors in these metabolic processes and, until the facts are known, it will be difficult to plan good experiments.

Immediate attention should be given to the use of the intact cell technique in comparative metabolism studies. Interesting results using rat liver cells have begun to appear and a recent report describes a system using both liver and kidney cells to reconstruct the entire metabolism of a drug from its oxidation and conjugation with GSH to the production of the corresponding mercapturic acid (52). These cells have been shown to resemble the microsomal oxidase system in enzyme activity and substrate specificity. They also appear to contain the conjugation systems of the liver (53-58), and to demonstrate the effect of inducers (52, 57, 59). Hepatocytes have also been prepared successfully from pig and human liver (60). Methods for the preparation of hepatocytes are described by Mouldes et al. (51).

## Abstract

In addition to the usual doubts about the use of in vitro methods to replace or support those conducted in vivo, their use in comparative biochemistry encounters other uncertainties. These arise from the genetic, behavioral, morphological, and physiological differences among species. There is a need for evidence that, in spite of these special difficulties, in vitro methods can be reliable in detecting metabolic differences between species.

The best method of establishing the reliability of data obtained in vitro is to compare the results with those from in vivo experiments performed on the same species. Another test of reliability is to determine how different laboratories rank the same species in terms of their relative enzyme activity. Up to the present time there are only a few reports which permit the use of either of these methods of evaluation. A critical examination of such data indicates that reliable comparisons of xenobiotic metabolism can be made in vitro providing a number of precautions are taken.

In vitro studies of species differences are of two types, those in search of quantitative relationships and those seeking qualitative information. There will be fewer problems in studies of the first type if the investigator uses the more complete in vitro systems such as the tissue explant or slice or, in the case of small animals, the low speed centrifugal fraction of the tissue homogenate. When the experiments are qualitative in nature, the more highly defined but less complete sub-cellular fractions are recommended.

Special problems arise in the study of wild species. These include: lack of information regarding the relationship between enzyme activity and age or stage of development; sites of metabolic activity; species differences in temperature of optimum enzyme activity; the presence of endogenous inhibitors of metabolic enzymes; and unpredictable environmental effects on metabolic activity. Another problem encountered in all comparative work but most acute in studies of wild species is the lack of a suitable basis of reference for comparing metabolic activity. The practice of comparing activities on the basis of protein content appears to be the best that can be devised at present, but its limitations should be understood. It is recommended that an additional system of reference be used in most species comparisons.

Carefully planned in vitro experiments can be very useful in comparative studies, especially those involving wildlife species which are difficult to rear or manage. The methods should also be useful in screening programs for new drugs and pesticides and in studies of drug metabolism by humans.

Research needed to expand the use of these methods includes studies of the use of hepatocytes and other intact cells as substitutes for tissue explants and slices and for sub-cell fractions. Additional information on the age dependency of metabolic enzymes and on conditions affecting in vitro assays for other enzymes such as the carboxyesterases, epoxide hydrase, and the conjugating enzyme systems is also needed.

## Literature Cited

1.  Gillette, J. R. in "Drug Metabolism: from Microbes to Man" (Parke, D. V. and Smith, R. L., Eds.) pp. 147-168, Taylor and Francis, London, 1977.
2.  Quinn, G. P., Axelrod, J., Brodie, B. B., Biochem. Pharmacol. (1958) 1, 152.
3.  Brodie, B., Maickel, R. P., and Jondorf, W. R., Fed. Proc. (1958) 17, 1163.
4.  Brodie, B. B., and Maickel, R. P., Proc. First Int. Pharmacol. Meeting (1962) 6, 299.
5.  Potter, J. L., and O'Brien, R. D., Science (1964) 144, 55.
6.  Adamson, R. H., Dixon, R. L., Francis, F. L., and Rall, D. P., Proc. Nat. Acad. Sci. (1965) 54, 1386.
7.  Creaven, P. J., Parke, D. V., and Williams, R. T., Biochem. J. (1965) 96, 879.
8.  Chakraborty, J., and Smith, J. N., Biochem. J. (1964) 93, 389.
9.  Schonbrod, R. D., Philleo, W. W., and Terriere, L. C., J. Econ. Entomol. (1965) 58, 74.
10. Chipman, J. K., Kurukgy, M. and Walker, C. H., Biochem. Pharmacol. (in press).
11. Sullivan, L. J., Chin, B. H., and Carpenter, C. P., Tox. and Appl. Pharmacol. (1972) 22, 161.
12. Chin, B. H., Eldridge, J. M., and Sullivan, L. J., Clinical Tox. (1974) 7, 37.
13. Hutson, D. H., and Hathway, D. E., Biochem. Pharmacol. (1967) 16, 949.
14. Donninger, C., Hutson, D. H., and Pickering, B. A., Biochem. J. (1972) 126, 701.
15. Chhabra, R. S., Pohl, R. J., and Fouts, J. R., Drug Metab. Disp. (1974) 2, 443.
16. Litterst, C. L., Mimnaugh, E. G., Reagan, R. L., and Gram, T. E., Drug Metab. Disp. (1975) 3, 259.
17. Whitehouse, L. W., and Ecobichon, D. J., Pest. Biochem. Physiol. (1975) 5, 314.
18. Machin, A. F., Rogers, H., Cross, A. J., Quick, M. P., Howells, L. C., and Janes, N. F., Pestic. Sci. (1975) 6, 461.
19. DeWaide, J. H. in "Metabolism of Xenobiotics," doctoral thesis, Univ. Nijmegen, Drukkerij Leijn, 1971.
20. Castro, J. A. and Gillette, J. R., Biochem. Biophys. Res. Com. (1967) 28, 426.

21. Terriere, L. C. and Yu, S. J., Pestic. Biochem. Physiol. (1977) 7, 161.
22. Yu, S. J. and Terriere, L. C., Pestic. Biochem. Physiol. (1975) 5, 418.
23. Yu, S. J. and Terriere, L. C., Insect Biochem. (1978) ( in press ).
24. Benke, G. M. and Wilkinson, C. F., J. Econ. Entomol. (1971) 64, 1032.
25. Benke, G. M. and Wilkinson, C. F., J. Econ. Entomol. (1972) 65, 1221.
26. Fyffe, J. and Dutton, G. J., Biochim. Biophys. Acta (1975) 411, 41.
27. Pohl, R. J., Bend, J. R., Guarino, A. M., and Fouts, J. R., Drug Metab. Disp. (1974) 2, 545.
28. Burns, K. A., Marine Biol. (1976) 36, 5.
29. Elmamlouk, T. H. and Gessner, T., Comp. Biochem. Physiol. (1976) 53C, 57.
30. Buhler, D. R. and Rasmusson, M. E., Arch. Biochem. Biophys. (1968) 103, 582.
31. Fouts, J. R. and Brodie, B. B., J. Pharmacol. Exp. Therap. (1957) 119, 197.
32. Terriere, L. C., Schonbrod, R. D., and Yu, S. J., Bull. W.H.O. (1975) 52, 101.
33. Bend, J. R., James, M. O., and Dansette, P. M., Ann. N. Y. Acad. Sci. (1977) 298, 505.
34. Elmamlouk, T. H. and Gessner, T., Comp. Biochem. Physiol. (1976) 53C, 19.
35. Krieger, R. I. and Wilkinson, C. F., Biochem. J. (1970) 116, 781.
36. Brattsten, L. B. and Wilkinson, C. F., Comp. Biochem. Physiol. (1973) 45B, 59.
37. Gilbert, M. D. and Wilkinson, C. F., Comp. Biochem. Physiol. (1975) 50B, 613.
38. Schonbrod, R. D. and Terriere, L. C., Pestic. Biochem. Physiol. (1972) 1, 409.
39. Terriere, L. C. and Yu, S. J., Pestic. Biochem. Physiol. (1976) 6, 223.
40. Jordan, T. W. and Smith, J. N., Int. J. Biochem. (1970) 1, 139.
41. Kamataki, T. and Kitagawa, H., Biochem. Pharmacol. (1973) 23, 1915.
42. DeWaide, J. H. and Henderson, P. T., Comp. Biochem. Physiol. (1970) 32, 489.

43.   Malins, D. C., Ann. N. Y. Acad. Sci. (1977) 298, 482.
44.   Gruger, E. H., Wekell, M. M., Numoto, P. T., and
      Craddock, D. R., Bull. Environ. Contam. Toxicol.
      (1977) 17, 512.
45.   Yarbrough, J. D. and Chambers, J. E., Life Sci. (1977)
      21, 1095.
46.   Payne, J. F. and Penrose, W. R., Bull. Environ.
      Contam. Toxicol. (1975) 14, 112.
47.   Payne, J. F., Marine Poll. Bull. (1977) 8, 112.
48.   Yawetz, A., Agosin, M., and Perry, A. S., Pestic.
      Biochem. Physiol. (1978) 8, 44.
49.   DeWaide, J. H., Comp. Gen. Pharmacol. (1970) 1, 375.
50.   Harper, C., Drew, R. T., and Fouts, J. R., Drug
      Metab. Disp. (1973) 3, 381.
51.   Moldeus, P., Hogberg, J., and Orrenius,  S., Methods in
      Enzymology (1978) 52, 60.
52.   Moldeus, P., Jones, D. P., Ormstad, K., and Orrenius,
      S., Biochem. Biophys. Res. Comm. (1978) (in press).
53.   Inaba, T., Umeda, T., and Mahon, W. A., Life Sci.
      (1975) 16, 1227.
54.   Vadi, H., Moldeus, P., Capdevila, J., and Orrenius, S.,
      Cancer Res. (1975) 2083.
55.   Grundin, R., Moldeus, P., Vadi, H., and Orrenius, S.,
      in "Cytochromes P-450 and b$_5$" (Cooper, D. Y., Rosenthal,
      O., Snyder, R., and Witmer, C., Eds.) Plenum Pub.
      Corp., New York, N.Y., 1974.
56.   Erickson, R. R., and Holtzman, J. L., Biochem.
      Pharmacol. (1976) 25, 1501.
57.   Wiebkin, P., Ery, J. R., Jones, C. A., Lowing, R., and
      Bridges, J. W., Xenobiotica (1976) 6, 725.
58.   Burke, M. D., Vadi, H., Jernstrom, B., and Orrenius,
      S., J. Biol. Chem. (1977) 252, 6424.
59.   Moldeus, P., Grundin, R., von Bahr, C., and Orrenius,
      S., Biochem. Biophys. Res. Comm. (1973) 55, 937.
60.   Belfrage, P., Borjesson, B., Hagerstrand, I., Nilsson,
      A., Olsson, A., Wiebe, T., and Akesson, B., Life Sci.
      (1975) 17, 1219.

RECEIVED December 20, 1978.

# INDEX